Renjie Shi · Lihua Zher
Editors

Diagnosis and Treatment of Anal Fistula

Chemical Industry Press Co., Ltd. Springer

Editors
Renjie Shi
Department of Anorectal Surgery
Affiliated Hospital of Nanjing
University of Traditional
Chinese Medicine
Nanjing, Jiangsu, China

Lihua Zheng
Department of Proctology
China-Japan Friendship Hospital
Beijing, China

ISBN 978-981-16-5806-8   ISBN 978-981-16-5804-4 (eBook)
https://doi.org/10.1007/978-981-16-5804-4

© Chemical Industry Press 2021

Jointly published with Chemical Industry Press
The print edition is not for sale in China (Mainland). Customers from China (Mainland) please order the print book from: Chemical Industry Press.
This work is subject to copyright. All rights are reserved by the Publishers, whether the whole or part of the material is concerned, specifically the rights of reprinting, reuse of illustrations, recitation, broadcasting, reproduction on microfilms or in any other physical way, and transmission or information storage and retrieval, electronic adaptation, computer software, or by similar or dissimilar methodology now known or hereafter developed.
The use of general descriptive names, registered names, trademarks, service marks, etc. in this publication does not imply, even in the absence of a specific statement, that such names are exempt from the relevant protective laws and regulations and therefore free for general use.
The publishers, the authors, and the editors are safe to assume that the advice and information in this book are believed to be true and accurate at the date of publication. Neither the publishers nor the authors or the editors give a warranty, express or implied, with respect to the material contained herein or for any errors or omissions that may have been made. The publishers remain neutral with regard to jurisdictional claims in published maps and institutional affiliations.

This Springer imprint is published by the registered company Springer Nature Singapore Pte Ltd.
The registered company address is: 152 Beach Road, #21-01/04 Gateway East, Singapore 189721, Singapore

Preface

This book deals with the diagnosis and treatment of anal fistula, a difficult anorectal disease. This book is an elaboration and discussion on the history of anal fistula, anatomy and physiology related to anal fistula, etiology and pathology of anal fistula, examination, diagnosis, treatment principles, surgical procedures and their evaluation, conservative treatments, academic disputes, and other aspects. The research and progress of the diagnosis and treatment of anal fistula at home and abroad are comprehensively and deeply expounded on. It contains the author's long-term research accumulation and clinical experience. This book provides an overview of both the history and current situation of the disease, pays close attention to new research trends, combines closely with clinical practice, is comprehensive in content and rich in information, and has excellent practicability. It is suitable for all researchers, graduate students, and clinical medical personnel engaged in anorectal specialty to learn from and reference.

Nanjing, China	Renjie Shi
Beijing, China	Lihua Zheng

Acknowledgements

I would like to thank Joanna song (Oxon) and Junfang song for their help in language edit. I also would like to thank my family for their support, especially my daughter Yunyang Shi, for her help in language edit.

Contents

1. **History of Cognition and Treatment of Anal Fistula** 1
   Renjie Shi and Feng Jiang

2. **Anatomy and Physiology of Anal Fistula** 11
   Renjie Shi, Dong Yang, and Min Zhang

3. **The Etiology of Anal Fistula** 35
   Renjie Shi, Feng Jiang, and XiaYong Yang

4. **Clinical Manifestations of Anal Fistula** 43
   Renjie Shi and Hongsheng Mao

5. **Common Methods of Examination for Anal Fistula** 47
   Renjie Shi and Lihua Liu

6. **Classification and Diagnosis of Anal Fistula** 89
   Renjie Shi and JinHui Gu

7. **The Therapeutic Principle of Fistula-in-Ano** 101
   Renjie Shi and Lihua Zheng

8. **Surgical Treatment of Anal Fistula** 109
   Renjie Shi and Lihua Zheng

9. **Nonoperative Treatment of Anal Fistula** 173
   Renjie Shi and YiXin Zhang

10. **Diagnosis and Treatment of Special Anal Fistula** 181
    Renjie Shi and Fang Liu

11. **Controversial Problems in the Diagnosis and Treatment of Anal Fistula** 223
    Renjie Shi and Yu He

Contributors

Jinhui Gu Suzhou Hospital of Traditional Chinese Medicine, Affiliated to Nanjing University of Chinese Medicine, Suzhou, Jiangsu, China

Yu He People's Hospital of Suzhow New District Hospital, Suzhou, Jiangsu, China

Feng Jiang Affiliated Hospital of Nanjing University of Traditional Chinese Medicine, Nanjing, Jiangsu, China

Fang Liu Sixth Affiliated Hospital, Sun Yat-sen University, Guangzhou, Guangdong, China

Lihua Liu Nanjing Jiangbei Hospital, Nanjing, Jiangsu, China

Hongsheng Mao Jingjiang People's Hospital, Jingjiang, Jiangsu, China

Renjie Shi Department of Anorectal Surgery, Affiliated Hospital of Nanjing University of Traditional Chinese Medicine, Nanjing, Jiangsu, China

Dong Yang Affiliated Lianyungang Hospital of Xuzhou Medical University, Lianyungang, Jiangsu, China

Xiayong Yang Taizhou Hospital of Traditional Chinese Medicine, Taizhou, Jiangsu, China

Min Zhang People's Hospital of Deyang, Deyang, Sichuan, China

Yixin Zhang Affiliated Hospital of Xuzhou Medical University, Xuzhou, Jiangsu, China

Lihua Zheng Department of Proctology, China-Japan Friendship Hospital, Beijing, China

History of Cognition and Treatment of Anal Fistula

Renjie Shi and Feng Jiang

Abstract

The names of anal fistula and perianal abscess have been recorded in Chinese literature more than 2000 years ago. For the treatment of anal fistula, historical documents of anal fistulectomy and internal medication could be found. In the Sui Dynasty, it was believed that the cause of anal fistula was related to the body as a whole. The treatment method of inserting medicine into fistulas to corrode fistulas was proposed in the Song Dynasty. In the Yuan Dynasty, the seton therapy of anal fistula based on gravity and medicated thread was developed. Since then, this therapy has been continuously improved and optimized in terms of materials and methods and is still widely used in clinical practice at present. Modern medicine has recognized the etiology, examination methods, and treatment principles of anal fistula since the time of Hippocrates more than 2000 years ago. However, the role of the anal gland in the pathogenesis and treatment of anal fistula was not recognized until 1958,

R. Shi (✉)
Department of Anorectal Surgery, Affiliated Hospital of Nanjing University of Traditional Chinese Medicine, Nanjing, Jiangsu, China

F. Jiang
Affiliated Hospital of Nanjing University of Traditional Chinese Medicine, Nanjing, Jiangsu, China

and it has been possible to cure anal fistula since then. Currently, the treatment of anal fistula is developing in the direction of protecting anal function and improving the cure rate.

Keywords

Anal fistula · Chinese medicine · History
Name of the disease · Pathogen · Pathology
Treatment · Seton therapy

1.1 The Knowledge and Treatment History of Anal Fistula in Chinese Medicine

In the ancient Chinese literature, "abscess," "fistula," or other terms were first put forward in the "Shan Hai Jing," which was written in the Western Zhou Dynasty. For example, an extract in "Shan Hai Jing • Zhongshan Jing" details, "there were many Teng Fish in He River which can be eaten to get carbuncle and treat fistula."

Next, hemorrhoids were classified into four categories: male piles, female piles, pulse piles, and blood piles in the "Prescriptions of Fifty-Two Diseases," which was written in the Western Han Dynasty (206 BC–AD 8). The symptoms of male piles were the anus having snail-like, rat-nipple like prolapses. The prolapses were small tumors on the surface of which there were often erosions, ulcers, and mouthwashes. The symptoms of female piles were half-inch of hemorrhoids in the anus shaped like a horn. Hemorrhoids that prolapsed and bled during defecation or female pile had several orifices, and many white mites came out of the orifice. Oral medicine, fumigation treatment, and surgical treatment for male piles and abscess were also written in this book. The treatment methods for male piles and abscess were mainly external, such as smoking, dressing, and ironing. For example, when treating male piles, "Quickly burn the base of the hemorrhoids to make it necrotic, and use ointment made from rice and ashes to apply to the wound. The patients who had male piles with multiple orifices should eat the fat from the cooked sheep meat and three buckets of rice. If Male piles are located on the external edge of the anus, about the size of the nucleus of jujube, sometimes itchy, sometimes painful, if it can be cut, it should be cut. If not, mix turtle's brain and bile worms into an application or iron the hemorrhoids with small cobblestones after burning with vinegar. When treating Male piles without fistula, cook a bucket of dates, a bucket of ointment, make four buckets of medicine solution and pour it into a tub for a sitz bath, so that pinworms can run out by themselves."

The book recorded that "Male piles are located outside the anus, the size of larger ones like a jujube and the size of smaller ones like a nucleus of jujube. When treating these kinds of male piles, it is effective to use a small cupping to pull the nucleus out for two measures of rice cooking time, pull out the cupping, ligature the nucleus with a thin wire, and then use a knife to peel off it. There will be a small block of blood clots in the nucleus, and the operation is completed after peeling it off." This is similar to the incision and drainage of the perianal abscess.

Under the section for female piles, there was a record: for patients with deep rectal rectum, kill a dog, take the dog's bladder, put it on a bamboo tube, insert it into the anus and inflate it, pull the lesion out of the anus, and slowly cut the lesion with a knife under direct vision. After the operation, the powder of *Scutellaria baicalensis* was applied to the patient for recovery. This is likely to be an incision treatment of the anal fistula.

The earliest record of abscess was found in the "Huang Di Nei Jing," "Ling Shu • Yong Ju": abscess occurs on the buttocks that are red and swollen, named pilonidal disease. "The patients need to be treated immediately, if not, the patient will die in 30 days." Pilonidal disease may be the earliest name in Chinese medicine for an anorectal abscess. The earliest record of a fistula is found in the article "Su Wen • Sheng Qi Tong Tian Lun": the coldness is deep in the veins and stays in the muscles and the movement of blood and Qi is not smooth, resulting in stagnation. As time progresses, it becomes a scab.

The term of "hemorrhoid and fistula" was seen in the "Shen Nong's Herbal" firstly. It documented the main cause of the diseases carbuncle sore and hemorrhoid fistula. Hemorrhoid fistula refers to hemorrhoids, fistula, and other anorectal diseases. A total of 365 kinds of effective drugs were collected in this book before the Han Dynasty, and there were more than 50 types of involuntary diseases involving anorectal diseases, 21 types can be used to cure hemorrhoids such as astragalus, acacia, clam, hedgehog skin, beehives, and so on, and 14 kinds of them can cure fistulas such as oysters and scorpions. There are astragalus, realgar, and other four types that can be used to cure hemorrhoids and fistulas together.

Gong Qingxuan in the Southern and Northern Dynasties wrote "Liu Juan-zi's Gui-Yi-fang" (AD 499), which is the earliest existing surgical monograph in China. In this book, the dialectical treatment of perianal abscesses, such as "Yun Ju" and "Chi Shi," is discussed in detail.

The etiology, pathogenesis, and syndrome differentiation and treatment of hemorrhoid fistula were recorded in "Zhu Bing Yuan Hou Lun" (AD 610), which was written by Chao Yuanfang in the Sui Dynasty. In the "Zhi Bing Zhu Hou," he proposed seven categories: male piles, female piles, pulse piles, intestinal piles, blood piles, Qi piles, and alcohol piles. The etiology and pathogenesis of these were also expressed vividly in the book. The male pile is a description of the symptoms of anal fistula, which are rat-like, nipple-like scorpions that grow next to the anus and always have outflows of pus and blood. In the section of "Earthworm fistula": "earthworm fistula … Its roots are in the large intestine, and it is swollen and purulent." In "Gu Dao Sheng Chuang Hou": "anal symptoms are the reaction of the large intestine and the deficiency heat of in the large intestine gathers in the anus, resulting in the anus sore and ulcer." It is recorded that the etiology of anal sores lies in the deficiency of heat in the large intestine. The notion of the fistula evolved from the unhealed abscess and was put forward in this book. As described about "chronic abscess": "coldness which stops in the meridian and blood which flows unsmoothly accumulate to be the carbuncle. When heat and toxic pathogens have not completely dissipated and at the same time the patient is infected by the cold wind, resulting in all kinds of evils clogging each other, the fistula begins to develop over time."

Due to the prosperity of the economy and culture in the Tang Dynasty, medicine also developed rapidly, and the understanding of hemorrhoids and fistulas became more in-depth. "Valuable Prescription for Emergencies" (AD 652) written by Sun Simiao is a clinical book representing the medical levels of the Tang Dynasty. In the book, there are special articles on anorectal diseases, such as Volume 18, "The Big Intestines" and Volume 23, "The Hemorrhoid and Fistula," which records a large number of anorectal specialist content. In "The Hemorrhoid and Fistula • Five Hemorrhoids," the classification, syndromes, and main drugs for hemorrhoids are systematically discussed, organically linking to disease differentiation, syndrome differentiation, and treatment. It clearly proposed the main drugs for five hemorrhoids, such as turtle shell, hedgehog skin, beehive and Serpentis Periostracum, and so on. It is another major advancement in the treatment of anorectal diseases. There is a record in "Valuable Prescription for Emergencies" that "hedgehog skin is useful for Male pile which is swollen for 5–6 days after rupturing and with outflows of pus." In AD 752, Wang Tao's "Wai Tai Mi Yao" made a certain contribution to the collection and preservation of ancient medical books. The book also expounds on treatment methods with the use of animal organs for the treatment of hemorrhoid and fistula diseases, such as the use of squid soup, the treatment of hemorrhoid with the sheep spinal cord, the treatment of prolapse of anus with pig liver, and the method of treating constipation with saltwater enema by bamboo tube.

In the Song Dynasty, there were many new contents in the "Tai Ping Sheng Hui Fang • Zhi Zhi Gang Bian Sheng Shu Ru Zhu Fang" (AD 982–992). The book puts forward the methods of "internal elimination" and "expelling pathogens by strengthening vital Qi," and the therapy in which arsenic was dissolved in yellow wax, twisted into slivers and absorbed in hemorrhoid fistula orifices, was the earliest recorded homogeneous treatment. At the same time, the book also listed hemorrhoids and fistula in two chapters, indicating that they are different diseases. "Tai Ping Sheng Hui Fang • Zhi Zhu Lou Zhu Fang" also pointed out: "the poisonous evil produced by hemorrhoids gathers on the edge of the anus to form a sore or rat-like, nipple-like sputum. After the perforation is broken, the fistula does not heal. There is always pus and blood flowing out, the anus is swollen and painful. If it does not heal for a long time, it will form an anal fistula." The etiology and symptoms of anal fistula are more clearly discussed. In addition, the prescription of Sophoricoside pill was also described, and the contents on internal treatment methods are also abundant.

At the end of the Southern Song Dynasty, Chen Ziming named the perianal abscess "Yong" for the first time in "Wai Ke Jing Yao" (AD 1263), saying: "the carbuncle located in front and rear of the anus is known as the Uvular Abscess."

"A-B Classic of Acupuncture and Moxibustion" recorded the method of using acupuncture to treat anorectal diseases such as hemorrhoids, prolapse of anus, and chronic dysentery. This was written by Huang Pumi in the Jin Dynasty. In the section of "Channel-of-Foot-Tai Yang Dong Fa Xia Bu, hemorrhoid and prolapse of anus," there is a record that the prognosis is very poor in patients with anal diseases connected with the pudendal part. This is the earliest record of anorectal diseases combined with vaginal fistula and urethral fistula. They were unable to cure this disease effectively limited to the conditions at that time.

In the Yuan Dynasty, "Shi Yi De Xiao Fang" (1337) and "Yang Lao Shou Qin Xin Shu" also included some dietary therapies for anal fistula and five hemorrhoids.

The principle and method of treating uvular abscess have been clearly put forward in the "Wai Ke Jing Yao" by Xue Ji in the Ming Dynasty. This established the basic treatment principle of dissipating at the beginning, expelling pus and expressing toxin at the stage of abscess formation, and invigoration and expressing toxin after abscess formation.

In the Ming Dynasty, Xu Chunpu's "Gu Jin Yi Tong" quotes the hanging therapy for anal fistula from the famous medical book, "Yong Lei Ling Fang," written in the Yuan Dynasty, which is lost now. The book points out that the indications for hanging line therapy are patients with a long course of disease with an internal orifice in the intestinal cavity and an external orifice in the buttocks and can be felt with the shape of the fistula. The method of making the medicine string is to cook a common turnip with the string. The method of operation is reaching the top of the internal orifice with grass, then threading the string into the internal orifice, out of the external orifice, tie a knot outside the anus, and hang a plumb to speed up the curative effect. The mechanism in how it works is that the string, which can drain the pus, cuts the sphincter down and the muscle above grows into the lumen below in order to heal the fistula without any damage. The course of treatment depends on the distance between the wound and the anus and is usually around ten days to half a month, no more than 20 days. It can be seen that the process of hanging therapy for anal fistula was very comprehensive even then, and details are abundant.

In the "Experience Book of Chuangyang • Hemorrhoid Fistula and Illustration" (AD 1569), the anal fistula is called leakage ulcer and single leakage. The cause, pathogenesis, and treatment were specifically discussed, and the genetic factors of anorectal disease were first recognized here. The book recorded that patients who cannot drink alcohol but suffer from hemorrhoids were caused by weakness of zang-fu viscera. This happens when the blood of the mother and the essence of the father are deficient. It is another progress in the understanding of the cause of anorectal disease in Chinese medicine. On the basis of the five hemorrhoids, they were further divided into 25 hemorrhoids in detail and illustrated with pictures, which fully reflected the meticulous and in-depth research on hemorrhoids fistula at that time. There is also a record of "single leakage" in "Experience Book of Chuangyang." For example, it detailed on the left or right side of the anus that there is a fistula called a single fistula that excretes out pus and blood. This is similar to the simple anal fistula in modern medicine.

In the Ming Dynasty, Shen Douyuan's "Wai Ke Qi Xuan" (1604) introduced the method of making drugs and the principles of the application method and changing the medicine.

The famous medical doctor Chen Shigong's book "Wai Ke Zheng Zong" (AD 1617) summarized the academic achievements of the previous generation in a comprehensive way and wrote the articles such as "Zang Du Theory" and "Hemorrhoid Theory." The etiology, pathogenesis, and syndrome differentiation of diseases such as hemorrhoids, fistulas, and abscess were comprehensively discussed. The theory, method, prescription, and medicine are all complete and scientific and have had a great influence on later generations. They are still effectively used in clinics now. "Wai Ke Zheng Zong • Hemorrhoid Theory" recorded San Ping Yi Tiao Qiang can cure 18 kinds of leaks (San Ping Yi Tiao Qiang is used to treat the hemorrhoids and fistulas by means of 100 g of alum, 60 g of arsenic trioxide, 24 g of realgar, and 12 g of olibanum, refined, ground into powder, simmered into a line, drying it, and then inserted into the hemorrhoid hole). "Zang Du Theory" recorded that in patients with a chronic cough, the sputum and fire condenses into a corn-sized mass on the anus. If the mass breaks, a fistula will be formed. If it is prolonged and does not heal, patients will have a poor prognosis after the exhaustion of Qi and blood.

Qi Kun's "Wai Ke Da Cheng" (AD 1665) detailed descriptions of anus carbuncle or abscess, hemorrhoid, anal fistula, anal fissure, and anorectal cancer. "Xia Bu Shuo" recorded hanging pain in the perineum, behind the scro-

1 History of Cognition and Treatment of Anal Fistula

tum, and in front of the anus. At the beginning of the course, the size of it is like a pine nut. During the progress period, the size becomes like a lotus seed. After a few days, this part begins to redden, swell and heat up, and is eventually swollen like a peach. Shang Ma Carbuncles are on the buttocks near the right side of the anus. Xia Ma Carbuncles are on the buttocks near the left side of the anus. It specifically described what is known as the site and syndrome of the anal anterior space abscess and the ischial rectal abscess. The perianal fistula is divided into ten categories with large amounts of information on internal treatment. The book first proposed the treatment principle that the complex anal fistula should be divided into ten types. All patients with complicated anal fistulas treated with thread-hanging therapy should only treat one fistula at a time and then treat another fistula in a few days. The fistula in "Wai Ke Da Cheng • Zhi Lou Fu Yu" was divided into eight types, including the anal fistula with complex bending fistula, such as the anal fistula of the scrotum that is difficult to deliver drugs to the base of the lesion because of its curved sinus tract. Patients with complex anal fistula must have multiple sinus tracts if they find that the skin around the lesion becomes hard and the color darkens. It described in detail the appearance of complex anal fistulas.

"Gu Jin Tu Shu Ji Cheng • Yi Bu Quan Lu" (AD 1723) systematically organized the relevant theories of doctors in the past and established a special book on hemorrhoid and fistula diseases, which was used to cure the disease. There were more than ten kinds of methods such as internal treatment, withering hemorrhoid, ligation, fume wash, iron stick, medication, acupuncture, hanging, drainage, etc. (Fig. 1.1), among which the most comprehensive prescription was internal treatment, containing 559 oral prescriptions.

"Yi Zong Jin Jian" (AD 1742) written by Wu Qian systematically discussed hematochezia, diarrhea, anal anus carbuncle and abscess, hemorrhoids, and other anal diseases from the aspects of etiology, pathogenesis, and syndrome differentiation. It was illustrated with drawings, among which 24 hemorrhoids depicted graphic images. Gao Bingjun's "Yang Ke Xin De Ji" (AD 1809) is a major influential surgical monograph. There are some articles, such as Bian Tuo-Gang-Zhi-Lou Lun, Bian Gang-Men-Yong-Zang-Tou-Du-Tou-Fen-Shu Lun, Bian Tun-Yong-Qi-Ma-Yong Lun, and so on. In the etiology, pathogenesis, and syndrome differentiation of anal diseases, the relationship between viscera, meridians, and Qi and blood was highlighted, and syndrome differentiation and disease differentiation were combined.

It has been recorded in "Wai Ke Shi San Fang" from the Ming Dynasty that San Ping Yi Tiao Qiang was inserted into the fistula and out of the canal, and it described a method to cure anal fistula out of the canal with salmiacum and red arsenic as the main medicines.

The medical instruments for the treatment of anal fistula in the Qing Dynasty were further developed. For example, the scimitar, hook knife, lancet, silver wire, and anal needle drawn in the "Wai Ke Tu Shuo" are all instruments for treating anal fistula. Gao Wenjin's "Wai Ke Tu Shuo" (AD 1834) recorded the diagnosis and treatment equipment of hemorrhoids and fistulas used in the past, including machete, hook knife, lancet, penknife, pointed scissors, small iron, anal tube, anal needle, etc. Many of these instruments are unique in design, compact, and practical and have been used ever since.

Zhao Qian's "Yi Men Bu Yao" (AD 1883) advocated to fix the medicine wire with a thin copper needle, insert the needle into the fistula with the right hand, insert the thick bone needle into the anus with the left hand, catch the needle and the medicine wire, hit a buckle, gradually tighten, and then tie the button to the medicine wire and keep the button suspended. The luminal, open after seven days, should be sprinkled with Sheng Ji powder, and the wound heals in a month. The probe was used for the hanging therapy, and knotting and tightening methods were improved. Moreover, the surgical methods of foreign body entering the anus and congenital analepsia were further improved, which reflected the new progress of hemorrhoid and fistula in the Qing dynasty. The name of anal fistula was first recorded in the "Wai Zheng Yi An Hui Bian."

Fig. 1.1 Commonly used external treatment methods in the treatment of hemorrhoids and fistulas in Chinese medicine

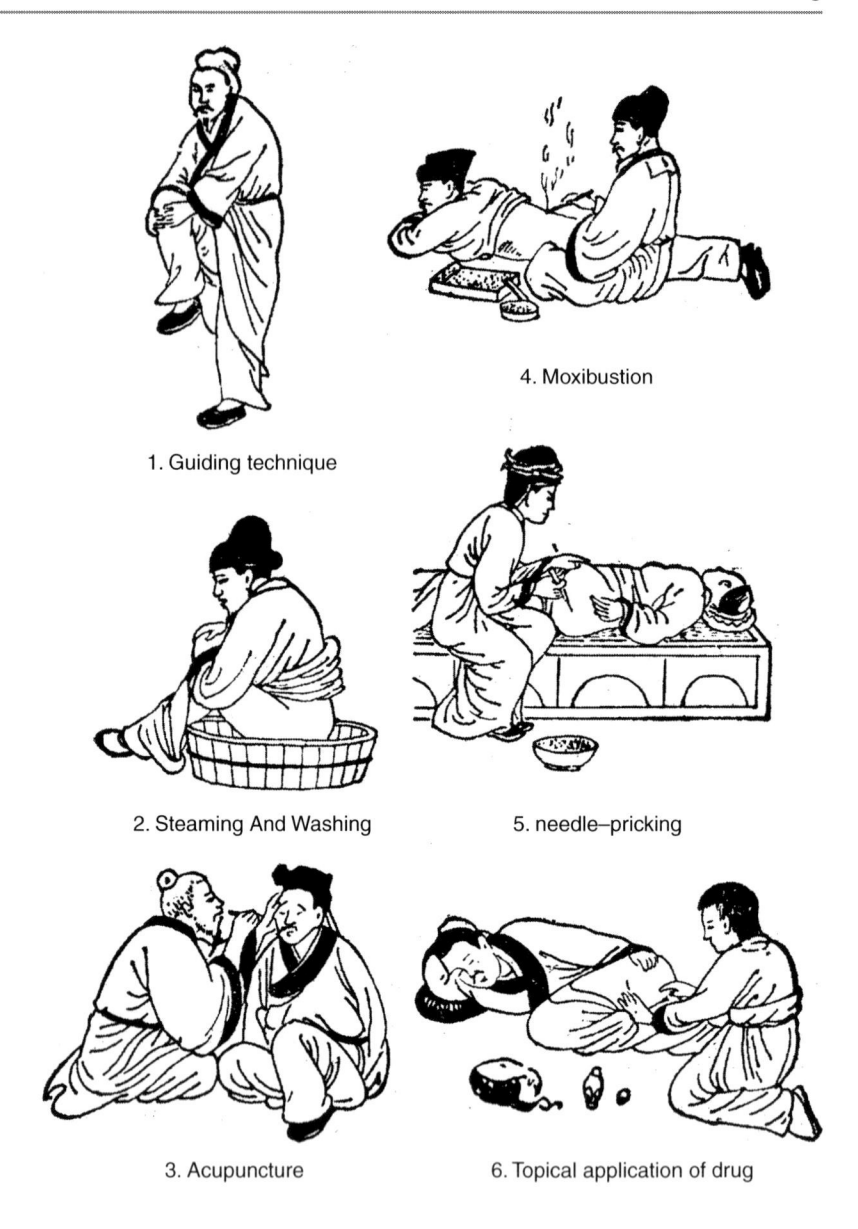

1. Guiding technique
2. Steaming And Washing
3. Acupuncture
4. Moxibustion
5. needle–pricking
6. Topical application of drug

For more than one hundred years (AD 1840–1949), due to historical reasons, the anorectal doctors of Chinese treatment mostly were folk practitioners, and their academics mostly relied on family members or teachers passing it down to them. They each have different opinions; in order to earn a living and beat rivals, there was basically no communication between doctors, so the progress of academics and improvement were relatively slow.

After the founding of the People's Republic of China, under the leadership and care of the government, Chinese medicine has been valued and developed. Many traditional Chinese and Western medicine anorectal disease monographs have been published continuously. In 1953, Zhang Qingrong published "Practical Anorectal Surgery." In 1955, Huang Jichuan's "Treatment of Hemorrhoids and Fistulas" was published. The book inherited and carried forward the legacy of traditional Chinese medicine treatment and introduced the author's own clinical experience and secret recipe for treating hemorrhoids and fistulas. It was sold quickly at home and abroad and was valued by Premier Zhou Enlai. In 1956, Wang Fanglin's "Clinical Hemorrhoids and Fistulas" was published, which combined personal experience, kept the characteristics of traditional Chinese medicine and combined the advantages of Western medicine treatment, and summarized the clinical experience of diagnosis and treatment. Before and after 1985, there were Yu Dehong's "Anorectal Surgical Diseases Q&A," Cao Jixun's "Chinese Hemorrhoids and Fistulas," Shi Zhaoqi's "Chinese Large Intestine Anal Diseases," Li Runting's "Anorectal Disease," Hu Bohu's "Practical Hemorrhoids and Fistulas," and Li Yunong's "Chinese Anorectal Diseases." These books provided a comprehensive introduction to the new knowledge, new technologies, and clinical experience in understanding and preventing anorectal diseases in China, and they were representative works at the time. Published in 1996 by Huang Naijian, a compilation of domestic famous anorectal experts, "Chinese Anorectal Disease," was a comprehensive and systematic summary of previous academic research results and achievements in anorectal diseases.

After the founding of the People's Republic of China, academic communications were valued by the government, and academic communication activities on anorectal diseases continued to increase. In 1956, the Institute of Traditional Chinese Medicine established the Research Group. In 1964, the Chinese Academy of Traditional Chinese Medicine was commissioned by the Ministry of Health to hold the first national scientific research conference in Beijing and officially formulated the diagnosis and treatment standards for anorectal diseases. In 1966, the Ministry of Health held a ministerial-level meeting of hemorrhoid fistula results attended by 24 units in Beijing and officially affirmed the achievements in the treatment of high complex anal fistula with incision drainage and seton therapy method, ligation method, and Withering hemorrhoids method in the treatment of internal hemorrhoids.

In recent decades, with the rapid development of science and technology, the traditional methods of treating anal fistula by Chinese medicine have been well explored and inherited and have been innovated on constantly, forming many new unique treatments for treating anal fistula. These include incision drainage and seton therapy operations, the internal orifice sutures and the medicine twists to detach the tube operations, virtual drainage of anal fistula operations, open and suture anal fistula operations, anal fistula preservation sphincter operations, and so on. They all raised the level of diagnosis and treatment of anal fistula to a new level.

1.2 The History of Anal Fistula and Treatment in Western Medicine

The record of Western medicine begins with Hippocrates (460 BC–377 BC). Hippocrates is called the "father of medicine" in the West. Hippocrates proposed the etiology, examination method, and treatment principle of anal fistula in his famous book on fistulas. He believed that anal fistula is caused by trauma or injury during horse riding or rowing because blood accumulates near the anus in the buttocks. The nodules are formed, and then the abscess ruptures into fistulas. He advocated draining the abscess before it ruptures. He used stirrups and twine for seton therapy. The purpose of using the stirrup is that it does not break due to pus soaking and decaying. Cersus C (25 BC–5 BC) recommended in his book that the anal fistula should be treated with a knife. For anal fistulas with multiple external orifices, patients were treated with suture and incision.

In 1370, John Arderne, a British surgical authority, performed fistulectomy with the help of seton and grotched probes and applied ointment made of egg yolk or egg white to replace the dressing after surgery. In his works, the discussion of anal fistula is close to the modern view. He had learned that ischiorectal abscesses far from the anus could eventually form an anal fistula. He argued that the abscess should be cut in order to drain pus before it ruptures. His treatment of anal fistula is a method of corroding the fistulas. It is said that this method of treating anal fistula failed to gain the trust of the court at that time. Because of this, the English monarch Henry V who was troubled by anal fistula did not turn to the famous doctor.

In November 1686, surgeon Felix and his assistant Bessier used a special "ball-end probe knife" tip probe to extend into the fistula from the external orifice without anesthesia and pulled it out from the internal orifice to quickly cut the fistula. This is a standard open fistulectomy. The success of the operation greatly changed the views of dignitaries of the time.

Louis XIV (AD 1636–1715) was a famous French bourbon king who suffered from anal fistula. In order to cure the king's anal fistula, court doctors and quacks discussed together and worked out a series of treatment plans. They selected a group of voluntary anal fistula patients to do test trials, but the results were not ideal. In the late seventeenth century, Felix M, a famous French surgeon, successfully cured the anal fistula of the French king Louis XIV with a special scalpel.

Hunter J (1728–1793) advocated that the anal fistula pipeline should be completely open from the external orifice to the internal orifice. He believed that the high anal fistula should be located near the inner opening, at a higher position than the outer opening. In 1765, in his book on the treatment of anal fistula, Sir Pott especially emphasized the importance of accurate definition and correct naming of diseases. "A clear and precise definition of a disease, and a name based on its true nature, is far more important than generalizations. Incorrect or imperfect definitions and naming may lead to incorrect or imperfect concepts. With this misconception, it can only be the wrong treatment." His insightful conclusion is a valuable motto for anorectal doctors and even the medical community as a whole.

In 1740, Hugier emphasized the "V" shape of the wound after fistula incision to facilitate drainage. In 1765, Pott indicated that the hardened fistula should be completely removed. In 1852, Chassaignac advocated suturing the wound after cutting the anal fistula.

In the nineteenth century, the German scholar Chiari (1878) and the French scholars Desfosses and Hermann respectively proposed the hypothesis that the morphology of the anal gland and the anal gland may have some connection with tissue infection around the anus. In the anal fistula operation, Salmon in London made a vertical auxiliary incision at the lateral end after opening the fistula tube so that the wound was in the shape of "7," so as to delay the healing of the external wound to avoid the formation of a pocket-shaped false passage. Later, this auxiliary incision evolved into a racquet-shaped incision at the external opening, which is more conducive to drainage and healing. In 1873, professor Diitel of Vienna introduced the use of elastic rubber strips for strangulation ligation of anal fistula. This was the earliest record of the Mark's Hospital in London. This method was studied, and a paper was published in 1874, reporting its success in treating 60 anal fistulas.

In 1835, Salmon founded a "poor relief hospital" with only seven beds, specializing in the containment and treatment of anal fistulas and other rectal disorders. By 1854, the hospital had expanded to 25 beds and was officially named St. Hospital. Under the leadership of Salmon, St. Mark's Hospital has cultivated a generation of anorectal surgery masters, whose outstanding theoretical research and clinical practice have promoted the development of anorectal surgery all over the world. In 1870, Goodsall and Miles W.E., who worked at St. Mark's Hospital, wrote the book *Anorectal Diseases*. In the chapter "Anal Rectal Fistula" of this book, the morphology, etiology, symptoms, examination, and treatment of anal fistula were described in detail. In particular, his observations on the position of the internal and external orifices of the anal fistula and the direction of the fistula were described in more detail. Later generations referred to his rules as "Goodsall's Law."

Over the past 100 years, our understanding of the important role of the anal sinus and anal gland in the infection of the anorectal area has been expanded. At the same time, there has been a breakthrough in the understanding of the etiology and pathology of anal fistula. The treatment of anal fistula has also been greatly improved. In 1958, Eisenhammer proposed the theory of anal crypt and gland infection and performed internal sphincter and anusotomy. In 1961, British scholars Parks et al. proposed the surgical method of thoroughly removing the infected anal rectum, anal gland duct, and anal gland and not cutting the anal sphincter of anus to dig out the anal fistula, which has become the basis of modern treatment of anal fistula and preserving the sphincter. Later, scholars from various countries continued to improve on this method so as to improve the overall treatment of anal fistula.

Suggested Reading

1. Huang Naijian. Chinese Anorectal Diseases. Jinan: Shandong Science and Technology Press, 1996, 1–26.
2. Cao Jixun. Chinese dropout. Chengdu: Sichuan Science and Technology Press, 2015, 1–30.
3. Colon and Rectal Surgery (5th edn). Beijing: People's Medical Publishing House, 2009, 1–24.
4. Zhang Shaojun, Yang Wei. Development and thinking of ancient anal fistula hanging thread. Jiangsu Journal of Traditional Chinese Medicine,2012,44(4): 6–62.
5. Yang Bolin, Ding Yijiang. Treatment of anal fistula line. Journal of Colorectal and Anal Surgery, 2005, 11(1): 7–81.
6. Chen Liang. Anal fistula of Louis XIV. All circles, 2013, (7): 77

2. Anatomy and Physiology of Anal Fistula

Renjie Shi, Dong Yang, and Min Zhang

Abstract

The rectum is derived from the endoderm, and the anal canal is derived from the ectoderm, and they are connected and fused at the anus tooth line. The tissue structure, blood circulation, innervation, and lymphatic regurgitation are different in the upper and lower tooth lines. According to the histology of the epithelium, the tooth line is anatomically defined as the upper limit of the anal canal. However, based on the function, the rectal column line is defined as the upper limit of the anal canal in surgery. The anal gland open in the anal sinus and is related to most of the infections around the anus and rectum. The functions of defecation, levator, and supporting pelvic organs are completed by the cooperation of internal sphincter, external sphincter, levator ani muscle, and longitudinal muscle. The damage of these muscles would affect the function of anal sphincter. The perirectal space is an important place for infection spread and development.

Keywords

Anatomy · Physiology · Histology · Anal canal · Rectum · Anal sphincter · Anal gland Perirectal space · Nerve · Lymph nodes

2.1 Anorectal Genesis

The digestive tract and the digestive glands are both evolved from the original intestinal tube that is rolled and folded at the top of the yolk sac. The original intestine originates from the endoderm at the top of the yolk sac. The digestive tract develops earlier. On the 20th day, when the blastoderm is folded into a cylindrical embryo body, the endoderm (the top of the yolk sac) is also folded into a tube, with blind ends on both the head and tail. The head end is the foregut, the tail end is the hindgut, and the middle part that connects with the yolk sac is called the midgut. The foregut develops into the first 2/3 of the pharynx, esophagus, stomach, and duodenum; the midgut develops into the posterior 1/3 of the duodenum, jejunum, ileum, cecum, appendix, ascending colon, and front 2/3 of the transverse colon. The hindgut develops into the posterior 1/3 of the transverse colon, descending colon, sigmoid

R. Shi (✉)
Department of Anorectal Surgery, Affiliated Hospital of Nanjing University of Traditional Chinese Medicine, Nanjing, Jiangsu, China

D. Yang
Affiliated Lianyungang Hospital of Xuzhou Medical University, Lianyungang, Jiangsu, China

M. Zhang
People's Hospital of Deyang, Deyang, Sichuan, China

© Chemical Industry Press 2021
R. Shi, L. Zheng (eds.), *Diagnosis and Treatment of Anal Fistula*,
https://doi.org/10.1007/978-981-16-5804-4_2

colon, rectum, and the part above the dentate line of the anal canal.

The urinary septum appears in the cloaca of the hindgut during the sixth week of the embryo. This septum is formed by the mesenchyme between the hindgut and the allantoic, which divides the cloaca into the dorsal rectum and the ventral urogenital sinus. The cloaca membrane is also divided into the anal membrane and the urogenital sinus membrane. The outer periphery of the anal membrane forms a nodular bulge with a central depression, and this is called the original anus. The anal canal develops from two parts, the upper part is formed from the end of the rectum, and the lower part is formed from the original anus. The epithelium of the original anus is derived from the ectoderm, and the rectum is derived from the endoderm. At the eighth week, the anal membrane ruptures, and the epithelium that forms the anal inner and ectoderm meet at the anal canal. The dentate line represents the fusion of the endoderm and the ectoderm. At the tenth week, the dorsal side of the anal nodules (a pair of ectodermal bumps surrounding the anal canal) fuse to form a horseshoe-like structure, and the perineal body is formed at the front. The cloacal sphincter is divided into the urogenital part and the anal part (external anal sphincter) by the perineal body. The internal anal sphincter is formed in the 6th to 12th week of the embryo. The sphincter noticeably migrates during their development, the external sphincter migrates to the head side, and the internal sphincter moves to the caudal side. At the same time, the longitudinal muscles descend into the intersphincter plane. Various congenital anal fistulas and anorectal malformations are related to abnormalities in the development process mentioned above.

2.2 Anal Canal and Rectum

2.2.1 Anal Canal

The anal canal is the anus. The upper end is connected to the rectum, and the lower end opens at the edge of the anus. The anal canal is usually tightly closed. The front wall is slightly longer than the back wall. It forms an angle of approximately 90° downward and backward to the rectum. During defecation, the anal canal expands into a tube with a diameter of about 3 cm and is shorter in length.

The anal canal is divided into anatomical anal canal and surgical anal canal (Fig. 2.1). Anatomical anal canal (anatomical anal canal) refers to the part covered by the anal epithelium, that is, the part from the tooth line to the anal edge. Surgery anal canal (surgical anal canal) refers to the part surrounded by the anal sphincter, that is, from the upper edge of the puborectalis muscle to the lower edge of the outer sphincter skin (anal verge). It is easier to understand the former as the sphincteric anal canal and the latter as the epithelial anal canal.

Dividing the anal canal into anatomical anal canal and surgical anal canal has certain practical significance. The anal canal in surgery is mainly confirmed by the anal sphincter, which has the same structure and function. Its upper boundary is the upper edge of the levator ani muscle, which can be confirmed by digital examination. For anal fistula, rectal cancer, and other treatments involving sphincter lesions, the definition of surgical anal canal is more convenient and more targeted. However, the upper boundary of the anal canal in surgery is the upper edge of the levator ani muscle, which cannot be confirmed by the naked eye. It needs to be diagnosed by digital examination. For patients with a weak front sphincter, the upper edge of the levator ani muscle is difficult to palpate. At the same time, the histological composition of the upper part of the anal canal in surgery is also diverse. Squamous epithelial carcinoma occurs in the rectum, adenocarcinoma occurs in the anal canal, and there are cases where malignant melanoma, leiomyoma, etc. occur. For qualitative benign and malignant tumors, it is difficult to explain clearly using the concept of surgical anal canal at this time, but it is easier to understand using the concept of anatomical anal canal.

On anatomy, the upper edge of the anal canal is the tooth line, and the lower edge is the anal edge, which can be clearly identified by the naked eye. The boundary is clear, and the observing

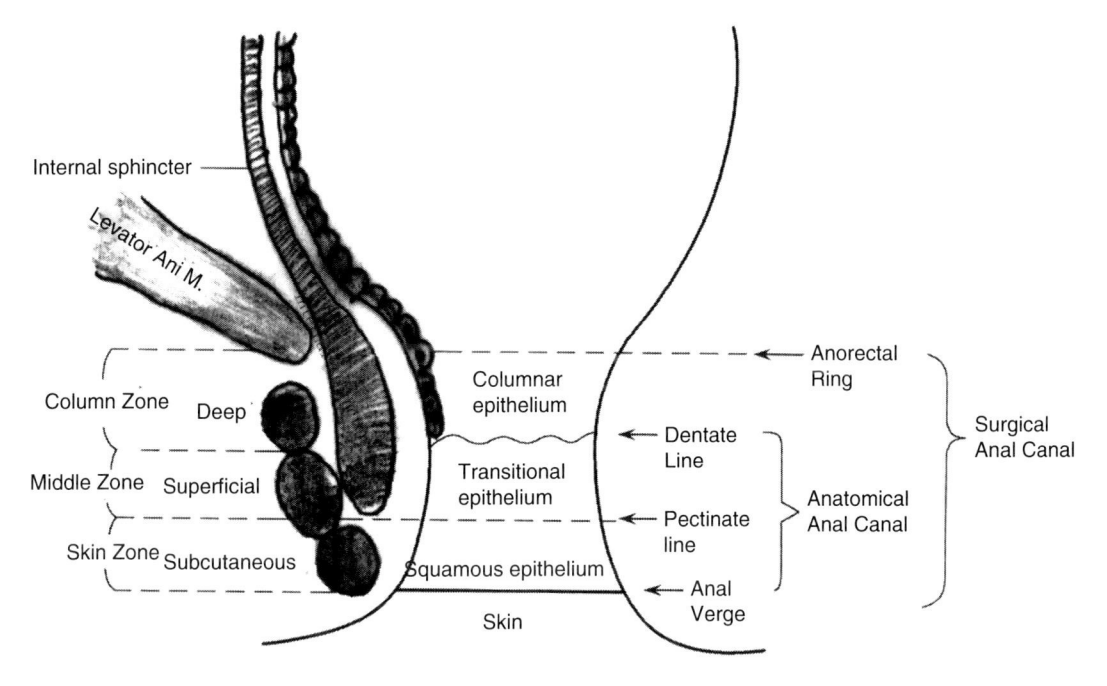

Fig. 2.1 Anal canal (from Masahiro Takano)

with the naked eye is consistent with histological performance.

The length of the anal canal in surgery is 3.2 cm for males and 2.9 cm for females, with an average of 3 cm. The length of the anal canal is 1.8 cm for males and 1.7 cm for females, with an average of 1.8 cm. On both sides of the anal canal is the ischiorectal fossa, the front of which is the urethra and prostate, the female has the vagina, and the rear is the tailbone. The perianal skin is mainly squamous epithelium, with abundant sweat glands and sebaceous glands, and sometimes dermatitis and eczema can occur. The causes of chronic perianal dermatitis and eczema include exudate caused by anal and rectal lesions, anal dampness, abrasions, and an unclean anus. Whenever the perianal skin and subcutaneous tissue become inflamed, and the swelling of the tissue subsides, the anal margin or perianal skin becomes loose or uplifted, and external hemorrhoids will form skin tags on the anal margin. In addition, it is easy to form skin tags on the outer end of the anal fissure wound when stimulated by secretions from an anal fissure wound.

The anal epithelium lacks sweat glands and sebaceous glands and is a thin and smooth stratified squamous epithelium. The anal canal has less subepithelial soft tissue, and the anal canal epithelium is surrounded by hard and poorly extensible internal sphincter and is fixed to the white line of the anus. It has poor mobility and is therefore vulnerable to injury and tear during defecation, resulting in anal fissure.

The epithelium covering above the dentate line is stratified cubic epithelium, and the migration epithelium is stratified columnar epithelium. The migration epithelium is slightly purple, and its width is reported to be 0.64–1.27 cm. Moving upward is the rectal mucosa covered by a single layer of pink columnar epithelium.

Being the upper boundary of the anal canal in anatomy, the tooth line is wavy. It is the junction of the endoderm and ectoderm, the dividing line between the flat epithelium and the columnar epithelium, and the division of the somatic nerve (sensory nerve) and the autonomic nerve (vegetative nerve).

On boundaries, internal hemorrhoids above the tooth line are painless because they occur in the area innervated by autonomic nerves. The inner sphincter is innervated by autonomic nerves, and the outer sphincter is innervated by somatic nerves. The vascular system is also bounded by this. There is an internal hemorrhoidal venous plexus that injects into the superior rectal artery upward, and an external hemorrhoidal venous plexus that flows to the middle and inferior rectum veins downward (Fig. 2.2). The return of lymph fluid also serves as the dividing line, but it is not absolute. Malignant tumors in the anal canal can move up to the root of the inferior mesenteric artery, laterally to the pelvis, and lower to the groin.

The dentate line is the dividing line between the internal and external hemorrhoids, and the branches of the joint longitudinal muscles, which Parks calls the so-called mucosal suspensory ligament, are attached here to distinguish the rectum from the anus. The epithelium is also divided into two parts: the upper part is the submucosal space, which contains the internal hemorrhoidal venous plexus, and the lower part is the perianal space, which contains the external hemorrhoidal venous plexus. There is very little blood flow between these two spaces. When swelling occurs, although the upper and lower parts are swollen, the boundary is fixed and causes blood circulation obstacles. Therefore, when the hemorrhoids are incarcerated, a deep groove can be seen there.

The shape of dentate line is a zigzag, and the upper part of the upward protruding area is the anal column, and the anal column has a rectal column of Morgagni (Fig. 2.3), of which there are about 8 to 14. The sunken between the anal columns is called anal sinus, and the epithelium on its lower edge is pocket-shaped or bowl-shaped, called the anal valve. The protruding part on the tooth line is called the anal papilla. When the anal papilla grows due to chronic inflammation, it is called anal papillary hypertrophy, also known as anal polyps.

The sunken on the inside of the anal flap is called an anal recess, also referred to as an anal sinus. The Italian anatomist Giantatista Morgagni (1682–1771) first recorded anal crypts. The number of anal crypts ranges from 6 to 11 (8 on average), with the anus being the deepest at 1.0 mm, the front depth being 0.7 mm, and the left and right sides being 0.4 mm. Inflammation here is known as anal cryptitis, and its symptoms are persistent mild to moderate pain. When the anal crypt is inflamed, mild tenderness and induration can be palpated on the anal crypt using a digital examination. About 65% of anal crypts have an opening at the bottom of the anal gland, which is connected to the anal gland through an anal gland duct (Fig. 2.4). For ease of understanding, sometimes it is

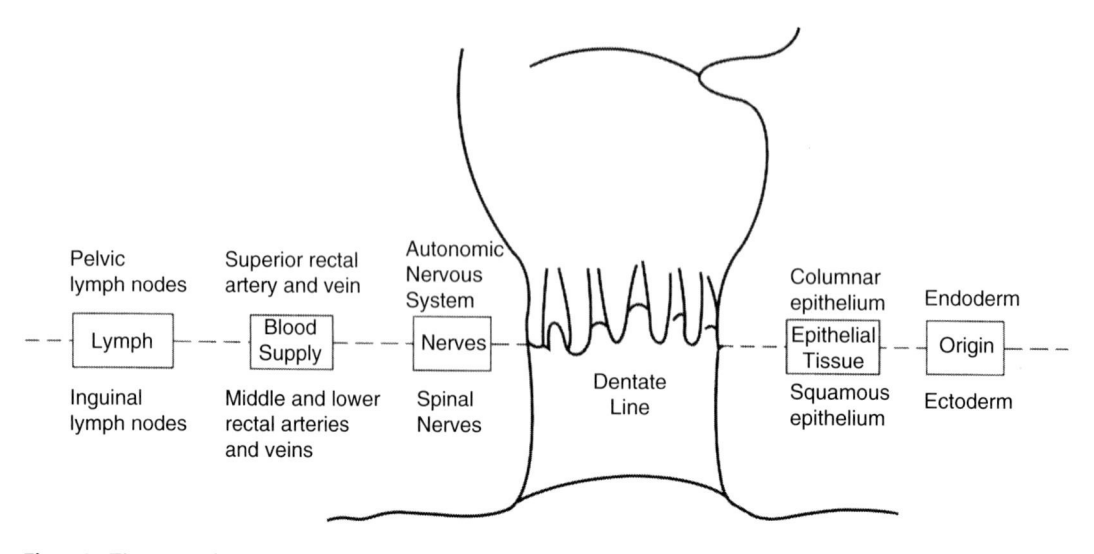

Fig. 2.2 The anatomical and clinical significance of dental line

2   Anatomy and Physiology of Anal Fistula

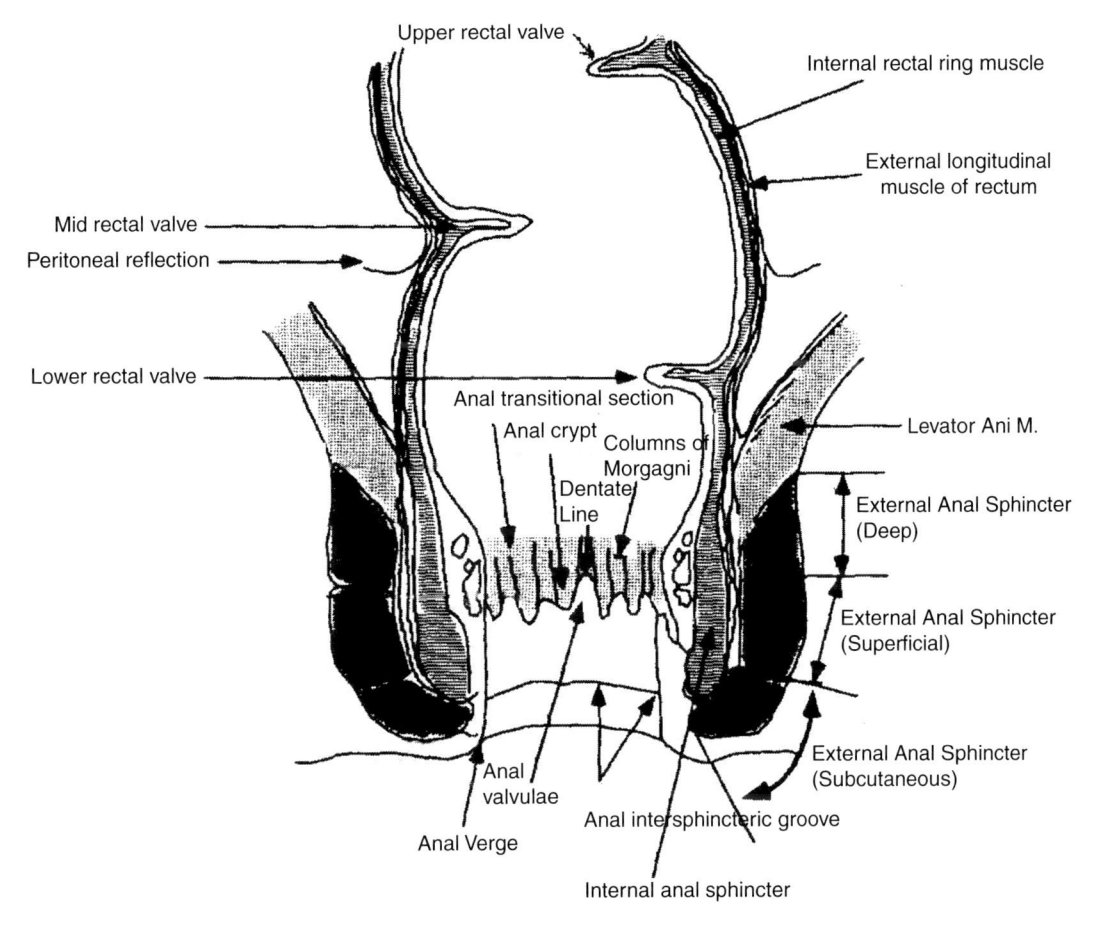

Fig. 2.3 Anal canal and rectum

Fig. 2.4 Anal gland and anal crypt

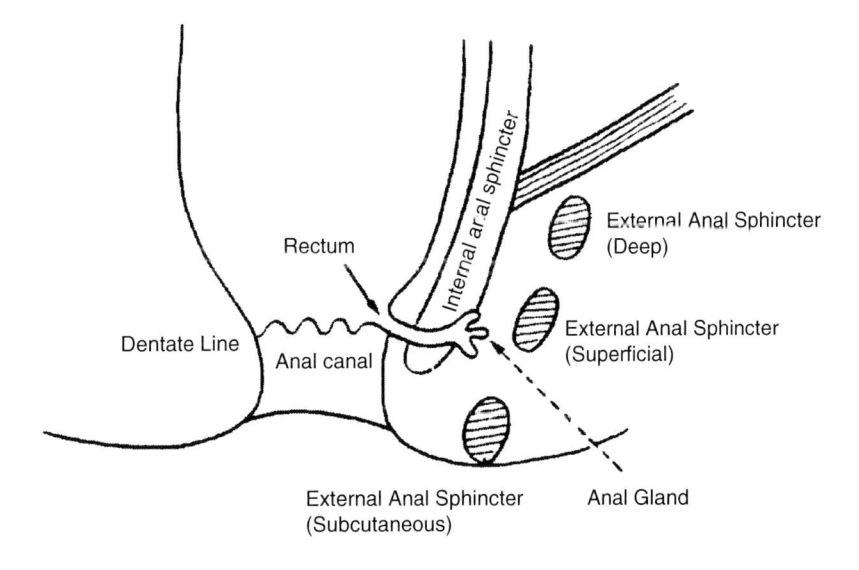

divided into three zones according to the four boundaries of the anal canal, namely the four lines and three zones (Fig. 2.1).

The four lines are the anal skin line, the anal white line, the dentate line, and the anorectal line. The anal skin line is the anal margin. The anal white line is equivalent to the boundary between the lower edge of the internal sphincter muscle and the underside of the external sphincter skin, that is, the position of the inter sphincteric grove. Because there are fewer blood vessels in this area, it may appear slightly off-white in some people. The anorectal line is the horizontal line of the upper edge of the anorectal ring, is located above the dentate line, about 1.5 cm from the dentate line, and is an imaginary line of the upper end of the rectal column.

The three zones are the column band, the hemorrhoid band, and the belt. The column band is the ring zone from the anorectal line to the dentate line. There is an anal column (i.e. rectal column) in between, and the surface is covered with a single layer of columnar epithelium. The hemorrhoid band is the ring zone from the dentate line to the white line of the anus. The sphincter is compressed into a ring-shaped bulge, where the surface is smooth and bright, and it is the transitional part of the mucous membrane and the skin. The dentate line changes from a single columnar epithelium to a stratified cubic epithelium and unkeratinized squamous (stratified flat) epithelium. The belt is the ring-shaped area from the white line of the anus to the edge of the anus, surrounded by the lower part of the external sphincter skin, and the surface is keratinized stratified squamous (stratified flat) epithelium.

Research by Gao Chunfang and Guo Maolin found that on MRI images, there is a clear anatomical interface between the rectum and its continuation and the pelvic floor; the anal canal can be divided into two parts: the anal canal and the perianal. It is composed of mucosal layer, submucosal layer, and anorectal smooth muscle layer. The rest is called the perianal region.

2.2.2 Rectum

The rectum is located above the anal canal and is about 10–15 cm long. It is connected to the sigmoid colon at the top and the anal canal at the bottom. The rectum descends along the front of the sacrum and coccyx and forms an angle of nearly 90° with the anal canal, called the anal right angle. The upper and lower ends of the rectum are narrow, and the middle is enlarged, called the rectal ampulla. Dilatation (rectal constipation), inflammation (ulcerative colitis, Crohn's disease), spasm (irritable bowel syndrome), and other diseases occur in the rectal ampulla. The upper part of the rectum migrates to the sigmoid colon, and its transition part is called the rectosigmoid junction (rectosigmoid) (Fig. 2.5).

There are three semi-moon-like rectal valves (rectal valves) on the rectal wall, which are called the upper rectal valve, the middle rectal valve, and the lower rectal valve. The lower rectal valve is about 5 cm from the anus, the middle rectal valve is about 8 cm from the anus, and the upper rectal valve is about 11 cm from the anus. The lower, middle, and upper rectal valves are located on the left, right, and left sides, respectively. The mid-rectal valve is called the Houston valve and is equivalent to the height of the peritoneal reflex. When treating rectal lesions above the Houston valve, it is easy to cause perforation to the abdominal cavity. PPH surgery in China may lead to perforation of the rectum and even death of the patient. Special attention should be paid to this.

The mucosal epithelium of the rectum is the columnar epithelium. The rectum is divided into the rectal mucosa, the inner ring muscle, and the outer ring muscle from inside to outside. The upper rectum is covered with peritoneum on the front and both sides, and the middle section is covered with peritoneum only on the front, and here it turns back into a rectovesical pouch or rectovaginal pouch. The distance between the peritoneal reflex and the anal margin is about 7.5 cm in men and 5.5 cm in women. Fascia surrounds the rectum below the peritoneal reflex.

2 Anatomy and Physiology of Anal Fistula

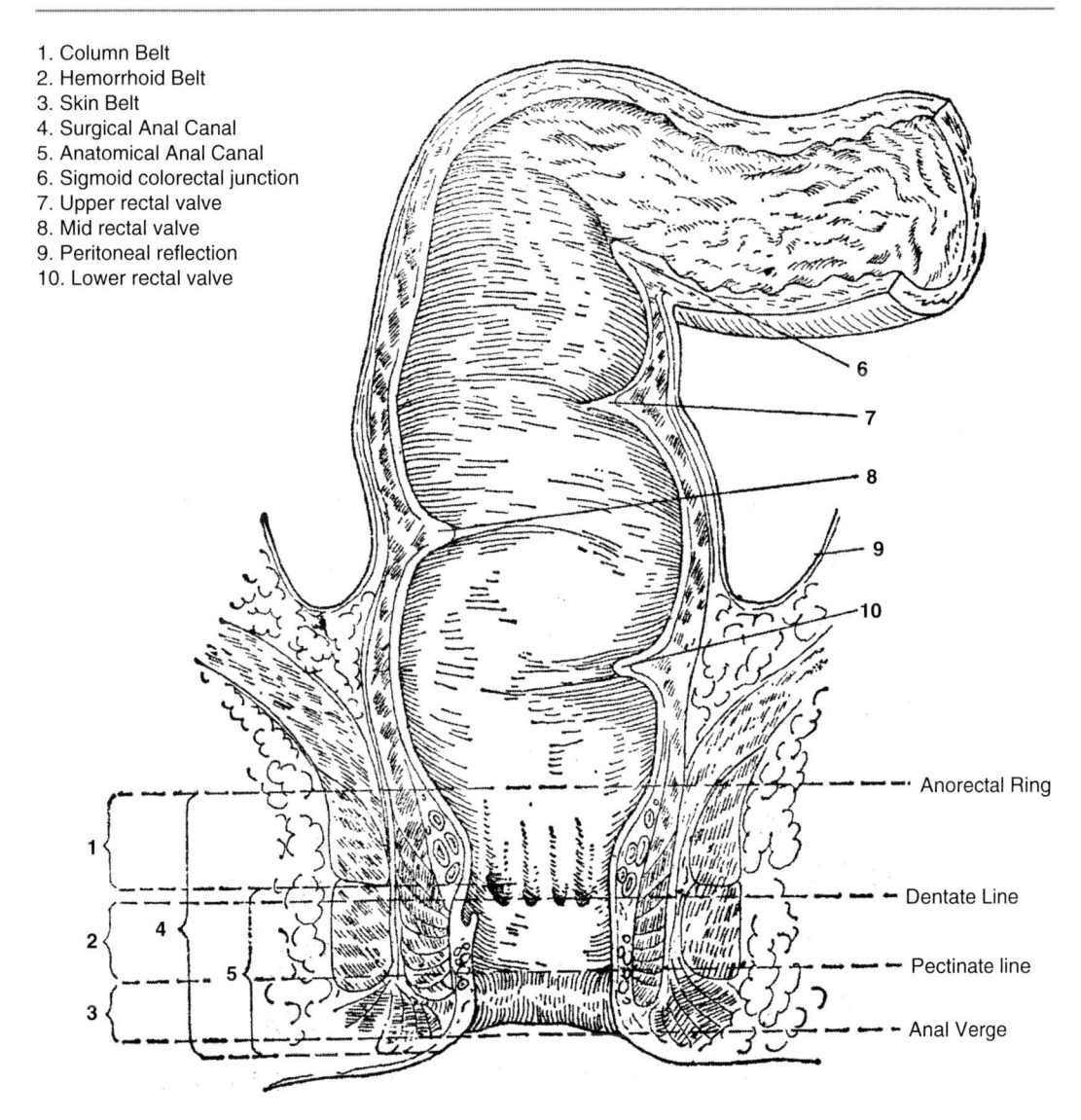

1. Column Belt
2. Hemorrhoid Belt
3. Skin Belt
4. Surgical Anal Canal
5. Anatomical Anal Canal
6. Sigmoid colorectal junction
7. Upper rectal valve
8. Mid rectal valve
9. Peritoneal reflection
10. Lower rectal valve

Fig. 2.5 Anal canal and rectum

The rectal mucosa is thick and rich in blood vessels. The mucosa is smooth, pink, and transparent, and large and small blood vessels in the submucosa can be seen. This characteristic "vascular morphology" disappears in patients with inflammatory diseases and melanosis. The rectal submucosa is loose and easily separated from the muscle layer and prolapses downward.

The rectal venous plexus is already formed under the rectal mucosa above the dentinal line when humans are born. With aging, the rectal venous plexus gradually expands and flexes and can develop into internal hemorrhoids. The venous plexus of external hemorrhoids exists in a ring shape at the anal margin and can develop into external hemorrhoids (Fig. 2.6). Because it is between the skin and the sphincter, the terminal fibers of the joint longitudinal muscle divide it into many small gaps (Compartment). Therefore, it is easy to produce blood circulation disorder and form thrombus. Such thrombus formation is accompanied by pain because it is located in the area where the sensory nerves are distributed.

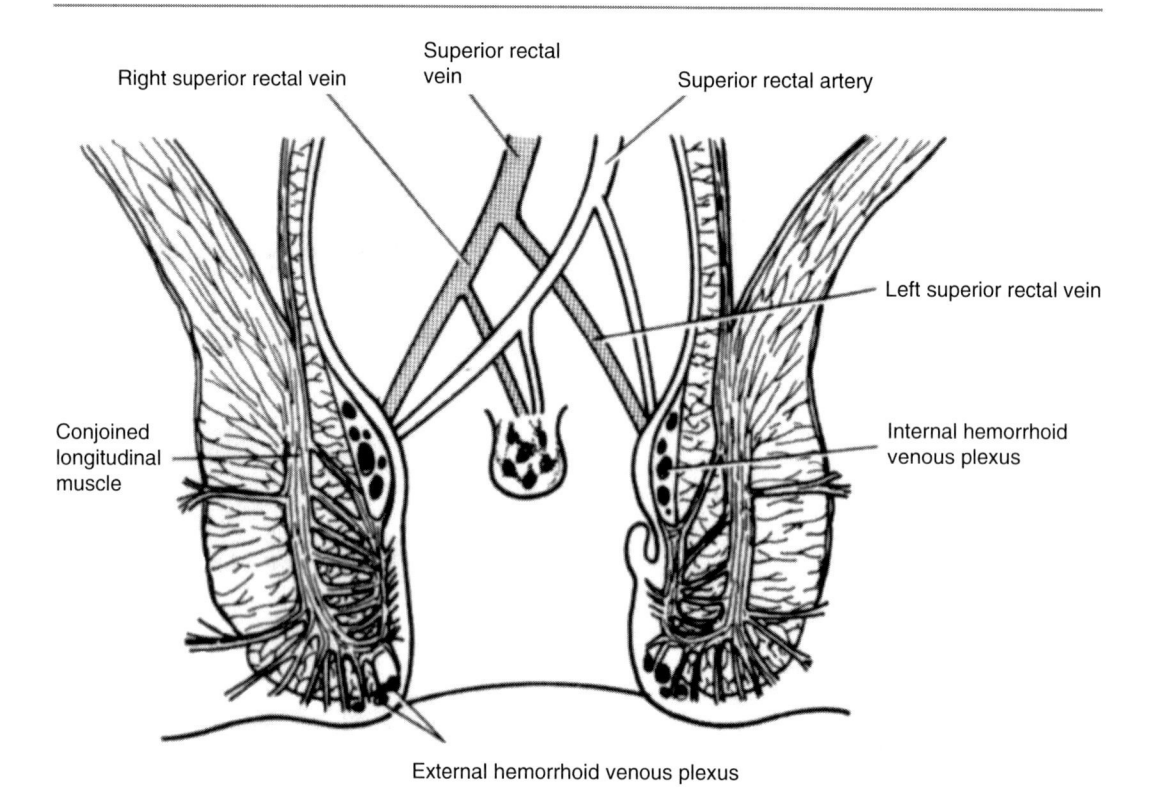

Fig. 2.6 Blood supply of hemorrhoids

The rectal muscle layer is an involuntary muscle, the outer layer is the longitudinal muscle, and the inner layer is the circular muscle.

In the front of the rectum, men have their prostate, seminal vesicles, vas deferens, bladder, and rectovesical pouch, and women have vaginas, cervix, uterus, and rectovaginal pouch (Fig. 2.7). There is the sacrum and the coccyx behind the sacrum. Blood vessels and the hypogastric nerve plexus on both sides are the sciatic bone, internal iliac artery, sciatic nerve, and ureter.

2.3 The Anal Gland

2.3.1 The History of Understanding the Anal Glands

In 1878, Hhiari of Germany first proposed the name of "anal gland." This structure was confirmed histologically by Hemauu and Desfosser in 1880, but they called it the "migratory intestinal gland." This was followed by F.D. Johson (1914, 1917) who used a large amount of materials to study the development of human embryos at various stages and further elaborated on the structure and location of anal glands and corrected the misconception that anal crypts are anal glands. British H.·A.·Harris (1929) also conducted further research and reports on the anal glands. In 1929, Lokhart-Mummery published a paper on the structure of anal glands and their relationship with infections around the anus. His understanding was valued by the medical profession at that time and was used clinically for the German medical community at that time.

However, it should be noted that in 1933 the etiological relationship between the anal gland and anal gland duct infection and perianal abscess and anal fistula was clearly recognized and valued in clinical practice. In 1993, Tucker of the American Academy of Proctology made a pathological anatomical observation on the structure of anal glands. The relationship between anal glands and anorectal inflammatory diseases was clearly

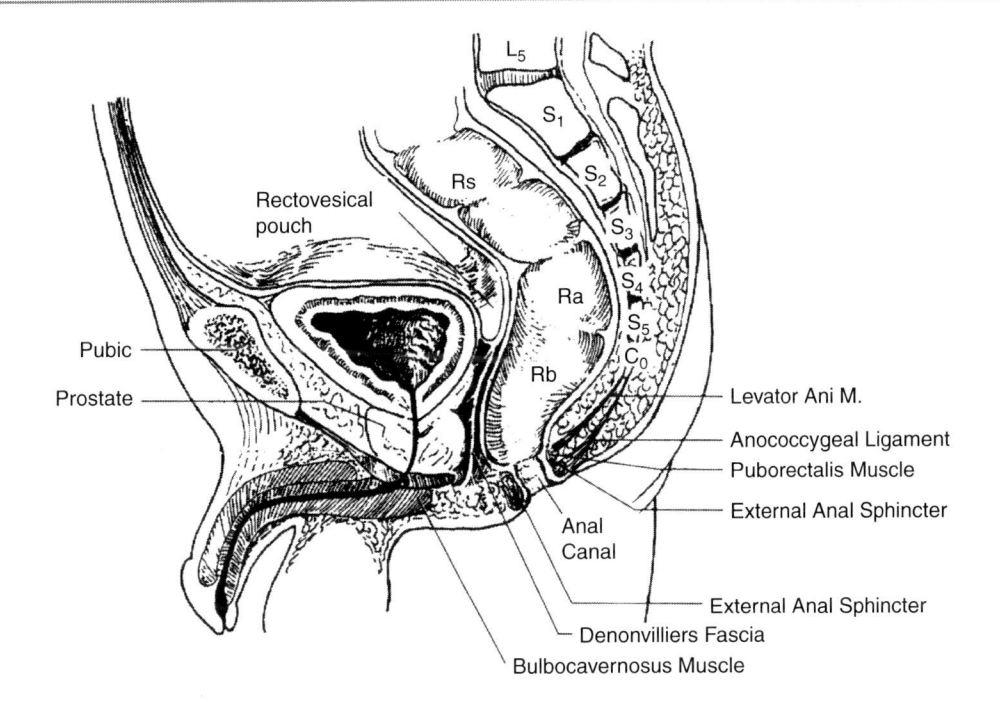

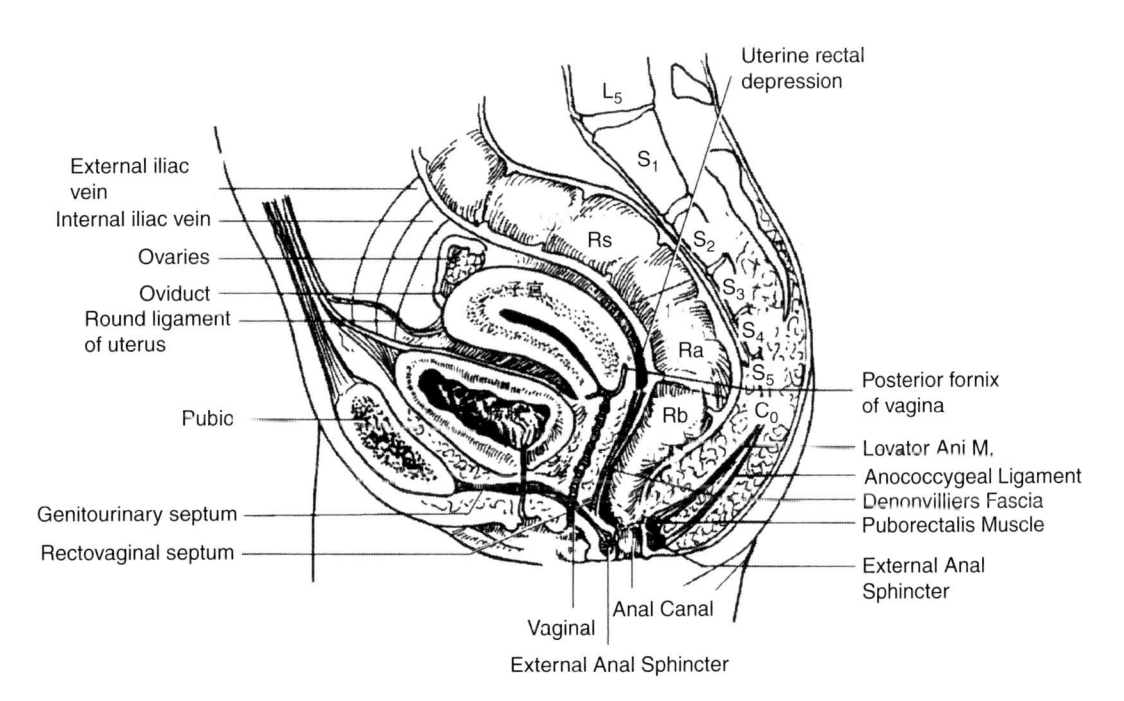

Fig. 2.7 Adjacent organs of the anorectum (male and female sagittal planes)

clarified so that the anal gland and its clinical significance were quickly paid attention to by more clinicians. In 1961, A. G. Parks proposed the theory of cryptoglandular infection on the mechanisms of anorectal infection. Parks believed that most anorectal abscesses and anal fistulas are caused by anal gland infection, and most anal gland infections originate from primary infections in the anal cryptsnal gland. Anal infections caused by blood and lymphatic circulation are generally rare. This study has been accepted or applied by most scholars and clinicians at home and abroad.

In my country, long before Parks put forward the "cryptic gland infection theory," the relationship between anal glands and the peri-anorectal abscess has been recognized and used to guide clinical practice. For example, Zhang Qingrong's report in 1957, based on his understanding that peri-anorectal infections all originate from infections of the anal glands and that their internal openings are mostly at the infected anal sinuses, proposed that the key to the treatment of anal fistula lies in the treatment of the infected foci of the anal glands. He reported 674 cases of anal fistula that were treated between 1951 and 1955, and the cure rate was as high as 98.8%.

In Japan, the understanding of anal glands and their clinical significance came relatively late and was tortuous. Although in 1907 the Osawa clan, followed in 1909 by the Taguchi clan and in 1931 the Ito Kazuki clan, Kono, Hashimoto, Shinkami, and Kagawa clan etc. all have done research into anal glands, they have all ignored the clinical significance of anal glands. At that time in Japan, as for the mechanism of peri-anorectal infection, some believed that it was mainly caused by bacterial invasion after rectal mucosal injury, some believed that it was mainly caused by tuberculosis infection, and some believed that it was caused by the anorectal wall or local infection of tuberculosis lesions.

2.3.2 The Distribution of Anal Glands and Their Clinical Significance

Regarding the distribution of anal glands around the anus, some people think that in children under five years old, they are irregular, while in adults, they are mostly concentrated near the posterior midline of the anal canal (84%), with less on both sides. However, it is believed that most of the anal glands are located in the posterior center, rarely in the anterior center, and none on both sides. Chen Qinglan, Jin Meifang, and others pointed out after observing 12 cases of anal canal and rectal specimens by continuous sectioning that 58% of the anal glands are located in the posterior half of the anal canal, and 42% of the anal glands are located in the front half of the anal canal.

In terms of clinical reports, many reports pointed out that the internal opening of anorectal abscess and anal fistula are located at the opening of the anal gland on the back of the anus. According to the observation of Sumikoshi, most of the fistulas of the ischiorectal fossa are caused by the formation of infection in the anal crypts on the back of the anus, and the inflammation further spreads to the ischiorectal fossa on both sides. Anal fistulas formed by anal gland infections in other parts rarely spread to other spaces even if they are infected again. If the infection starts in the posterior midline anal gland, it will form low and high intermuscular fistula and is easy to develop into ischiorectal fossa fistula. However, Sumakoshi believes that this is because the anal crypt in the middle of the anus is deeper, and there are more opportunities for fecal dirt to enter the anal crypt.

Some people think that anal cryptitis usually occurs in the posterior center and is related to the following factors: (1) the number of crypts in this area is large and obvious; (2) the posterior center of the anus is the weakest resistance in the tricyclic system of the external sphincter; and (3) the inferior rectal artery does not form arterial branches at the joint behind the anus, and the blood supply is relatively poor.

According to Wang's statistics, 68.6% and 69.7% of perianal abscesses and anal fistulas have the internal orifice behind the anus, with relatively few on both sides.

In short, the current understanding of the plane distribution of anal glands around the anus is still inconsistent.

Regarding the distribution of anal glands above and below the dentate line, Fujihara Akira pointed out through the morphological study of the anal recesses, anal glands, and anal glands of Japanese people that 65% of the anal gland ducts are arranged perpendicular to the dentate line, not with the dentate line. The vertical accounted for 35%, of which 28% had the catheter running under the dentate line and 4% were partly on the dentate line and partly under the dentate line. Zhou Liangyou et al. pointed out that the anal glands are mainly located near the dentate line and are distributed in the submucosa. A portion of the anal glands enters the internal sphincter, and none enters the external sphincter.

The understanding about the extension direction and distribution range of anal glands is also inconsistent. Eisenhammer in 1957 and Parks in 1961 reported that the vast majority of anal glands penetrated the internal sphincter and then traveled between the internal and external sphincter and did not distribute to the joint longitudinal and external sphincter. However, it was also pointed out that the anal gland can penetrate into the external sphincter, ischiorectal fossa, and levator ani to the pelvic cavity. Zhou Liangyou and Zhang Dongming also believed that the anal ducts are mostly confined to the submucosa in children and penetrate the internal sphincter in adults. It can reach as far as the junction between the internal sphincter muscle and the joint longitudinal muscle, and no further extension is found. He also believed that this situation can be explained by the genesis of the anal canal, that is, the anal canal is composed of two components of internal organs and the body, but is not intertwined, so the anal glands belonging to the visceral component cannot penetrate deeply into the external sphincter and the body component within the levator ani muscle. Therefore, it is considered that the report on the long-stroke anal duct is questionable.

The extensive direction and scope of anal glands are of great significance to the formation and treatment of anorectal infections. Based on the knowledge that the anal glands are mainly located in the internal and external sphincter, statistics found that 97% of perianal abscesses and anal fistulas occur between the internal and external sphincter, and a theory of "interanal fistula abscess" was put forward on the mechanism of perianal abscess. The idea of preserving the sphincter to cure anal fistula based on the distribution characteristics of the anal glands was also put forward and put into practice. However, due to insufficient treatment of the primary intermuscular lesions, the recurrence rate is high. This surgical method of preserving the anal sphincter to cure anal fistula was the first success for Parks. At present, the radical operation of anal fistula and peri-anorectal abscess preservation anal sphincter at home and abroad has also been proposed and developed based on Eisenhmmer and Parks' understanding of the structure and distribution of anal glands.

2.3.3 The Shape and Clinical Significance of Anal Glands

In order to further clarify the relationship between anal fistula and anal glands, Japanese scholars such as Akio Kurokawa and Hirokawa Kurokawa divided the anal glands into anal fistula group and nonanal fistula group for histopathological observation. Through the serial section and observation of the paraffin specimens of 41 cases of anal fistula group and 37 cases of nonanal fistula group, it was found that the anal glands consisted of glands and ducts opening in the anal crypts, which were divided into the straight type and the curved type according to different shapes. The glandular room type is composed mainly of glandular rooms; the mixed type has equal proportions of ducts and glandular rooms; and the cystic type has mucus retained as cysts. In the nonanal fistula group, the most common type of anal glands is duct-curved type, accounting for 37.9%, followed by mixed type, accounting for 21.6%; glandular room type, accounting for 18.9%; duct-straight type, accounting for 13.5%; and cystic type, accounting for 8.1%. In the anal fistula group, most of the anal gland types were ductal straight type, accounting for 85.3%, followed by mixed type, accounting for 9.5%; duct curved type, accounting for 4.9%; and glandular chamber type and cystic type not being found. Compared with the non-anal fistula group, there are significant differences between the two groups in the types of anal glands. Further observation found that 78% of the anal fistula group had a small amount of squamous epithelium in the anal glands, while 24.3% of the nonanal fistula group had a small amount of squamous epithelium. This is also very significant. Furthermore, Langerhaiis cells are often found in anal glands mixed with flat epithelium. As for why the anal glands of the anal fistula group and the nonanal fistula group have this difference and what their clinical significance is, they did not provide further explanation.

2.3.4 The Relationship Between the Obstruction of Anal Glands and the Occurrence and Development of Anorectal Infections

Many scholars believe that the obstruction of anal glands has a very important relationship with the occurrence of anorectal abscess and anal fistula. Yasuo Yamamoto (1980) believed that when the infected material enters the anal duct from the anal crypt and then retrogrades from the anal duct to the anal glands, the anal glands become infected, and the inflammation is aggravated due to the action of the acidic fluid in the glands. In turn, the gland cells are stimulated to promote the secretion of mucin. The secretion of mucin promotes further inflammation, forming an anal gland abscess, and part of the pus can be discharged through the anal gland duct. However, when this process occurs repeatedly, the inflammation causes the adhesion and occlusion of the anal gland ducts. The pus of anal gland abscesses cannot be discharged through the anal gland ducts and can only break through the surroundings, such as through submucosal and subcutaneous breakthroughs, or it will move along with the movement of the muscles along the joint longitudinal muscle fibers and spread up, down, left and right, forming various perianal abscesses and anal fistulas. Especially when the anal glands are within the internal sphincter or penetrate into the internal sphincter to reach the intersphincter, the anal glands are more likely to be blocked due to muscle compression. Therefore, Yamamoto believed that according to experience and pathology, once the inflammation spreads to the deep part, the anal glands are occluded and no longer communicate with the anal crypts. Therefore, Yamamoto advocated retaining the anal canal and rectal mucosa, including anal recesses, during anal fistula surgery.

Eisenhammer believed that the primary anorectal recessed adenomyosis (intersphincter) fistula abscess and every damage to the fistula stem from the spread of abscesses in the deep anal gland or perianal space. The spread of the abscess is due to obstructive infection of the duct that connects the gland to the anal recess at the dental line. At the same time, he also pointed out that this view that only obstructive infections can cause abscess formation is still controversial because anal cryptitis caused by nonobstructive infections is not uncommon, and infectious diarrhea and severe diarrhea are not uncommon disease factors.

As early as 1957, Zhang Qingrong pointed out that anal duct obstruction is closely related to the occurrence of anorectal abscess. He pointed out that when stool passes through the anal canal, it can sometimes send infectious material into the anal sinus and then pass through the duct to infect the anal glands. The infectious material accumulates in the ducts and acinars and finally causes the ducts and glands to inflame. The bubble swells and ruptures so that the infectious material directly invades the tissues around the anus and rectum, or indirectly spreads through blood vessels or lymphatic vessels, and finally forms an abscess around the anus and rectum.

Chen Qinglan et al.'s observation of 12 serial sections of anal canal specimens showed that there are closed glands in the deep layer of the anal canal in adults, and it is not uncommon. This kind of glandular cyst is mostly located at the end of the glandular duct and near the joint longitudinal muscle. No open duct is found to connect to the intestinal cavity, and there was even secretion in the glandular cavity. They believe that this kind of closed glandular cyst is one of the reasons for the loss of ducts. Inflammation causes internal sphincter spasm, oppresses the ducts, and occludes them, causing the secretions of the anal glands to be difficult to discharge, and thus cystic enlargement occurs. Once this saccular line is infected, a primary abscess between the sphincter will be formed. From a clinical point of view, some people think that the inner orifice of the anorectal abscess is mostly occluded. The reason may be the necrotic tissue has not liquefied and blocked the anal duct; the tissue around the anal duct is inflamed and occludes the orifice; and the duct is in the sphincter. The perianal inflammation causes sphincter spasm, which can in turn cause twisting and occlusion of the duct and high pressure in the abscess cavity of anal gland abscesses, compressing the duct or internal opening to seal it.

Eisenhammer reported that in only one-third of anal fistula cases, the anal gland duct is connected to the inner wall of the anal duct.

2.3.5 The Relationship Between Anal Glands and Sex Hormones and Their Clinical Significance

As a skin urologist, Gao Yuejin in Japan found that according to his observations in more than 50 years of clinical work, there is a clinical phenomenon that cannot be explained by the "anal crypt gland infection theory" that there are almost no babies in the early patient cases of anal fistula. There are two very similar peaks in the age distribution curve of male patients, adolescents, and the elderly, and these are in the neonatal infant period and the young adult period; the incidence rates of male and female are significantly different. The ratio of rates is 8–9:1, while in adults it is 5–6:1. Whether it is a newborn baby or an adult, male patients account for the vast majority of cases; the occurrence of anal fistula in a newborn baby tends to occur before the age of one year, and most of the onset sites are on both sides of the anus and are symmetrically distributed. In addition, most males have fistulas with more branches compared to female patients. Based on the genetic origin of the anal glands from the fat glands, combined with research on the cypress (showing that the adult anal glands are apocrine glands, and their contents sometimes contain fat),

he speculated that the anal glands may also resemble the fat glands, which are excellent target organ for hormones in males. However, the author failed to directly and clearly explain the role of male hormones in anal gland infections. The article mainly describes the relationship between fat glands and male hormones.

2.3.6 Histochemistry of Anal Gland Mucus and Its Clinical Significance

Research by Akio Kurokawa has shown that the production and nature of anal gland mucus have a certain relationship with the occurrence of anorectal infections.

Kurokawa found that the flat epithelial metaplasia of the anal gland epithelium can lead to a decrease in the ability of the anal glands to produce mucus, and the anal glands with flat epithelial metaplasia accounted for 81.5% of the anal glands in patients with anal fistula. This meant that they were flatter than the anal glands in non-anal fistula patients. The epithelial metaplasia rate is 28% higher. At the same time, it was found that the incidence of the squamous epithelium of the anal glandular epithelium increased with age, while the ability of the anal glands to produce mucus also decreased or declined. Further studies have shown that the anal gland epithelium (mainly mucus-producing columnar epithelium with a small amount of goblet cells) stained with AB-PAS, HID-AB, a layer of thiomucin can be found. This is true even in areas with squamous metaplasia. When observing the affinity of phytohemagglutinin to the surface membrane, it was found that some of the goblet cells were UEA-1 and PHA-positive, while the cell edges and cells with squamous metaplasia were VEA-1-positive. Therefore, it was believed that due to the flat epithelial metaplasia of the anal gland epithelium, the low ability to produce mucus is related to its immune function.

In short, most scholars currently believe that the anal glands play an important role in perianorectal infections. Once the anal glands are infected, an abscess is formed between the internal and external sphincter and then spreads to the surroundings. This is the main mechanism of the formation of peri-anorectal abscess.

However, Goligher believed that about 2/3 of the cases have nothing to do with anal crypts. He believed that some perianal abscesses are not derived from anal gland infections but directly from anal fissures, thrombotic external hemorrhoids, internal hemorrhoids, or after rectal prolapse injections. Also, some can come from direct trauma and so on. He believed that anal gland infection is not the only mechanism of infection around the anorectum.

2.4 Anal Muscles

The anal sphincter (anal sphincter) is divided into three layers: the internal anal sphincter, external anal sphincter, and levator muscle (Fig. 2.8).

2.4.1 Internal Anal Sphincter

The internal anal sphincter is the swollen part of the lower end of the internal rectal muscle, with a thickness of about 2 to 3 mm. The circular lower edge of the internal anal sphincter can be touched above the sphincter groove during digital examination of the anal canal. The internal anal sphincter is a smooth muscle that is innervated by autonomic nerves and cannot be arbitrarily innervated. It has moderate tension and plays the role of continuously closing the anus in the innermost part of the anorectum. As a smooth muscle that is continuously in contraction, it is the main force preventing the involuntary discharge of feces and gas. The maintenance of the anal canal's resting pressure of 50%–85% is provided by the internal anal sphincter and is the result of the combination of intrinsic myogenic and external autonomic neurogenic characteristics. Therefore, when the internal sphincter is cut, it becomes unconscious. Moreover, the function of closing the anus continuously will be lost, and symptoms such as wet and unclean anus will easily appear.

The internal anal sphincter lacks flexibility and is prone to become hard, fibrotic, and change in nature due to inflammation. When there is anal fissure, inflammation, sclerosis, and scarring of the epithelial and subepithelial connective tissue, it may spread to the internal sphincter, resulting in internal sphincter hypertrophy and anal stenosis. Therefore, in radical anal fissure surgery, the lower end of the hypertrophic internal sphincter must be cut off.

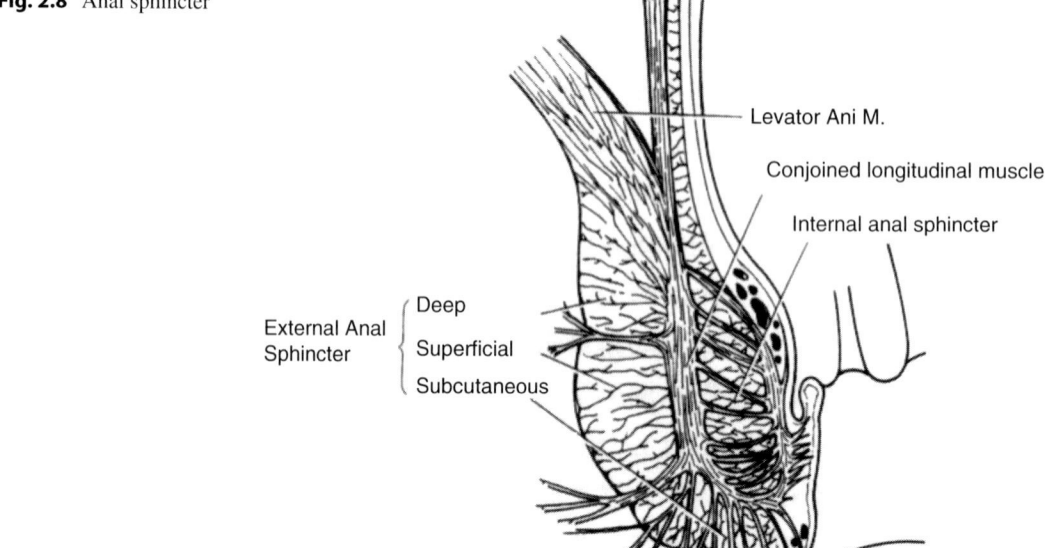

Fig. 2.8 Anal sphincter

The internal sphincter has a joint longitudinal muscle fiber running through it, called the Treitz ligament. The Treitz ligament has the function of supporting the venous plexus under the mucosa and preventing the development of hemorrhoids. During defecation and anesthesia, the internal sphincter can shift downward, flush the underside of the external sphincter skin, and even go beyond the underside of the external sphincter. Doctors should pay attention to such changes in the position of the internal sphincter when the internal sphincter is cut.

2.4.2 External Anal Sphincter

The external anal sphincter is divided into three layers: the subcutaneous, superficial, and deep external sphincter. These three muscles have different shapes.

2.4.2.1 Subcutaneous Sphincter

Subcutaneous sphincter is located under the skin of the anal margin and is composed of circular muscle bundles surrounding the lower part of the anal canal. There are a small number of muscle fibers attached to the central tendon of the perineum in the front of this muscle, and the posterior fibers are attached to the anus-caudal ligament. The upper edge of this muscle bundle is adjacent to the lower edge of the internal sphincter, forming an intersphincter groove, which can be touched during digital examination. Between the internal and external sphincter, there are fibers that unite the longitudinal muscles, and the internal sphincter is lowered and the external sphincter rises through traction and coordination during defecation. Golight noticed that during hemorrhoid ligation and resection, when the hemorrhoids were pulled out, the internal sphincter also slipped easily and was prone to injury.

2.4.2.2 Superficial Sphincter

Superficial sphincter is between the subcutaneous and deep parts of the external sphincter and is the flat muscle bundle. It is the most powerful muscle in the external sphincter. The posterior edge of the anal canal is divided into two bundles, which extend forward from both sides of the anal canal to surround the internal sphincter, meet in front of the anal canal, and stop at the perineal body. The superficial muscle bundles of the left and right external sphincters intersect anteriorly (decussafe) and attach to the central tendon of the perineum. The central tendon of the perineum in men is firm and reliable, while the central tendon of the perineum in women is relatively loose. This must be paid attention to during surgery. The superficial part of the external sphincter has a triangular gap at the intersection of the quadratus muscle bundles before and after the anus, which results in weaker muscle support in the anteroposterior position of the anal canal than on both sides. This is also an anatomical basic factor that is prone to anal fissure before and after the anal canal.

In addition, if the superficial part of the external sphincter is removed from the coccyx in the rear, it may cause the anus to shift forward. In general, avoid cutting the anal caudal ligament. However, due to inflammatory changes around the anal canal and rectum during anal fistula, when the superficial part of the external sphincter is excised from the coccyx, sometimes serious forward displacement of the anus may not actually occur.

2.4.2.3 Deep External Sphincter

It is a thick circular muscle bundle that surrounds the upper third of the internal sphincter. The upper fibers are fused with the fibers of the puborectal muscle immediately above, and some fibers are cross-attached to the opposite side, causing ischial tuberosity.

The external sphincter belongs to the striated muscle and is innervated by the somatic nerve and is a voluntary muscle. When the rectum is full of feces, the internal sphincter will relax. This is the anorectal reflex. The role of the external sphincter is to consciously tighten the anus at this time. In Hirschsprung disease, the rectal anal reflex disappears.

It should be pointed out that the division of the external anal sphincter has always been controversial. In 1979, Shafik classified the puborectalis muscle as the external anal sphincter. In 1999,

Rociu et al. conducted 100 cases of intra-anal coil MRI studies and confirmed that it is composed of two parts: the subcutaneous and superficial parts. The 39th edition of Grignard's Anatomy in 2005 also accepted the "fact" that the external anal sphincter has only two parts. In 2005, the conventional MRI study by Hsu et al. showed that the external anal sphincter is composed of three parts. In 2009, Guo Maolin et al. again confirmed that the external anal sphincter is composed of three parts. At the same time, they found that the blind area of the intra-anal coil MRI caused Rociu and others to misjudge it as two parts. The lower part of the external sphincter skin and the perianal skin form a skin muscle loop-like structure, sealed at the exit of the anal canal.

In addition, the mechanism of the three loops of the external anal sphincter proposed by Shafik had a great clinical impact. Based on the anatomical study of 59 pediatric cadavers, Cui Long and others believe that this mechanism is clinically misleading. Cui Long believes that the mechanism of the three loops of the external anal sphincter does not exist objectively, because in addition to the puborectalis muscle (attached to the inferior branch of the pubis) and the deep upper half of the external anal sphincter (attached to the perineal body), there is no solid support structure for attachment. The so-called "middle loop" refers to the external anal sphincter. The "superficial" part of the external anal sphincter does not exist. It is actually only a part of the muscle fibers of the deep lower edge of the external anal sphincter because these muscle fibers span the lower end of the anal canal and the mid-anal seam. The transitional part is turned back and up slightly, and there is better fascia tissue coverage on its surface during lateral anatomy observation, which can easily be mistaken for the spindle-shaped muscle bundle extending backward and downward to the tip of the tailbone by the external anal sphincter. There are only a few muscle fibers at the tip of the tailbone, and it is unimaginable to support the strong muscle strength of the "middle loop," the reverse muscle bundle. As for the "basal loop," the forward muscle loop has an attachment point on the skin of the midline of the perineum that can provide a firm support for it.

2.4.3 The Levator Ani Muscle

The levator ani muscle is the uppermost muscle of the anal canal. Because this group of muscles alone can roughly maintain the function of the anus, the levator ani muscle is the most important sphincter in the anal canal muscles. When the levator ani muscle is ruptured, separated, or weak, it will cause serious obstacles to the anal sphincter function and anal incontinence. The levator ani muscle constitutes the pelvic diaphragm and is innervated by the anal nerve or perineal nerve of the second, third, and fourth sacral nerves. Its function is to support the internal organs of the pelvis, fix the rectum, raise the pelvic floor and anal canal, keep the anal canal and rectum at a certain angle, open and close the anus at will, and help defecation.

The levator ani muscle is composed of three groups of muscles: the puborectalis muscle, the pubococcygeus muscle, and the iliococcygeus muscle.

2.4.3.1 Puborectal Muscle

It occupies the innermost part of the levator ani muscle, starts from the left and right pubic branches, bypasses the back of the anus, and ends at the contralateral pubic bone and is a "U" shape around the anal canal from the back of the anus (Fig. 2.9). The puborectalis muscle is a striated muscle. The muscle fibers are interwoven with the longitudinal muscle layer of the rectum to form a joint longitudinal muscle decline between the internal and external sphincter. Its muscle fibers are interwoven with the internal and external sphincter. In terms of innervation and the structure of muscle cells, it has the special effect of voluntary contraction.

Research by Guo Maolin et al. showed that the puborectalis muscle is a completely independent muscle bundle, which has a clear anatomical interface with the deep part of the levator ani

2 Anatomy and Physiology of Anal Fistula

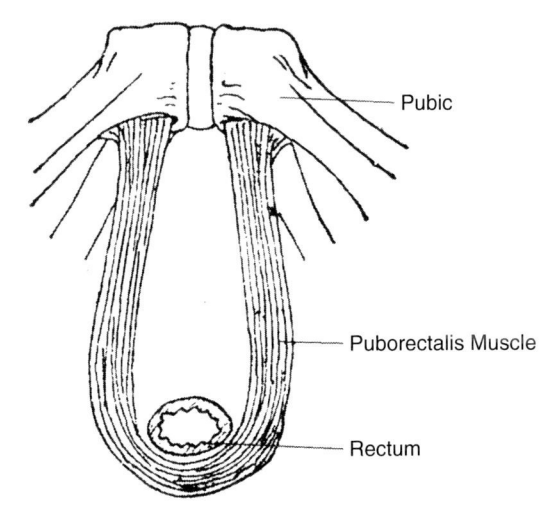

Fig. 2.9 Puborectalis muscle

muscle and external sphincter. CT defecation imaging shows that the puborectalis muscle also has the function of reducing urogenital hiatus, lift basin, and levator anus multiple functions. When the puborectalis muscle is shortened, the urethra, vagina, and rectum-anal junction will be squeezed, and these organs will be suspended forward and above. Therefore, the main functions of the puborectalis muscle are the contraction hole, pelvic lift, and levator anus.

2.4.3.2 Pubococcygeus Muscle

The pubococcygeus muscle is also known as the levator prostate in men. In women, it is also known as the pubic vagina. It starts behind the pubic branch and runs inward and downward. The medial muscle fibers form a U-shaped loop through the prostate or both sides of the vagina and urethra. Part of the fiber ends on its wall, and the other part ends at the central tendon of the perineum. The lateral muscle fibers end at the tip of the tailbone and the anterior sacral ligament and the anal-coccygeal ligament on both sides.

2.4.3.3 The Iliac Coccygeus Muscle

It is located on the outside of the puborectalis muscle, starting from the inner surface of the ischial spine and the back of the white line, going down and back to the opposite side and ending at the coccyx, sealing the anal triangle in the posterior half of the perineum to prevent the rectum coming out. Because the latter two are fixed to the tailbone, there is no sphincter function.

2.4.4 The Joint Longitudinal Muscles

The longitudinal rectal muscles are located at the junction of the anorectal canal and merge with some fibers of the puborectalis muscle and the upper and lower fascia of the pelvic diaphragm, interlacing each other to form a united longitudinal muscle (Fig. 2.8). The joint longitudinal muscle runs down between the internal and external sphincter, and its end is divided into many fiber bundles. The medial bundle obliquely penetrates the internal sphincter muscle to the submucosal muscle of the hemorrhoid ring, and the lateral bundle penetrates into the outer sphincter deep and shallow, outward and downward. Part of the end fiber bypasses the lower edge of the internal sphincter and ends at the white line of the anus; some fibers appear downward. The radial passes through the lower part of the external sphincter skin and ends at the corrugated skin muscle of the anus. Other fiber bundles pass through the lower and superficial parts of the external sphincter skin, attach to the ischial tuberosity forming a gap, and separate the space around the anus from the ischial rectal fossa. The joint longitudinal muscle binds the various tissues of the anal canal together to maintain the position and function of the anal canal. It penetrates into the muscle fibers of the internal sphincter, external sphincter, and levator ani to form a connective tissue network. When there is an infection in the sphincter space, it can spread along these fibers and generate various abscesses.

The combined longitudinal muscle plays an important role in lifting the anal epithelium and has a major relationship with the occurrence of hemorrhoids. Eils and Milligan (1942) called the end of the combined longitudinal muscle the corrugator cutisani. Because of the corrugator cutisani, the anus has radial wrinkles. The other terminal part of the combined longitudinal muscle forms a very thin muscle under the anal epithelium, namely the musculus submucosae ani.

2.4.5 Anorectal Ring

The anorectal ring is a muscle ring formed by the deep and superficial parts of the external anal sphincter, combined with longitudinal muscles, internal sphincter, and puborectal muscles around the anorectal junction, called anorectal ring (Fig. 2.10). The back of the ring is more developed than the front, and the front is slightly lower than the rear. During digital examination, the U-shaped muscle ring can be palpated behind and on both sides of the anal canal. The main function of this ring is to maintain anal sphincter function. If this ring is cut off by mistake during surgery, anal incontinence can be caused.

2.5 Perirectal Space of Anal Canal

The space around the anorectum includes the perianal subcutaneous space, ischiorectal space, posterior anal space, intersphincter space, submucosal space, pelvic rectal space, and retrorectal space (Figs. 2.11 and 2.12). After the anal gland is infected, the gap can become an important channel and place for anal gland abscess to spread to the surrounding.

2.5.1 Perianal Subcutaneous Space

The perianal subcutaneous space surrounds the lower part of the anal canal, the side is connected with the subcutaneous fat of the buttocks, and the middle extends to the sphincter space. The external hemorrhoidal venous plexus is located in the subcutaneous space of the perianal area and connects to the internal hemorrhoidal venous plexus at the dentate line. The perianal space is a common site for anal hematoma, perianal abscess, and anal fistula.

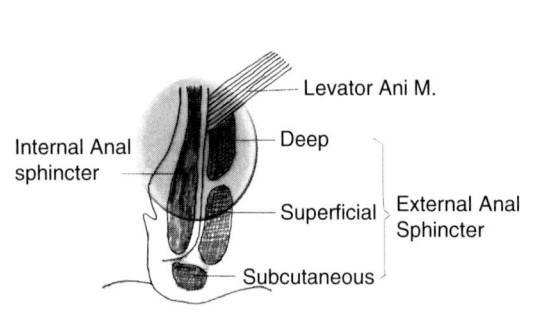

Fig. 2.10 Anorectal ring

Fig. 2.11 Anorectal space (Frontial view)

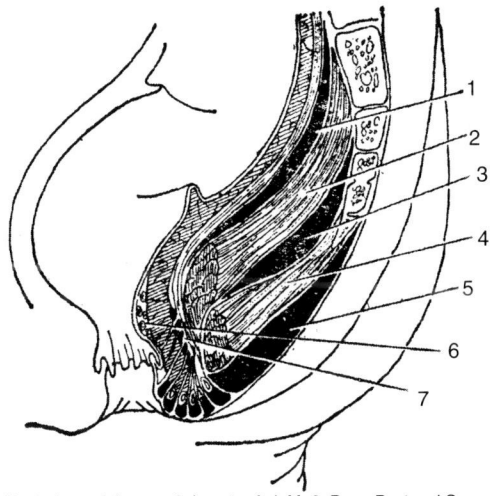

1. Posterior rectal space 2. Levator Ani. M. 3. Deep Postanal Space
4. Anococcygeal Ligament 5. Superfical Postanal Space
6. Internal anal sphincter 7. Intersphincter space

Fig. 2.12 Anorectal space (Lateral view)

2.5.3 Posterior Anal Space

The posterior anal space is located between the anal canal and the tailbone, the upper boundary is the levator ani fascia, the lower boundary is the posterior anal skin and the perianal fascia, and the superficial part of the external sphincter divides it into two parts: deep and shallow. The deep space is behind the anal canal, and the shallow space is behind the anal canal. The superficial posterior space of the anal canal is located between the anal caudal ligament and the skin, and the two sides are connected to the perianal fascia; the deep part is also called the Courtney posterior sphincter space, located between the anal caudal ligament and the anal suture, and its two sides are connected to the ischiorectal fossa. At the front is the inner sphincter and the deep part of the outer sphincter.

2.5.2 Ischiorectal Space

Its center is the anal canal and the lower rectum. The sides are the side walls of the pelvis. The front of the ischiorectal fossa is the urogenital diaphragm and perineal transverse muscle, and the back is the sacrotuberous ligament. The lower edge of the gluteus maximus, the top is the levator ani muscle, the pudendal nerve and internal blood vessels enter the pudendal canal (Aleock tube) on the upper side wall, and the perianal subcutaneous space is at the bottom. The sciatic rectal fossa is full of fat, blood flow is slow, disease resistance is weak, and abscess is easy to form. According to Goligher's observation, the fat particles in the upper gap of the ischiorectal fossa are large, while the lower fat particles are smaller. The sciatic rectal fossa contains fat, blood vessels, and nerves under the rectum.

Some people think that the ischial and rectal fossae are equivalent to the plane of the anal canal, not the plane of the rectum. More appropriately, the top is the levator ani originating from the obturator fascia, and the bottom is the perianal subcutaneous space.

2.5.4 Sphincter Muscle Space

It is the potential space between the internal and external sphincter muscles of the anus. Because the anal gland is located in this gap, the intersphincter gap plays an important role in the occurrence and development of anorectal abscess. After the anal glands are infected, intermuscular abscesses are formed between the sphincter muscles, and the intermuscular abscesses spread further around the anal canal and rectum, forming various abscesses and anal fistulas. The intersphincteric space connects to the pelvic rectal space. After the formation of intermuscular abscess after anal gland infection, pus can spread along the fibrous diaphragm to the surrounding spaces.

2.5.5 The Submucosal Space

It is located between the anal canal mucosa and the internal sphincter. It connects upward with the submucosa of the rectum and downward with the perianal subcutaneous space. The submucosal space is connected with the intersphincteric space through the internal sphincter muscles by fibers from the medial intersphincteric diaphragm. Abscesses that occur in this space are called submucosal abscess.

2.5.6 The Pelvic-Rectal Space

It is located in the pelvis, with the peritoneum above it, the superior pelvic diaphragm below it, and the rectum and lateral ligaments behind it. Males have the bladder and prostate in front, females have the uterus and broad ligament. There is loose connective tissue in the gap. Abscesses that occur in this space are called pelvic-rectal space abscesses.

2.5.7 The Posterior Rectal Space

It is located in front of the sacrum and behind the rectum, the upper part is the peritoneum, the lower part is the pelvic diaphragm superior fascia, and the pelvic rectal space is separated by the rectal ligament. An abscess in this space is called a posterior rectal space abscess.

2.6 Anorectal Arteries and Veins

2.6.1 Arteries

The blood supply of the anorectal canal is mainly provided by the superior rectal artery, inferior rectal artery, anal artery, and middle sacral artery. The superior rectal artery and the middle sacral artery are single branches, and the inferior rectal artery and anal artery are on the left and right in pairs.

2.6.1.1 Superior Rectal Artery
The superior rectal artery is the last segment of the inferior mesenteric artery and is the artery with the largest blood supply to the rectum. It passes through the pelvic cavity, across the left iliac artery, follows the rectum and descends into the sacral fovea, levels at the third sacral vertebra, divides into two branches, to the left and to the right, descends down both sides of the rectum, and diagonally forwards to the lower rectum into several branches from the muscular layer to the submucosa. It then enters the rectal column, and at the dentate line, it is divided into many small branches that are mutually anastomosed, supplying blood to the rectum above the dentate line, and in the submucosa anastomoses with the branches of the subrectal artery and anal artery.

The superior rectal artery is distributed in all the layers of the upper rectum and the entire rectal mucosa. There are important branches on the right anterior, right posterior, and the left side above the anal canal (that is, the lithotomy positions 11, 7, 3), which bleed after internal hemorrhoids. During digital examination, sometimes obvious arterial pulsations can be palpated in the upper right front, right back, and left hemorrhoids of the anus, especially in patients with severe internal hemorrhoids or mixed hemorrhoids; the pulsation of the suprahemorrhoidal artery is more obvious.

2.6.1.2 Inferior Rectal Artery
Stems from the internal iliac artery or internal pudendal artery, is located on both sides of the pelvis, reaches the rectum through the lateral rectal ligament, is mainly distributed in the lower rectum, in the submucosal layer, is anastomosed with the superior rectal artery and anal artery, and supplies blood the anterior rectal muscles and to the lower layers of the rectum.

2.6.1.3 Anal Artery
The anal artery originates from the internal pudendal artery, is on both sides of the perineum, is divided into several branches (2–3 branches) through the ischiorectal fossa, and is distributed to the levator ani muscle, internal sphincter, external sphincter, perineal skin, and dental line. The lower anal canal and the submucosa of the anal canal are anastomosed with the superior and inferior rectal arteries.

2.6.1.4 The Middle Sacral Artery
The posterior bifurcation is sent out above the bifurcation of the abdominal aorta, down to the sacral fovea, close down to the sacrum, and ends at the coccyx body. There are small branches dis-

tributed to the rectum and anastomosed with the upper and lower rectal arteries. However, it is not constant and has little effect on blood supply.

2.6.2 Veins

The anorectal veins are parallel to the arteries, including the superior rectal vein, inferior rectal vein, anal vein, and middle sacral vein. The first two are mainly composed of the internal hemorrhoid venous plexus, and the anal vein is collected by the external hemorrhoid venous plexus. The internal and external hemorrhoidal venous plexus connect to each other near the white line of the anus, connecting the portal vein system with the systemic vein system. In patients suffering from portal hypertension, the anal vein is one of the pathways for collateral circulation.

2.6.2.1 The Venous Plexus Within the Hemorrhoid

This is also known as the superior rectal venous plexus. Above the dentinal line, there is a sinus-like venous plexus, which originates from the tiny venous plexus in the submucosa, gathers in the veins of the rectal mucosa and forms several small veins, passes through the muscular layer in the middle of the rectum, and merges into the superior rectal vein and the portal vein. These veins have no valves and pass through the muscular layer in the middle of the rectum. They are susceptible to blood stagnation and expansion due to compression by muscles, which is one of the factors for internal hemorrhoids. This venous plexus corresponds to the arteries in the same part and is more prominent in the right front, right back, and left side of the anus. These three areas are the main parts of internal hemorrhoids, commonly known as the mother hemorrhoid area.

2.6.2.2 External Hemorrhoid Venous Plexus

This is also known as the anal venous plexus, inferior rectal venous plexus, or sinus venous plexus. Below the tooth line, in the subcutaneous tissue of the anus, a marginal vein trunk is formed along the outer edge of the external sphincter and gathers the veins of the anal canal. The upper part joins the inferior rectal vein and the internal iliac vein; the lower part joins the anal vein and the internal pudendal vein.

The anal canal and rectal mucosa have a large number of arteriovenous anastomoses, also known as sinus veins. There are small arteries directly injected into it so that the blood supply of the anal canal and lower rectal mucosa greatly exceeds its own metabolic needs. Due to the arterial and venous rectal anastomosis, the bleeding of internal hemorrhoids is often bright red, and it is also found to be arterial blood during blood gas analysis. The sinus vein wall has many glial fibers, muscular dysplasia, low tissue tension around the venous plexus and venules, and a lack of supporting elastic fibers. In addition, there is no venous valve from the superior rectal vein to the portal vein and its branches, which is not conducive to the backflow of blood in the venous plexus of hemorrhoids and can easily cause local venous congestion and expansion and blood in the stool. This is the anatomical basis of the "varicose vein theory" of hemorrhoids.

2.7 Anorectal and Lymphatic System

The lymphatic tissues of the anorectum can be divided into the upper and lower two groups, which are tightly connected by anastomotic branches.

The upper group is above the dentinal line, including the submucosa of the rectum, the muscle layer, and the lymphatic network under the serous membrane. They connect to each other and forms a lymphatic plexus outside the rectal wall, which drains upward, laterally, and downward. They go up along the upper rectal and lower mesenteric vessels to the posterior rectal lymph nodes and the sigmoid root lymph nodes, and finally to the lumbar lymph nodes in front and on both sides of the abdominal aorta. The anorectal lymph nodes that run along the subrectal vessels on both sides drain to the rectal lymph nodes in the rectal lateral ligaments, to the internal iliac lymph nodes, and then to the lumbar lymph nodes along the internal iliac blood vessels.

The lower group is below the dentinal line and gathers in the lower rectum, the anal canal and the internal and external sphincter muscles of the anus, and the subcutaneous lymph nodes around the anus, enters the inguinal lymph nodes through the perineum and scrotum, and then reaches the external iliac lymph nodes.

During the resection of anorectal and colonic malignant tumors, one should be familiar with the distribution of lymphatic tissue and its return route. Lymphatic metastasis is an important way for the metastasis of anorectal malignant tumors. When malignant lesions of the rectum begin, they can be transferred to distant lymph nodes from the lymphatic vessels on the top, bottom, and both sides. When performing radical surgery on malignant tumors of the anal canal and rectum, except for early cancers, the corresponding regional lymph nodes should be cleaned as much as possible. For anal canal cancer, when combined abdominal and perineal resection, inguinal lymph node dissection is usually required.

2.8 Anorectal Innervation

The anorectal nerve (Fig. 2.13), above the dentate line, is the autonomic nerve, and below the dentate line is the spinal nerve. Therefore, the lesions that occur below the tooth line are painful, while the lesions that occur above the tooth line are usually not painful.

2.8.1 The Nerves of the Rectum

The rectum is innervated by autonomic nerves, namely sympathetic and parasympathetic nerves.

2.8.1.1 The Sympathetic Nerve of the Rectum
Forms from the presacral nerve (i.e., the upper abdomen inferior plexus) and the pelvic plexus (i.e., the inferior abdomen plexus). The presacral nerve divides a pair of hypogastric nerves in front

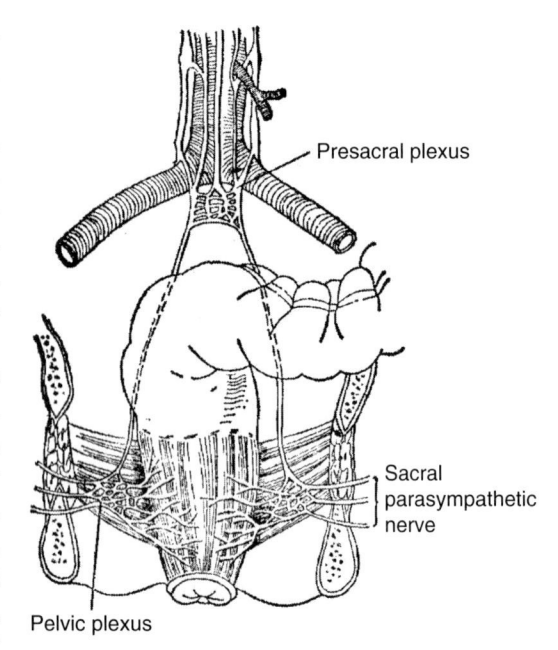

Fig. 2.13 Innervation of the colon, rectum and anal canal

of the fourth and fifth lumbar vertebral bodies and the first sacral vertebral body, goes down on both sides of the rectum and outward to the pelvic plexus behind the bottom of the bladder, and connects with the parasympathetic nerves. Nerve fibers, distributed to the rectum, internal anal sphincter, bladder, and external genitalia, have the effect of inhibiting intestinal peristalsis and contracting the internal sphincter.

2.8.1.2 Parasympathetic Nerves
They come from the sacral nerves (S2,S3,S4) and run to the side, front, and above, and sympathetic lower abdominal nerves are added to the pelvic plexus. From the pelvic nerve plexus, the mixed postganglionic parasympathetic and sympathetic fibers are distributed through the inferior mesenteric nerve plexus to the left colon and upper rectum and directly reach the lower rectum and upper anal canal. They play the role of increasing bowel movement, promoting secretion, and relaxing the internal sphincter.

The parasympathetic nerve is very important for the function of the rectum. Pain in the rectum is transmitted by the parasympathetic pelvic nerve and has nothing to do with the sympathetic nerve. It also has an awareness of defecation. Sensory nerve fibers control the effect of defecation and can sense the fullness of the rectum becoming filled or completely swollen with feces and can identify the urgency of defecation. The receptors in the rectum that cause the feeling of fullness are less in the upper part and more in the lower part. If too much rectum is surgically removed, defecation dysfunction is likely to occur, and anal incontinence may also occur in severe cases.

2.8.2 The Nerves of the Anal Canal

The internal anal sphincter is innervated by the sympathetic nerve (lumbar 5) and parasympathetic nerves (sacral 2, sacral 3, and sacral 4) through the same route as the rectal nerve.

The movement of the levator ani muscle is innervated by the sacral nerve roots (sacral 2, sacral 3, and sacral 4) from the pelvic surface and the perineal branches of the pudendal nerve below. The external anal sphincter muscles on both sides are innervated by the lower rectal branch of the pudendal nerve (sacral 2 and 3) and the perineal branch of the sacrum 4. Although the innervation of the puborectalis and external anal sphincter appears to be somewhat different, these muscles appear to function as an indivisible unit. After unilateral pudendal nerve resection, the function of the external anal sphincter remains because the nerve fibers cross each other at the level of the spinal cord.

The nerves that innervate the pelvic floor muscles mainly come from the pudendal nerve plexus. The pudendal nerve plexus is mainly composed of the anterior branches of the sacrum 2 to 4, and its branches are limited to the perineum. The inner part of the pudendal plexus is divided into the pelvic visceral nerve, levator ani muscle nerve, and coccygeal muscle nerve, which all run along the pelvic diaphragm and then distribute in the pelvic viscera and pelvic diaphragm. The lateral part runs under the pelvic diaphragm and separates the dorsal nerve of the penis, the perineal nerve, and the anal nerve (the three are collectively called the pudendal nerve)

and are distributed in the perineal muscle and the skin of the vulva. The anal coccyx nerve is a branch of the tail plexus, distributed in the skin from the coccyx to the anus. When the pudendal plexus nerve is overstretched and damaged, it will cause pelvic ptosis, rectal protrusion, rectal prolapse, and other diseases.

The upper part of the anal canal contains abundant, free, and orderly sensory nerve endings, especially near the anal valve. Ordered nerve ends include Meissner corpuscle (touch), Krause ball (cold), Golgi-Mazzoni body (pressure), and genital corpuscle (friction). Anal sensation is innervated by the inferior rectal branch of the pudendal nerve, which is believed to have the effect of restraining anal defecation.

2.9 Anorectal Physiological Function

The function of the rectum is to store and excrete feces.

Defecation is a complex reflex process. When the rectum is filled, it indirectly stimulates the distraction receptors located in the puborectalis muscles to produce afferent impulses. The impulses are transmitted along the afferent fibers of the sacral nerve or pelvic nerve and hypogastric nerve to the "defecation center" located in the sacral spinal cord. The signal from the pelvic nerve spreads along the parasympathetic fibers, causing the descending colon, sigmoid colon, and rectum to contract, and the internal anal sphincter relaxes. At the same time, the sacral spinal cord center sends out impulses via the sacral nerve and the pudendal nerve to relax the puborectalis muscle and external anal sphincter, the anorectal angle is straightened, the anorectum is funnel-shaped, and the feces are excreted. Generally, when the internal rectal pressure reaches 20–50 mmHg, the threshold is reached, which will cause bowel movements. Under normal circumstances, the defecation reflex process is carried out under the control of the cerebral cortex. On the one hand, the afferent impulse caused by the filling of the rectum is uploaded to the brain to cause defecation; on the other hand, with the participation of the higher brain center, the abdominal muscles and diaphragm contraction increases abdominal pressure and promotes defecation. When environmental conditions are not available, the brain can inhibit the defecation reflex process so that the defecation process can be subjectively controlled to a certain extent.

Suggested Reading

1. Masahiro Takano. Compiled by Shi Renjie. Essentials of Diagnosis and Treatment of Anorectal Diseases. Beijing: Biomedicine Branch of Chemical Industry Press, 2009, 1–21.
2. Cao Jixun. Chinese Hemorrhoids and Fistula. Chengdu: Sichuan Science and Technology Press, 2015, 13–30.
3. Huang Naijian. Chinese Anorectology. Jinan: Shandong Science and Technology Press, 1996, 1–26.
4. Colon and rectal surgery (5th edition). Beijing: People's Medical Publishing House, 2009, 1–24.
5. Zheng Zhitian. Gastroenterology (3rd edition). Beijing: People's Medical Publishing House, 2000, 8–13.
6. Gao Chunfang, Guo Maolin. New concepts of anal area and pelvic floor anatomy and physiology and their clinical significance. Journal of Medical Research, 2010,39(8):24–26
7. Chen Qinglan, Jin Meifang, etc.; Anatomical histological observation of anal crypts and anal glands Chinese Journal of Anorectal Diseases 1989(3): 27–29
8. Fujiwara Akira. The study of the morphology of the anal fossa, anal canal and anal glands in the Japanese. The Journal of Colon and Anus 1969 22(2) 18–19
9. Zhou Liangyou, et al. Histology and clinical significance of anal glands. Chinese Medical Journal 1981 6·(3) 27–29
10. Akio Kurokawa, Yukio Kawa. The histopathology of the anal glands. Anal Journal of the Large Intestine. 1986, 39 (5): 544
11. Nobori Takatuki. New Hemorrhoids and Fistulas, あたらしいアプノーチーホルモン and hemorrhoids ろう. Colon and Anus. 1985, 38: 40–46.
12. Akio Kurokawa. The study of histopathology in the sequence of the development of hemorrhoids. The Study of Histopathology in the Colon. 1989·42 (5): 878
13. Cui Long,Li Zhongren. The anatomical relationship of the perianal muscles and its role in defecation control and clinical application. Hainan Medicine, 2001,12(12):85–88.
14. Zhan Xuebin. Anal Anatomy and Physiology. Chinese Clinicians, 2005, 33(3): 9–10

The Etiology of Anal Fistula

Renjie Shi, Feng Jiang, and XiaYong Yang

Abstract

Chinese medicine considers the incidence of anal fistula to be related to irritating food, susceptible constitution, tuberculosis, bacterial infection, and local injury. These factors lead to the accumulation of toxins around the anus and rectum, resulting in the formation of perianal abscess and anal fistula. Anal fistula is a sequela of perianal abscess. Western medicine considers that most of the perianorectal infections originate from the infection of anal gland, and a few infections are related to trauma, inflammatory bowel disease, immune dysfunction, and so on. The theory of anal gland infection and the theory of central space infection are the main theories of perianorectal infection. The purulent infections of perianorectal space generally go through the early stage of abscess and the later stage of anal fistula. Incomplete treatment and poor drainage of anal gland abscess are important causes of anal fistula.

Keywords

Anal fistula · Perianal abscess · Pathogeny Immunity · Bacteria · Anal gland · The theory of anal gland infection · The theory of central space infection

R. Shi (✉)
Department of Anorectal Surgery, Affiliated Hospital of Nanjing University of Traditional Chinese Medicine, Nanjing, Jiangsu, China

F. Jiang
Affiliated Hospital of Nanjing University of Traditional Chinese Medicine, Nanjing, Jiangsu, China

X. Yang
Taizhou Hospital of Traditional Chinese Medicine, Taizhou, Jiangsu, China

3.1 The Pathogenesis of Anal Fistula in Chinese Medicine

The etiology of perianal abscess and anal fistula, scattered in the literature of the past in traditional Chinese medicine, can be summarized as follows:

1. Greasy and surfeit flavor that accumulates in the body will gather around the anus.

"Su Wen • Zhi Zhen Yao Da Lun" recorded that overeating fat meat and fine grain can cause the occurrence of abscess. "Wai Ke Da Cheng" elaborated that overeating fat meat and fine grain can cause the occurrence of abscess. It would also mean that *Rong Qi* is running poorly and retrograde into the muscles, which leads to the formation of carbuncles. *Rong Qi* is the *Qi* of the stomach. After eating, *Rong Qi* enters the stomach, moves to the spleen, and then enters the

© Chemical Industry Press 2021
R. Shi, L. Zheng (eds.), *Diagnosis and Treatment of Anal Fistula*,
https://doi.org/10.1007/978-981-16-5804-4_3

lung, which connects all vessels and hovers between the skin and muscle. After that, *Rong Qi* travels down the *Yang Dao* and deposits in the viscera, which can be reflected in the CunKou pulse. Overeating fat and fine grain generates an exuberant *Rong Qi*, which cannot hover between the viscera and the skin. Under these circumstances, *Rong Qi* travels down the *Yin Dao* and retrograde into the muscles, which results in carbuncle, and is caused by a block of excess *evil* in the muscles. An excessive diet can lead to deficient *Rong Q*i, which cannot hover between the viscera and the skin. The *Rong Qi* is short and deficient and gathers in the striae and interstitial space, resulting in abscess, and is caused by a block of deficiency *evil* in the muscles. "Wai Ke Zheng Zong" recorded that accumulation of poisonous substances in the viscera of the patients is usually the result of greasy and surfeit flavor. The poisonous substances accumulate in the body and will gather around the anus to form a lump.

2. Hyperactivity of *fire* due to *Yin* deficiency. The damp heat accumulates in the body and will gather around the anus.

"Xue Shi Yi An" recorded that uvular abscess is a disease of the loss of *Foot Three Yin*. "Yang Ke Xin De Ji" recorded that the patients suffering from this disease are all very weak, caused by the accumulation of damp heat resulting from the loss of Foot Three Yin.

3. Suffering from a consumptive disease such as long-term coughing. The *phlegm fire* that accumulates in the body will gather around the anus.

"Wai Ke Zheng Zong Zang Du Lun" recorded that patients who suffer from a consumptive disease, such as a long-term cough and the anus of whom is surrounded by the *phlegm fire* that accumulates in the body, can suffer from fistula if it ruptures.

4. Fatigue damage to *Qi* and blood. Damp heat and static blood accumulates in the body and will gather around the anus.

"Wai Ke Yi An Hui Bian" recorded that running with a burden, toiling, and overstraining when giving birth are all conditions that can cause depression resulting from deficiency of *Qi* and damp heat and static blood to block in the anus. Anal fistulas result from deficiency of *Qi* and blood in the liver, spleen, and kidney because of drinking and preference for spicy food, sleeping after drinking and eating, sprinting and sedentary habits, the cleavage of the muscles, and the injury of viscera.

5. The external *evils* entering the body, producing *heat evils*. The *Qi* and blood accumulate and block. The carrion flesh then progresses into an abscess.

"Ling Shu • Yong Ju" recorded the *cold stays* in the meridians, causing the flow of blood to be blocked. Obstruction of the movement of *Wei Qi* results in carbuncles. After the stagnation of the *cold*, it turns into *heat*. The excessive *heat* causes the carrion flesh to progress into an abscess. "He Jian Yi Xue Liu Shu" recorded that as *wind heat* does not evacuate and the *essence of water and grain* flows into the anus, the anus is/becomes swollen, and the size of the lump is as large as the core of a plum. In serious patients, this can develop into anal fistula.

6. Hemorrhoids being untreated for a long time can progress into anal fistula.

Chinese medicine has always had this type of understanding. "Qian Jin Yi Fang" pointed out that fistulas are the aftermath of abscesses. It recorded that abscesses with flowing pus become rat fistulas when it is *cold*. "Zhu Bing Yuan Hou Lun" recorded that hemorrhoids that do not heal will turn into anal fistula. "Yang Ke Jing Cui" recorded that hemorrhoids that do not heal for a long time due to the blockage of *damp heat* and blood stasis penetrate the intestinal wall, damage muscle, injure the marrow, and thus turn into anal fistulas. "Qi Xiao Liang Fang" recorded that if anal fistula is formed without treatment, the patients who form a fistula on the buttocks often have an internal orifice in the intestine, and feces will leak from the external orifice.

3.2 The Etiology and Pathogenesis of Anal Fistula in Western Medicine

3.2.1 The Cause of Anal Fistula

Currently, it is believed that most anorectal infections are caused by anal gland infection, and a small number of them are caused by trauma, anal fissure, postoperative infection after surgery or treatment, specific infection, inflammatory bowel disease, immune dysfunction, and so on. Foreign scholars have reported that 8.6 persons per 100,000 suffer from anal fistula (nonspecific anal fistula accounts for 90.4%, tuberculous anal fistula accounts for 0.2%, iatrogenic anal fistula accounts for 3.3%, anal fistula developed by anal fissure accounts for 3.3%, anal fistula complicated by ulcerative colitis accounts for 1.5%, and anal fistula complicated by Crohn's disease accounts for 1.3%). The average age of onset of anal fistula is 38.3 years, and the ratio of male to female is 1.8:1.0. Most patients younger than 15 years are male.

It should be pointed out that before the "anal gland infection theory" was proposed, the following factors were considered to be the main causes of anal fistula, including (1) injury of anus and rectum, such as enema and various trauma, foreign body injury in the digestive tract, hard discharge, and abrasions; (2) infection after surgery or treatment—this can be seen in hemorrhoid surgery, postpartum perineal suture infection, rectal, prostate, urethral surgery infection affected/affecting the anus and rectum, and hemorrhoid infection after injection; (3) tuberculosis infection of the anus and rectum— tuberculosis infection is considered to be one of the complications of tuberculosis; (4) other specific infections such as infections caused by *Pseudomonas aeruginosa*, actinomycetes, and Clostridium perfringen; (5) perianal abscess and anal fistula complicated by ulcerative colitis and Crohn's disease—this kind of abscess and anal fistula is different from general anal fistula and perianal abscess and has its special pathogenesis.

At present, perianal abscess and anal fistula are occasionally seen in patients with anal cancer or rectal cancer, which is related to the destruction of the barrier effect caused by tumor invasion and the decline of patients' own resistance. Patients with aplastic anemia, diabetes, leukemia, AIDS, and malignant tumors after radiotherapy and chemotherapy are also prone to infection around the anus and rectum due to their reduced resistance. In addition, presacral cyst or teratoma can also lead to infection and concurrent anal fistula due to puncture, surgery, and other reasons. The anal fistulas caused by these reasons are rare and different from common anal fistulas.

At present, there are many etiological theories about perianal abscess and anal fistula, among which the most important is "anal gland infection theory." In addition, there are others such as "central gap infection theory," "sex hormone theory," and "immune function decline theory." The theory of sex hormones has been described in Chaps. 2 and 10. "Immune function decline theory" states that a decline in the body's immune system causes the anti-infective ability to weaken, resulting in the body becoming prone to infection. This is however not the direct cause of infection around the anus rectum; the incidence is accidental, so the author thinks that this cannot constitute a "theory" so is not further discussed in this chapter.

3.2.1.1 Anal Gland Infection Theory

The theory of anal gland infection was first proposed by French anatomists Hermann and Desffosses in 1880 and later confirmed and reported by famous scholars such as Lockhart-Mummery (1929), Tucker and Hellwing (1934), Gordon-Waston and Dodd (1935), Hill, Shryoch, and Rebell (1943), and Parks (1956, 1958, 1961). Klosterhalfen and colleagues performed routine staining and immunohistochemical staining on 62 necropsy specimens and confirmed that there was anatomic relationship between the glands in anal muscle and anal fistula. Parks confirmed through careful histological examination that half of the anal sinuses had no glands entering, the openings of glandular ducts were often irregular, and the most common trend was submucosal prowl. Of particular interest was his observation that two-thirds of the specimens had one or more branches going into the anal sphincter and half of the branches passing completely through the internal sphincter and terminating in the longitudinal layer. However, no branch of the anal gland was found to pass through the external sphincter in his study. He reported that in only 8 of the 30 cases, the anal glands that caused the infection were clearly pathologically confirmed to have caused the saccular dilatation. He suggested that the anal glands in the remaining cases may have been destroyed during the formation of abscesses.

"Anal gland infection theory" means that when the bacterium in the bowel is invaded by antral sinus, it causes the anal gland infection to form an anal gland abscess. The spaces between the internal and external sphincter are composed of loose connective tissue; consequently, the primary anal gland abscess between the internal and external sphincter muscle is easy to expand and form an abscess between the muscles. When the accumulation of pus in the intermuscular abscess between the sphincters increases and the pressure in the abscess cavity increases, the abscess will spread and develop to form different types of abscesses. Finally, the abscess cavity is reduced, and anal fistula is formed after the abscess is discharged through incision or self-rupture. Through the ultrasonic examination of 50 cases of upper intermuscular abscess, 36 cases of ischiorectal fossa abscess, and 21 cases of ischiorectal fossa fistula, Takano Masao found that in the formation of perianal abscess and anal fistula, intermuscular abscess was first formed after the anal gland was infected and then developed in all directions through the weak places. Some cases formed upper intermuscular abscess and upper intermuscular fistula along the internal and external sphincter, while some cases were reduced to lower intermuscular abscess and lower intermuscular fistula. There was also a break through the external sphincter deep into the posterior anal space, forming a horseshoe-shaped ischial rectal socket abscess and ischial rectal socket fistula centered on the posterior anal space.

The opening of the anal gland in the infected anal recess is called the primary opening, and the abscess between the internal and external sphincters is called the primary abscess or primary lesion. It is considered that the obstruction or infection of the anal duct is an important condition for the formation of inter sphincter abscess after infection of the anal gland. Due to the occlusion of the anal gland duct, the pus that causes the primary abscess of the anal gland cannot be discharged through the anal crypt and then spreads in multiple directions. When the abscess collapses or cuts the pus, the pressure in the abscess is reduced, the abscess is gradually reduced, and a wall is formed around the abscess, gradually forming an anal fistula.

On the other hand, Goligher's investigation on the perianal abscess and anal fistula found that not all patients could find inter-sphincter abscesses, and only 8 out of 28 cases of perianal abscess and 8 out of 32 cases of anal fistula could find intermuscular abscesses. Especially in sciatic rectal abscess, inter-muscular abscesses can be seen in only 7 of the 20 cases in the acute abscess stage, while in the chronic anal fistula, only 1 of the 8 cases can see an inter-muscular abscess. Takano Masao also believed that not all anal fistulas form abscesses between internal and external sphincters.

However, from Park's treatment of anal fistula with the method of excising the internal sphincter, it can be confirmed that the anal gland has an important relationship with the continued development of anal fistulas. Ghostushiji emphasizes that it is impossible to cure anal fistula without understanding the "crypt theory of crypt infection." It is believed that clearing the internal opening and primary lesions is the most basic prerequisite for curing anal fistula.

3.2.1.2 Central Gap Infection Theory

The concept of central gap and the theory of central gap infection were proposed by Shafik (1979), an Egyptian scholar.

Shafik believed that the rectal longitudinal muscles pass through the pelvis, blending the puborectalis, levator ani, and the fascia and deep fibers of the external sphincter. They travel down the internal and external sphincters, the internal longitudinal muscle fibers that go through the internal sphincter tubing attached to the skin and mucous membrane, the upper part of the medial longitudinal muscle that is located between the medial longitudinal muscle and the deep part of the external sphincter, the lower half stops at the central tendon between the internal and external sphincters, and the lateral longitudinal muscle that is the deep extension of the external sphincter and puborectalis. Between the deep part of the external sphincter and the central longitudinal muscle, the lower edge of the internal sphincter stops at the central tendon. The central tendon is located in the central gap and is made up of rubber fibers, elastic fibers, and a small amount of muscle fibers and adipose tissue. It gives many small fibers insulation in the external sphincter circular gap between subcutaneous part, inward to the lower part of anal canal skin, outward into the sciatic rectum, down to perianal skin. There are six muscle gaps between the layers of the combined longitudinal muscles, namely the medial and lateral septum of the anus, the medial and lateral septum of anus sphincter, and longitudinal muscle of the lateral and medial septum. Except for the branch of the lateral septum of the anus, which enters the external sphincter and the ischial rectal space and the medial septum of the sphincter between the internal sphincter and the medial longitudinal muscle, the rest stops at the central tendon. The space around the lower portion of the anal canal between the lower end of the conjoint longitudinal and the subcutaneous portion of the external sphincter is called the central space. The central tendon is located in it and directly or indirectly connects with other spaces through its fibrous septum. It reaches the ischial rectal space outward, reaches the submucosal space inward, reaches the sphincter gap upward, and communicates with the pelvic rectal space and the rectal posterior space downward into the perianal subcutaneous space.

The central gap infection theory believes that the occurrence of perianal abscess is mainly due to the infection of the anal canal epithelium injury. This happens when bacteria invade the central space to form a central space abscess, and other parts of the abscess can also enter the central space to form a central space abscess. After the formation of the central space abscess, it spreads to other interstitial spaces to form various types of abscesses.

3.2.2 The Pathology of Anal Fistula

Anal fistula and perianal abscess are two pathological stages of purulent infection in the perianal space, respectively. The acute stage is perianal abscess, while the chronic stage is anal fistula. After the perianal abscess becomes pus, the perianal skin or anorectal mucosa is broken or cuts out pus. After pus fluid is drained adequately, the purulent cavity subsequently gradually shrinks, the purulent cavity wall connective tissue enlarges, causing the purulent cavity to contract and form a straight or curved conduit, which then becomes an anal fistula. A few anal fistulas show no obvious acute abscess and show a state of chronic development. In general, it can be said that anal fistulas are the result of the development of perianal abscesses, and their etiology is basically consistent with that of perianal abscesses.

The main reasons for the formation of anal fistula in perianal abscess are as follows:

1. The internal orifice and the primary infection lesions continue to exist. Although the abscess is ulcerated or incised and drained, anal cryptitis and anal gland infection that form the primary infection still exist, and the intestinal contents can continue to enter from the internal orifice.
2. Because feces, intestinal fluid, and gas in the intestinal cavity continue to enter the fistula, forming long-term chronic inflammation and repeated infection, the connective tissue of the wall becomes hyperplasia, forming a fibrotic tube wall. The tube wall is difficult to close and the tube is often curved and narrow, resulting in poor drainage.
3. The fistula can pass through the anal sphincter at different heights, and local inflammatory

stimulation can cause anal sphincter to spasm, hinder the drainage of pus in the lumen, and thus adversely affect the healing of the fistula.
4. The external orifice is narrow and small, sometimes closed and sometimes collapsed, resulting in the uneven drainage of the abscess cavity. The accumulation of pus may lead to the recurrence of abscesses and pierce the skin to form a new branch tube.

A typical anal fistula consists of three parts: the internal orifice, the fistula, and the external orifice.

1. The internal orifice is the infection of the anorectal rectum, and there is a distinction between the primary internal opening and the secondary internal opening. About 95% of the original internal orifice is located in the anal crypt near the dentate line. About 80% of it is located in the median line and on both sides of the posterior anal canal. It can also be in the lower part of the rectum or any part of the anal canal. The majority of secondary internal orifices are iatrogenic, among which the most common causes are probe examination and improper operation, and a few are caused by the spread of infection and abscesses that ruptures into the rectum and anal canal. The secondary internal orifice is located on the dentate line and may also be located anywhere in the rectal membrane above the tooth line. Generally, a fistula has only one internal orifice, and very few patients have more than two internal orifices for an anal fistula.
2. The fistula is the canal connecting the internal orifice and the external orifice of the anal fistula and can be divided into the main pipe and branch pipe. The main pipe is the pipe connecting the original internal orifice and external orifice. Some of the main pipes travel straight, while others travel curved. Most of them are related to personal constitution, external forces that squeeze, pull, and so on. A fistula formed by purulent infection of the anal gland in the front of the anal canal, usually in the same direction as the internal orifice, will be a short, shallow, and straight fistula. Branch pipe is the pipe connecting the main pipe to the secondary external orifice. Due to poor drainage of the main pipe, or closure of the external orifice, infections recur and spread to the surrounding areas. Blind tubes are formed when no skin or mucous membranes are penetrated elsewhere. If the inflammation is controlled after the formation of a new abscess, the abscess fluid is absorbed or flows out through the original internal orifice, resulting in multiple recurrence and formation of multiple branches by foreign body reaction. Generally, the inner wall of anal fistula is composed of nonspecific inflammatory granulation tissue, and there are a lot of fibrous tissues in the outer layer of the wall. Because the fistula is directly connected to the rectal and anal canals, feces can often enter into the fistula. As a result, the fistula tissue often has reactions of foreign body multinucleated giant cells and more monocytes, some of which have more eosinophilic granulocytes. Tuberculous anal fistula can be seen in the wall of the tuberculous granuloma and is composed of epithelioid cells, lymphocytes, and Langerhans giant cells, and some caseous necrosis can also occur. Foreign bodies of foreign body multinucleated giant cells often show the presence of foreign bodies, no nodules are formed alone, and no caseous necrosis occurs.
3. The external orifice is the opening from a fistula to the perianal, which is the wound of the abscess around the rectum or the incision of the abscess and is located on the skin around the anus. Some of the external orifices are closer to the anus, and some are farther away. Some anal fistulas have no external mouth and are called external blind fistulas. Most anal fistulas have external, and some even have multiple external orifices. The shape and size of the outer mouth are different, and some may have granule connective tissue hyperplasia to form a prominent hillock, some are concave, and some just coincide with the skin. Most anal fistulas can overflow purulent blood secretion from the external orifice when squeezed.

The external orifice is divided into the primary external opening and secondary external orifice. The primary external orifice is the opening of the first sputum or incision of the perianal abscess, which is the end of the main fistula. If the infection is secondary, causing a secondary abscess, the opening of the sputum or the incision of the abscess is called the secondary mouth, which is often the end of the branch.

Clinically, we can predict the approximate position of the anal fistula according to the shape and size of the external orifice, the distance from the anal verge, and the number. If the external orifice contraction is small, no more than 3 cm from the anal verge, the location of the general fistula is relatively shallow; if there is more granulation tissue in the external orifice, the fistula may be deeper. If the external orifice is large, the edge sneaks, and the granulation is swollen, then it will often be considered a tuberculous anal fistula. If the secretion of the external orifice is mucus, it is necessary to be alert to the possibility of cancer.

Suggested Reading

1. Takano Masahiro. Shi Renjie compiled. Anorectal disease diagnosis and treatment essential. Beijing: Chemical Publishing House Biomedical Branch, 2009
2. Cao Jixun. Chinese dropout. Chengdu: Sichuan Science and Technology Press, 2015, 145.
3. Huang Naijian. Chinese Anorectal Diseases. Jinan: Shandong Science and Technology Press, 1996, 729–766.
4. Liu Li, Guo Yaohui. A Survey of Anal fistula and its treatment. Chinese and Foreign Health Digest, 2010, 7 (11): 151–153
5. Zhu Rui, Zhang Pingsheng, Shen Lin et al. Research progress in diagnosis and treatment of anal fistula. Chinese Integrative Medicine, 2011,03(3):156–161,166.
6. Zhang Yuxiang, Wang Huasheng. On Zhang Dongyue's cognition of anal fistula in Chinese and Western medicine. Journal of Traditional Chinese Medicine and Pharmacy, 2006, 14 (8): 58–60
7. Mao Hong. Understanding of the incidence of perianal abscess in Chinese and Western medicine. Chinese Medicine Modern Distance Education, 2013, 11(14): 138–140.
8. The etiology of acquired perianal infection and anal fistula formation. Chinese Journal of Pediatric Surgery, 1996, 17 (1): 28–30.

Clinical Manifestations of Anal Fistula

Renjie Shi and Hongsheng Mao

Abstract

The main symptoms of anal fistula in the active stage are itching, swelling and pain, anal dampness, pruritus, poor defecation, and sometimes fever. The anal fistula caused by Crohn's disease and tuberculous infection has its own specific symptoms. The symptoms of anal fistula in the resting stage are relatively insignificant. The typical anal fistula consists of the external opening, the fistula, and the internal opening. The external opening is the opening of anal fistula around the anus. Some anal fistulas have no external opening, and some have multiple internal openings. The fistulas could be straight or circular, and some have one or more branches. One fistula usually has only one internal opening, and different fistulas can have different internal openings.

Keywords

Anal fistula · Purulence · Swelling · Pain
Anal dampness · Itching · Constipation
External opening · Internal opening

R. Shi (✉)
Department of Anorectal Surgery, Affiliated Hospital of Nanjing University of Traditional Chinese Medicine, Nanjing, Jiangsu, China

H. Mao
Jingjiang People's Hospital, Jingjiang, Jiangsu, China

4.1 Symptoms

4.1.1 Pus Outflow

The amount and nature of pus discharge are related to the time of fistula formation, the length, thickness, and the size of the internal aperture of the fistula. The newly formed anal fistula has more pus, thick pus, and odor and is of yellowish color. After that, pus gradually decreases; sometimes there will be pus, and sometimes not. After the external opening is closed, the purulent flow stops.

If the pus suddenly increases, it indicates that there is an acute infection focus or an acute attack of anal fistula. If there is local swelling and an increase in temperature, indicating that the infection is more serious, then lesions have developed. At this time, the previously closed external orifice may burst again or form another new one. After the pus overflows through the external orifice, the mass will gradually shrink. If the internal orifice and fistula are large, sometimes feces or gas may flow out from the external orifice.

In submucosal fistulas, ulcerations mostly in the anal sinus, pus often flows out from the anus. Internal blind fistulas also often have purulent blood secretion from the anus or symptoms such as feces with purulent blood or bloodstains.

Common anal fistula pus is more yellow or grayish-white, tuberculous anal fistula pus is more dilute or rice-water, and Crohn's disease anal fistula secretion is usually more dilute. If there is mucus in pus, it may be intestinal fluid flowing out through the fistula and will more likely mean mucinous adenocarcinoma. In this case, clinical attention should be paid.

4.1.2 Pain

When the external orifice of the fistula is open and pus can flow out through the external orifice, the patient usually has no pain and only feels moist and uncomfortable in the anus area. If the external orifice is closed, sometimes the local effect of the lesion is slightly painful. Severe pain will gradually increase when pus in the fistula accumulates more, and local anal pain or jumping pain may appear. There will be obvious tenderness during defecation or anal finger examination. Rectal submucosal fistulas can cause obvious anal bulging or pain. Anterior fistulas can also cause dysuria or even retention of urine.

4.1.3 Moisture and Itching

The skin around the anus of patients with anal fistula can be irritated by pus from the fistula, which can cause the anus to become moist and itchy and even cause perianal skin erosion, papules, and more seriously mossy-like changes.

4.1.4 Dysdefecation

Most patients with anal fistula usually have no influence on their defecation. However, high complex anal fistula or horseshoe-shaped anal fistula, due to chronic inflammatory stimulation, causes fibrosis of the anal and rectal ring. Or if the fistula is around the anal canal, forming a semicircular fibrous ring and affecting the contraction and relaxation of the anal sphincter may also result in dysdefecation. When the anal fistula develops infection, suppuration, and an acute attack, this can lead to anal swelling and pain; defecation will also become noticeably painful and more difficult.

4.1.5 Systemic Symptoms

Common anal fistulas usually have no systemic symptoms, but complex anal fistulas and tuberculous anal fistulas often manifest as emaciation, anemia, constipation, and difficulty in defecation due to the long duration of the disease and decades of illness. During an acute inflammation period, the infection is festering again, the systemic symptoms of abscesses will appear. Tuberculous anal fistula is often accompanied by low fever, night sweats, cough, and other manifestations. Anal fistula in Crohn's disease can be accompanied by mild or severe intestinal symptoms.

There are different clinical manifestations of anal fistula in active and static stages. During the resting period of anal fistula, the internal orifice is temporarily closed, the pipeline is drained smoothly, and the local inflammation is dissipated. There will be no symptoms or only slight discomfort. However, the primary lesion has not been eliminated and can recur under certain conditions. During the chronic active period of anal fistula, the infection will be persistent due to the continuous entry of infections from the internal orifice or poor drainage of the canal. There will be typical symptoms of anal fistula such as pus, anus dampness, itching, and so on. During the acute inflammation stage of anal fistula, the external orifice is closed or the drainage is not smooth and the infection enters continuously from the internal orifice and the pus accumulates. The symptoms and signs are similar to those of abscesses, with fever, local redness, swelling, fever, pain, and other symptoms. When the abscess re-bursts or after incision and drainage, the symptoms of swelling and pain can be relieved immediately.

4 Clinical Manifestations of Anal Fistula

4.2 Signs

The typical anal fistula consists of three parts: the external orifice, the fistula tract, and the internal orifice (Fig. 4.1). Usually, the external opening is connected with the hard rope-like canal, which goes straight or obliquely to the anus. There are often scleroma and tenderness in the internal dental line of the anus. Sometimes the external opening closes and sometimes bursts. In the inactive period, the external orifice of anal fistula is closed and there is no evident purulence (Fig. 4.2). When the external orifice bursts, purulent secretions may flow out from the external orifice. In the acute attack period, there may appear light or heavy perianal swelling and protuberance (Figs. 4.3, 4.4, and 4.5). See Chap. 5 for details.

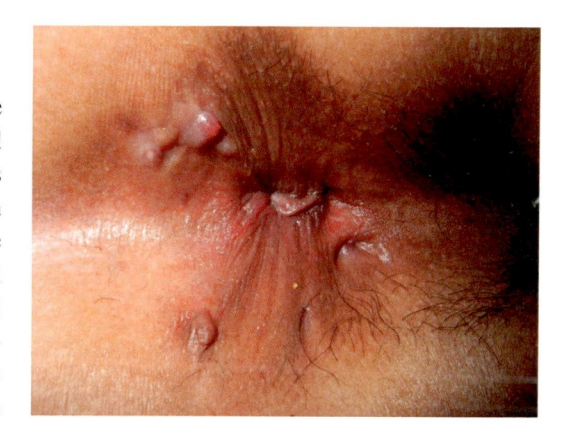

Fig. 4.2 Multiple anal fistula rest period

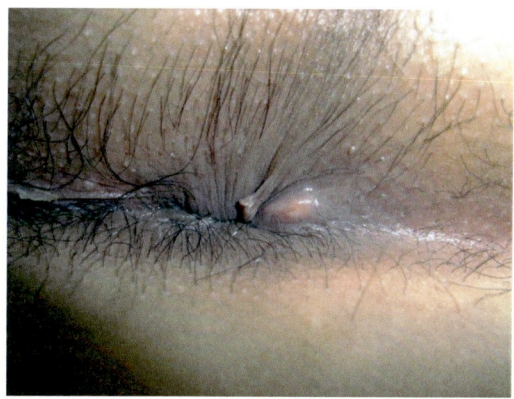

Fig. 4.3 Anal fistula mildly active period

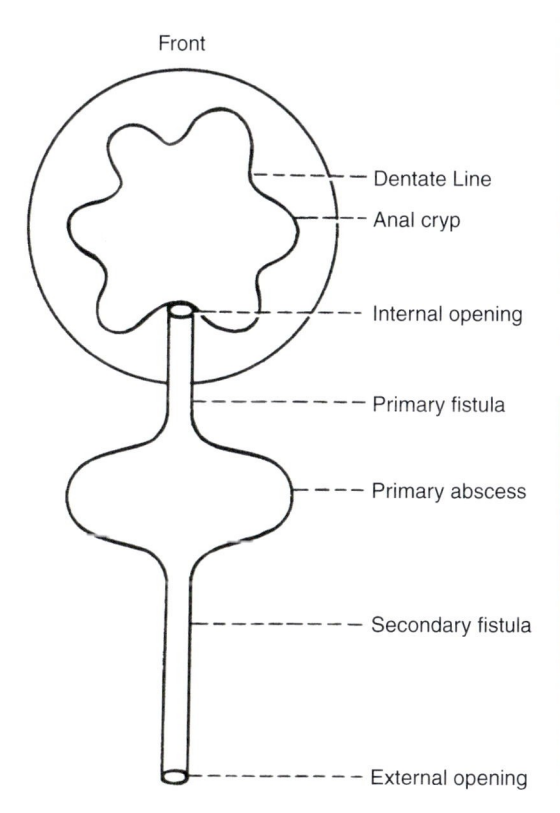

Fig. 4.1 The basic shape of anal fistula

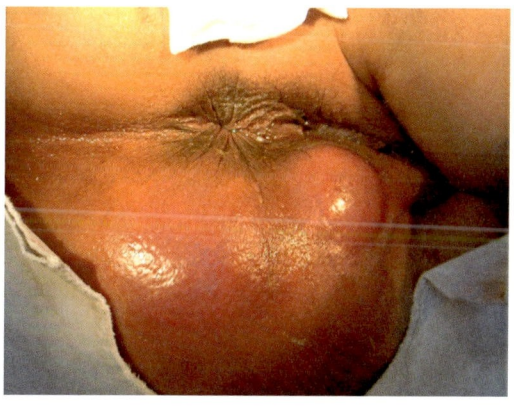

Fig. 4.4 Anal fistula moderate active period

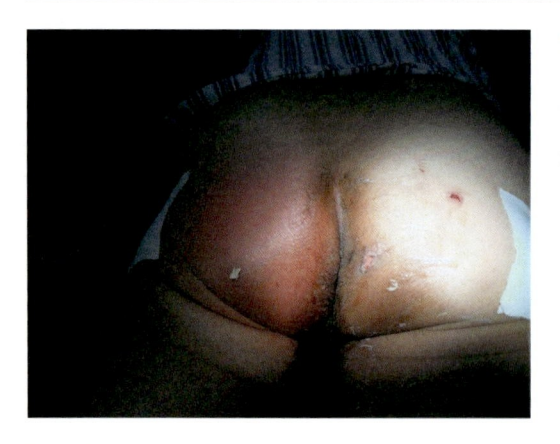

Fig. 4.5 Anal fistula severe period

Suggested Reading

1. Naijian Huang. Chinese Anorectal Diseases. Jinan: Shandong Science and Technology Press, 1996.
2. Yin Yu, Traditional Chinese Medicine Diagnosis of Anal Fistula. World Health Digest, 2011, 08 (8): 405–406.

Common Methods of Examination for Anal Fistula

5

Renjie Shi and Lihua Liu

Abstract

The lateral position is widely applied for anal fistula examination. The first step is observing the external opening around the anus and checking its amount, location, shape, distance from the anus, the characteristics of secretion in the external opening, the color of the skin around the anus, and the absence of defects in the anal canal. In the palpation, the exterior of anus is touched firstly, and then the interior of anus, and, if necessary, a combination of internal and external palpation should be done. The keypoints of palpation are the direction of fistula, the location of internal opening, and the integrity and elasticity of the anal and rectal ring. Probe exploration helps to understand the direction of fistula and the condition of the internal opening and should be conducted gently. The staining examination of fistula is helpful to confirm the location of internal opening and penetration of anal fistula. Ultrasonic examination and MRI examination are the most important test methods of anal fistula examination, as they are effective in determining the direction and location of anal fistula, in exploring the relationship between fistula and sphincter, and in finding the internal opening of anal fistula. In addition, in the diagnosis of anal fistula, bacterial culture, histopathology, fistula angiography, colonoscopy, and other means are necessary sometimes. The common methods of anal function examination and evaluation before and after anal fistula surgery are anorectal pressure measurement, ultrasonic examination, MRI, pelvic floor electromyography examination, anorectal sensory function examination, anal function scale evaluation, and a questionnaire survey of patient life's quality.

Keywords

Anal fistula · Inspection · Body position
Visual examination · Palpation · Exploration
Ultrasonic · Magnetic resonance imaging
CT · Colonoscopy

R. Shi (✉)
Department of Anorectal Surgery, Affiliated Hospital of Nanjing University of Traditional Chinese Medicine, Nanjing, Jiangsu, China

L. Liu
Nanjing Jiangbei Hospital, Nanjing, Jiangsu, China

In order to make a definite diagnosis of anal fistula, and to know the type, location, number, course, relationship with anal sphincter, the possible nature of anal fistula, and the presence or absence of concurrent lesions of anal fistula, it is necessary to make some examinations. The examination of anal fistula can be divided into two categories: systemic examination and local examination. This chapter mainly discusses the local examination methods for anal fistula, including general specialist examination without special equipment and auxiliary examination with special equipment.

Prior to examining a patient, the patient's medical history needs detailed inquiry, and a preliminary diagnosis should be considered based on the patient's age, gender, and chief complaint, followed by a focused and targeted examination. If the patient complains that the anus is often swollen and painful or moist and discharges pus with months or even years of intermittent attacks, the initial diagnosis should be considered as anal fistula. Afterward, specialized examination combined with visual examination, digital rectal examination, probe inspection and anoscopy, endoanal ultrasound, and MRI of rectoanal canal can be performed as needed.

The purpose and significance of examination should be briefly explained to the patient before the specialist examination. For patients who are nervous and afraid of the examination, appropriate comfort should be offered, and their understanding and cooperation should be obtained.

The medical history of patients with anal fistula should include the following contents: previous treatment history of the patient, history of drug allergies, history of women's pregnancy and menstruation, and whether there are any other medical histories of hypertension, cirrhosis, heart disease, blood disease, hepatitis, nephritis, etc. Colonoscopy should not be performed in the following patients: women during pregnancy and menstruation, patients with mental illness, and those with severe heart or brain diseases. For these patients, even undergoing anoscopy should be done with caution. Radiological examination is prohibited for pregnant women. Patients who have been taking anticoagulants must stop using anticoagulants for one week before they can undergo colonoscopy and other examinations.

Before examination, necessary preparations should be made. For example, before anal digital examination and rectal examination, patients need to empty their bowels and urinate, and before colonoscopy and barium enema examination, the bowel should be cleaned.

Also, be careful to palpate gently. Care should be taken to protect patient privacy. When male doctors examine female patients, female doctors, nurses, or family members should be present in principle. For children or those who cannot take care of themselves in life, family members should accompany and assist them.

5.1 Special Examinations of Anal Fistula

5.1.1 Common Positions

Clinically, an appropriate body position can be chosen according to the examination method and the patient's physical condition when undergoing physical examination of anal fistula. The usual positions are the following three.

5.1.1.1 Lateral Position
The patient lies on his side, bends his hip, and exposes his hip. This is a common examination and treatment position. The advantage is that it is simple and convenient; even for the disabled and infirm, this is an easy position to take. This position is suitable for outpatient examination and minor surgery. The disadvantage is that the anus of obese patients is not fully exposed, so it is often needed for the patient to use his hand to pull the nonimplantation side of the hip to help expose the anus.

5.1.1.2 Knee-Chest Position
The patient lies prone with chest close to the bed and kneels down on the bed. The advantage is the abdominal wall of the patient naturally sags and does not compress the bowel cavity. This position is suitable for observing the intestine during a sigmoid colonoscopy. It is a common position for rectal cancer and sigmoidoscopy. The disadvantage is that this position is not easy to do and patients can become tired very quickly, especially for the elderly, infirm, or overweight.

5.1.1.3 Lithotomy Position
Also called the bladder lithotomy position. The patient lies on his back, moves his hips to the

edge of the operating table, and places his two legs on the two leg racks on both sides. During operation, the lower limbs placed on the leg racks need to be properly fixed. The advantage of this position is that the anus is exposed and the field of vision is good, convenient for examination and surgery, and so it is the commonly used position of anorectal examination and surgery. Its disadvantages are long preparation time, complete exposure of genitals, and easy for the operator to become tired and is difficult position for the assistant. When maintaining this position for a long time, it is easy to oppress the veins and nerves of the patient's lower extremities and occasionally causes certain complications.

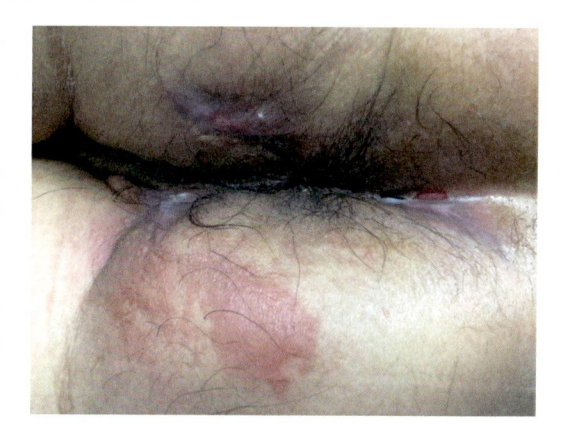

Fig. 5.1 Appearance of anal fistula recurrence

5.1.2 Inspection Methods

5.1.2.1 Visual Examination

Visual examination is to use the eyes to observe the changes in the following contents: the shape of the anus, the scope of lesions, the position of the external opening of the anal fistula, the number, the shape, and the characteristics of the secretion.

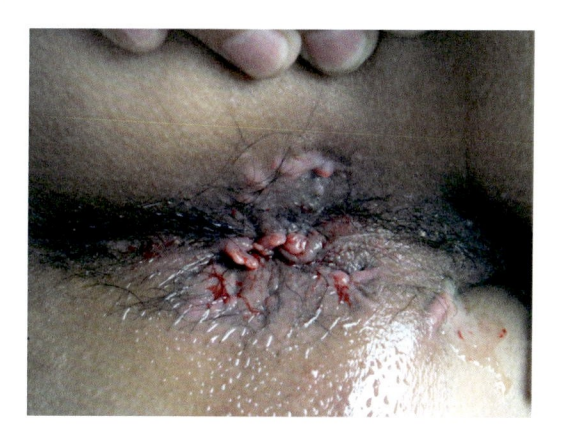

Fig. 5.2 Perianal of patients with Crohn's disease and anal fistula

Appearance of Anus

Anal fistula can often lead to perianal local or irregular swelling. The perianal tissue defects, depressions, and bumps are often seen in patients with anal fistula surgery (Fig. 5.1). Some patients have anal relaxation after anal fistula, and even a little traction can be seen in the rectal mucosa, suggesting the presence of anal incontinence. These patients are often accompanied by anal moisture, overflow, perianal skin redness, or even erosion. The perianal skin of Crohn's disease patients is typically moist and shiny (Fig. 5.2).

External Openings of Anal Fistula
1. **The Number of External Openings of Anal Fistula**

    There can be one or more or even dozens of external openings of the anal fistula. However, there are also some patients who do not have any obvious external opening, and these are termed the external blind fistula. Simple anal fistula has only one external opening, and those with more than two external openings are mostly complex or multiple anal fistulas. When there is more than one that breaks either sides or rear of the anus, it is often a horseshoe fistula. Most of the fistulas with an anterior external opening are not connected with each other, and most of them belong to different fistula groups. When the anal fistula with an anterior external opening is far from the anus, it is often possible to invade the scrotum subcutaneously. If many external openings locate on one or both sides of anus, most of the pipelines are complex, and the diagnosis is complex anal fistula. In patients with extensive lesions of complex

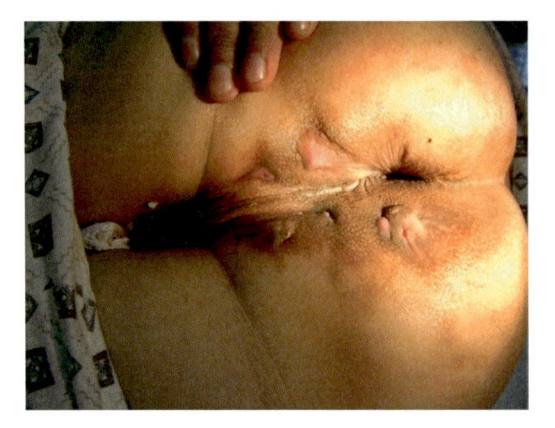

Fig. 5.3 Appearance of complex anal fistula

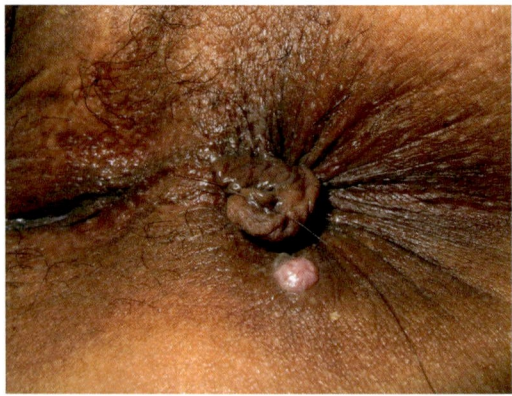

Fig. 5.4 The external opening of anal fistula may bulge due to repeated inflammation

anal fistula, the skin surface can be uneven, and the number and shape of external openings are different (Fig. 5.3).

2. **The Distance Between the External Opening and the Anus**

    Generally, if the external opening is close to the anus, the tract is straight. If it is distant from the anus, the pipeline is curved and is more complex. There are some exceptions; although in some patients the external opening is close to the anus, the pipeline is however curved, and the position is deeper. Some external openings are so far apart from the anus, the pipeline is actually quite straight, and the surface is shallow.

3. **Appearance of the External Opening**

    For the elderly with a long history of anal fistula, due to the repeated purulent swelling, hyperplasia of the tissue, and uplift, the external openings are often nodular, and there are also scar depressions. There is a fistula in the central area of the tubercle or depression (Fig. 5.4). The external opening with nodular uplift is mostly anal fistula caused by general inflammation. If the outer edge of anal fistula is curled inward, the granulation tissue is gray and bright, and most of them are diagnosed as tuberculosis anal fistula.

    When the anal fistula is in the static stage, the external opening is often closed. In the attack stage, the external opening of the anal fistula is often broken (Fig. 5.5), and secre-

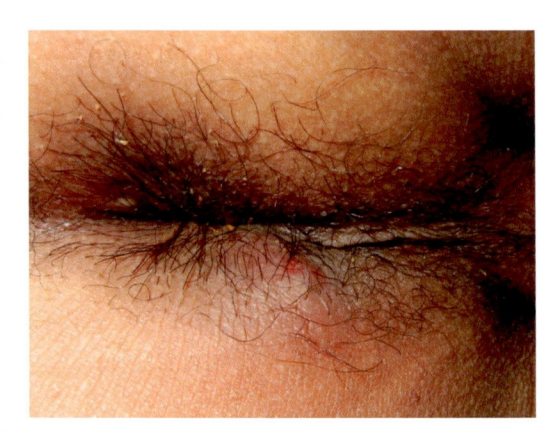

Fig. 5.5 Appearance of anal fistula active period

tions such as pus and blood often flow out of the opening.

Secretions

If the pus from the external opening of anal fistula is gray or golden, the thick texture is mostly caused by common bacteria. If the pus is mixed with blood or light red, it usually breaks up soon or is in the acute inflammation stage. If the pus is gray-white or yellow-white and accompanied by a heavy odor, it is mostly caused by *E. coli* or *Staphylococcus aureus* infection. If the pus is green, there is likely to be a *Pseudomonas aeruginosa* infection. When the pus has uniform yellow particles, this suggests actinomycetes infection. When the pus is either thin or like the water that cleans out rice, it may be caused by

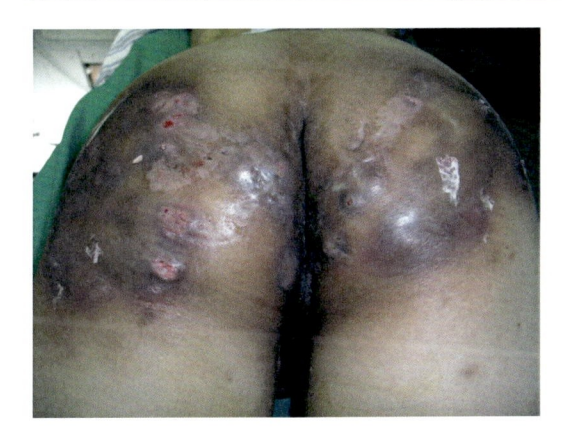

Fig. 5.6 Suppurative apocrine inflammation complicated by anal fistula

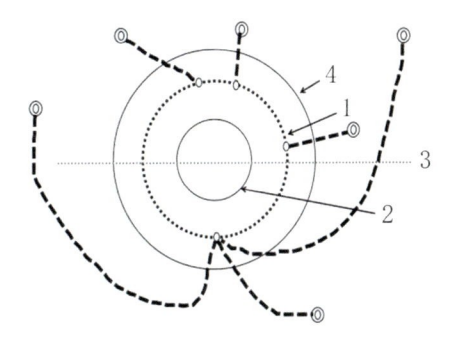

1. Dentate Line 2. Anorectal Ring 3. Transverse line 4. Anal Verge

Fig. 5.7 Solomon's law

tuberculous anal fistula or inflammatory bowel disease. The possibility of malignant tumors, such as mucinous adenocarcinoma, should be considered if there is transparent gelatinous or coffee-colored bloody mucus in the exocrine secretions.

Skin Color Changes in the Anal Fistula Lesion Area

In common anal fistula, the perianal skin often has no obvious changes, but the color of perianal skin can also be deepened in patients with long-term nonhealing of ulceration (Figs. 5.3 and 5.4). In tuberculous anal fistula, there is often a brown round halo around the external opening. If the skin in the duct area presents a diffuse dark brown, or there is normal skin color between the changed skin colors, or there is an obvious or dull brown halo, the subcutaneous cavity is often empty, the space may be single or more, or a honeycomb structure, and this situation is more common in perianal suppurative hidrosadenitis (Fig. 5.6). Anal fistula suppurative sweat adenitis is often accompanied by anal fistula.

The Relationship Between the Location of the External Opening and the Trend and Type of Anal Fistula

1. Salmon's Law: when a horizontal line is drawn in the center of the anus, if the outer opening of the fistula is in front of the line and no more than 5 cm away from the anus, the pipe is straight and the internal opening is on the same dentate line as the external opening. If the external opening is located behind this line, the pipeline is more curved, and the internal opening does not correspond to the external opening. The internal opening is mostly located at the middle dentate line behind the anus (Fig. 5.7).

2. Goodsall's rule: when a horizontal line is drawn in the center of the anus, if the external opening of the fistula is in front of this line or on the horizontal line of the anus, and the distance from the anal margin is within 2.54–3.81 cm, the pipeline is straight and the internal opening occupies the area of the dentate line. If the external opening is behind the line, the main pipe is bent and the internal opening is behind the middle dentate line. If the distance between the external opening and the anal border is more than 2.54–3.81 cm, the main wall bends backward and medially, regardless of whether the external opening is in front or behind this line (Fig. 5.8).

In addition, Parks marks eight areas of the anus and perineum as the center according to natural anatomy. These are namely the anterior midline area, left anterior area, left posterior area, left posterior area, posterior midline area, right posterior area, right area, and right anterior area. The area 3–5 cm outside the anal fold is called the inner band, and the area 3–5 cm outside the anus is called the outer band. The lesion is named

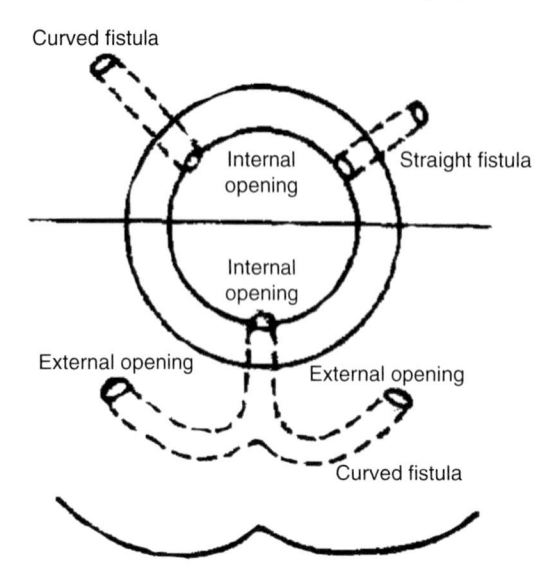

Fig. 5.8 Goodall's rule

according to its location, such as the right external fistula, left posterior internal fistula, etc. For example, if the fistula is located in the inner band, the direction of the pipeline is radial and vertical; most of the inner bands are located in the corresponding anal recess, and most of the anal fistulas in the inner band are confined to the anterior anal region. If the external opening of fistula is located in the external band, the tube is curved, and most of the internal opening is located in the posterior midline area.

5.1.2.2 Palpation

Palpation has a special significance for the diagnosis of anal fistula. Through palpation, the direction of the anal fistula, the position and number of fistula, the relationship between the fistula and the sphincter, the integrity of the anorectal ring, and its elasticity can be directly detected. The methods of palpation in anal fistula can be generally divided into the following.

External Anal Palpation

External palpation of the anus should be performed by way of sliding palpation, that is, pressing the finger on the perianal skin and slowly sliding to feel the changes of subcutaneous tissues, fistulas, and other lesions (Fig. 5.9).

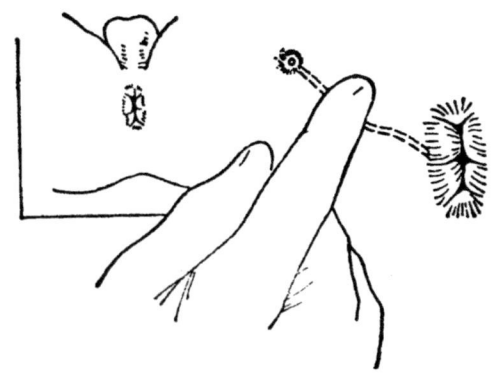

When palpating an anal fistula, slide the fingertips to palpate the cord-like fistula

Fig. 5.9 Palpation of anal fistula

Anesthesia will affect the accuracy of palpation, so palpation should be carried out before anesthesia. Apply paraffin oil or grease to gloves before palpation.

During the attack of anal fistula, the lesion site is repeatedly inflamed, swollen, and purulent, and it usually can be hard to the touch and like a tough cord that leads from the external opening to the anal cavity. When the larger mass can be touched below the external opening of anal fistula, the presence of purulent cavity is more suggestive. Anal fistula pipeline is often relatively small when anal fistula rarely attacks. However, the sensation of hard cord in the pipeline is often not obvious when tuberculous anal fistula is palpated.

If several external openings are located on the same side or the opposite side of the anus, the pipeline often has branches; one should pay attention to touch the branch and its direction. When anal fistula occurs repeatedly because the lesion area is often hard and tough and uneven, it is difficult to know the branch and direction of the pipeline, so care and experience are needed.

In low anal fistula, because of its shallow position, the boundary between the hard cord and the surrounding tissue is obvious, so it is easy to be touched. However, because of the high anal fistula's deep pipeline, external anal palpation is often not satisfactory, it is often difficult to touch the deep hard cord, and only the isolated indentation of the external opening area can be felt.

Anal Internal Palpation

After anal external palpation, the internal anal palpation is performed. After the finger is inserted into the anus, it should touch the areas from shallow to deep to further understand the direction of the fistula, the location of the internal opening, the relationship between the fistula and the anal sphincter, and the integrity and elasticity of the anorectal ring.

1. **The Path and Direction of the Fistula**

    The direction of the fistula is determined according to the extension of fistula in external palpation of the anus, and the fistula direction in the anus is further explored during internal palpation. The posterior anal fistula often extends upward in the back of the anus and then extends to both sides in the anorectal ring plane, forming a high horseshoe fistula. In some cases, the fistulas extend upward to the high muscle or submucosa, where there may be strips of cable in the high muscle or submucosa, and some of the ends are enlarged or irregularly upheavaled.

2. **The Internal Opening**

    The internal opening of anal fistula is mostly located in the dentate line, digital rectal examination can touch the definite small knot in the dental line, and most patients have significant palpitation pains. The internal opening of simple anal fistula is mostly in the same position as the external opening in the dentate line of the anal canal. The internal opening of horseshoe fistula is mostly in the posterior median dentate line of the anal canal. The recurrent anal fistula is hard at the internal opening; the hard knot is large and easy to be touched. The anal fistula soon after the formation of an abscess is not obvious, and it is not easy to be touched.

    Under anesthesia, the scleroma of the internal opening of many anal fistula patients is often not obvious; however, the scleroma of the internal opening is obvious before anesthesia, so palpation examination and positioning of the internal opening are best performed before surgery. If other examination methods such as intraoperative probe fail, clamp the external opening of anal fistula or the fistula wall suspected of being the external opening, pull outward, and touch the position of anal canal dentate line with the fingers. There is a traction feeling accompanied by depression of traction position or depression of traction position seen under an anal microscope, and this can be considered as the location of the internal opening.

3. **Anorectal Ring**

    Attention should be paid to the elasticity and integrity of the anorectal ring when touching the high anal fistula. When the anorectal ring becomes hard, physicians can use their fingers to hook the anorectal ring backward and instruct patients to contract and relax the anus. If the anorectal ring has good adaptability and strong contraction, it suggests that the anorectal ring has good elasticity and function. If the anorectal ring cannot arbitrarily relax and contract or has poor adaptability, this indicates that the anorectal ring is hardened, the elasticity is poor, or the scar tissue is large, or there is a fistula that is hardened and thick.

    When the anorectal ring is defective or incomplete, it indicates that the previous anorectal surgery may have caused great damage to the anorectal ring, and it is necessary to avoid and minimize further damage to the anorectal ring during the re-operation so as to avoid further aggravating the injury and further damaging anal function. If the anus function is incomplete, no further surgery should be carried out.

Bimanual Examination

Sometimes, when simple palpation outside the anus or finger examination inside the anus is not satisfactory alone, the overall appearance of the anal fistula can be grasped by palpation outside the anus and inside the anus at the same time, and by the subtle sense of the position and shape change of the fistula perceived when fingers touch each other inside and outside. This kind of examination method is usually better than the simple examination or palpation of the anus with fingers alone.

5.1.2.3 Probe Examination

The purpose of probe examination is to clarify the relationship between the path, length, depth of the fistula, the relationship of anal sphincter, and the position of the internal opening. Since the probe is prone to cause pain during examination, it should be fully explained to the patient before examination to explain its importance so as to obtain patient cooperation.

The probe is made of silver alloy, copper, stainless steel, and other alloy materials. The probe has different shapes, and the ball-head rod probe is often used to examine the fistula and its internal opening. A sickle-shaped grooved wire hook probe is often used for intraoperative wire hook. There are also sickle probes with blades that can be used to probe and open fistulas directly.

When inspecting, apply lubricant to the glove or finger sleeve, and insert the index finger of one hand into the anus, the other hand should take the appropriate probe depending on the thickness (usually using a silver or aluminum alloy ball-shaped rod probe), based on the initial impression of the fistula obtained by visual palpation. The probe is to be gently inserted into fistula along the direction of the fistula, and the fistula is gently penetrated. Through perception and guidance with the finger in the anus, the direction of the tube, the location of the internal opening, whether the inner port is unobstructed, and the relationship and distance between fistula and muscle tissue are explored (Fig. 5.10).

In the process of exploration, the pipe should be gently plunged into the direction of the fistula, the action should be as meticulous and gentle as possible, and it should not be harsh to prevent perforation or artificial openings. The examination should ensure that the patient does not feel obvious pain, and there should be no bleeding. During the exploration, the probe direction should be repeatedly adjusted according to the direction of fistula. If there is resistance, the probe should be withdrawn, and the bending degree should be adjusted properly before further exploration. If the bent part of the probe cannot be penetrated into the entire fistula after repeated adjustment, it may be due to tube narrowness or occlusion, and no forced forward exploration is to be allowed.

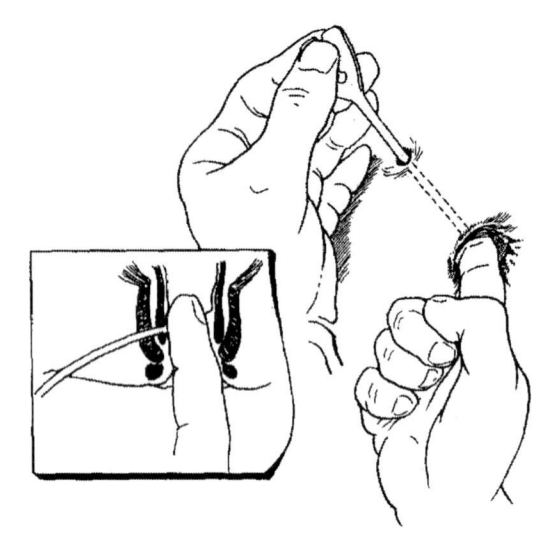

Fig. 5.10 Anal fistula detection method

For complicated anal fistula with a deep fistula location and a long fistula, it is sometimes difficult to reach the bottom with a probe. In this situation, probes can be inserted from different external openings for exploration at the same time. For example, if the probe touches somewhere in the pipeline, it indicates that the branches of fistula converge here and the two external openings are connected. When the probe is inserted into the anus through different external openings, experienced doctors can easily perceive the relationship between the probes and the path and the position of the fistula through the touch of the finger placed in the anus.

5.1.2.4 Anoscope Examination

Tube and Horn Anoscope

Before examination, ask the patient to empty the stool. The surgeon holds the handle of the anal mirror in the left hand and use the thumb to press the core. The mirror body and the head of the anal mirror are coated with paraffin oil, and the right hand should assist in exposing the anus. First, gently massage the anal edge with the top of the anoscope, and ask the patient to open the mouth to breathe, so that the anus is relaxed. Then, insert the anoscope slowly into the anus.

The direction of the lens should be facing the navel first and then facing the sacral tail after passing through the anal canal. After reaching the ampulla of rectum, the core should be pulled out to observe whether there is adhesive mucus or blood on the top of the core. After adjusting the light to directly illuminate the visual field in the tube, carefully observe the color of the mucosa at the lower end of the rectum, whether there are tumors, polyps, ulcers, foreign bodies, secretions, etc. Then, slowly withdraw the mirror body from the anus, and observe whether there are internal hemorrhoids, anal nipple hypertrophy, anal sinusitis, or anal fistula opening near the dentate line. Below the dentate line, look for cracks, growths, etc. (Fig. 5.11). In order to observe the lesion carefully, it is sometimes necessary to insert the lens several times. Note: during the examination, if further observation is required or the rotating mirror body is required, the core must be inserted again before operation to prevent injury to the anal canal and rectal mucosa.

In patients with anal fistula, there is often congestion and swelling in the internal opening in the dentate line, or there are red, inflamed pits and protruding nodules. Because the anal canal is dilated, the fistula wall is compressed; sometimes, pus can be seen flowing from the internal opening to the intestinal cavity. At this time, if methylene blue is injected from the external opening of fistula, the overflow of methylene blue from the internal opening can be seen, or the gauze placed in the anus will have methylene blue.

Leaf Anoscope

Before anoscopy, ask the patient to empty his stool. The surgeon should hold the handle of the anoscope in his left hand, close all the leaves of the leaf anoscope, smear paraffin oil on them, insert them into the anus, and then open them up. The lesion is observed by using the space between the leaves (Fig. 5.14). Note: during the examination, do not suddenly pull up the leaf anoscope to prevent the injury of intestinal mucosa and do not force to push in order to prevent stabbing the intestinal wall.

5.1.2.5 Inspection of Anal Crypt Hook

Crypt hook examination is an important method to examine the internal opening. There are two kinds of hooks commonly used: the hooks are 0.5 cm and 1.0 cm, respectively. When using the crypt hook probe, first take the small hook, probe the suspicious lesion area of the anus under the microscope, and then slowly explore the rest of the anal fistula along the dentate line. If necessary, take the hook to explore again. In general, the normal crypt can be probed by the crypt hook, but the hook is shallow. If the hook is deep, the location of the internal opening should be highly suspected; if the direction of the hook is consistent with the direction of the anal fistula, the location of the internal opening can be clarified. The

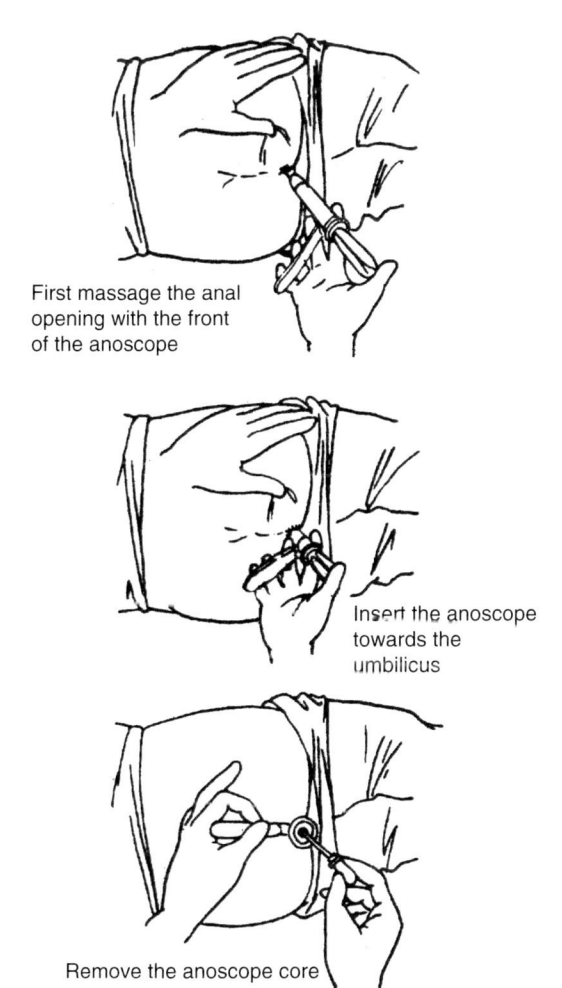

Fig. 5.11 Anoscopy method

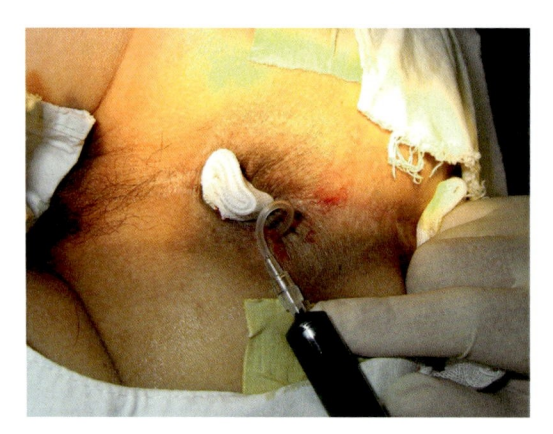

Fig. 5.12 Staining examination of anal fistula

lower fistula is then inserted with a probe from the external opening. If the two meet and touch, it indicates that the explored internal opening and fistula are interlinked, and the anal crypt is where the internal opening is.

5.1.2.6 Methylene Blue Staining Examination

The staining agent is injected into the fistula from the external opening of the anal fistula to stain the wall of the fistula so as to show the position of the internal opening and determine the range, course, morphology, and number of fistula (Fig. 5.12). The commonly used staining agent is 2% methylene blue or 2% methylene blue mixed with 1% hydrogen peroxide. Specific examination methods are as follows:

Fill the Gauze Roll in the Anus
Take the anus mirror and apply lubricant and insert it into the anus, extract the lens core, and then put the rolled yarn roll into the anus, and then slowly take out the anus mirror so that the gauze roll is placed in the anal canal. During the operation under anesthesia, the gauze can be directly put into the anus.

Dye Injection
Use a 5-ml syringe to extract 2–4 ml of methylene blue, cut off the needle of the scalp needle hose, connect the syringe to the scalp needle hose, insert the hose through the external opening into the fistula for more than 1–2 cm, and press on the external opening to prevent methylene blue from spilling out of the external opening. Inject methylene blue slowly. After infusion, continue to press the external opening to prevent methylene blue from spilling out, and then lightly press and knead the fistula for observation.

Observation of Staining Area
The observation of the internal opening staining area can be divided into direct observation and indirect observation. At the same time as injecting the liquid, direct observation is made by opening the anus and looking directly at the colored spot, while indirect observation is made by identifying the colored area of the yarn coil. When the anal plug gauze rolls out, first observe whether there is any color or not. If there is staining, it indicates that the internal and external opening of fistula is on the same path. The position of the internal opening can be determined by observing the position of the shading area, and the corresponding area of the shading area is the position of the internal opening. However, when the internal opening is large, the stain will overflow more, and it is difficult to accurately identify the location of the internal opening. In the case of internal opening atresia, although no staining agent is spilled from the anus, sometimes blue dye can be seen in the anal mucosa, so the location of the internal opening can also be determined.

In addition, the anoscope can also not be removed during the staining examination to observe whether the dye spills from the internal opening. This method is often used for intraoperative examination of the internal opening.

5.2 Auxiliary Examination of Fistula

5.2.1 Ultrasonic Examination

Ultrasound examination is a method to diagnose diseases by utilizing the information generated by the interaction between the physical characteristics of ultrasound and the acoustic characteristics of human organs and tissues and by receiving, amplifying, and processing the information to form graphics, curves, or other data. Because it is painless, inexpensive, and portable equipment, it is widely used in the clinic.

5.2.1.1 Equipment
There are two types of transanal ultrasound: linear and radial. The radial examination function can observe the pathological changes of the anus within a range of 360°, and the whole perianal image can be better displayed by using the urethra as the 12-point position (Fig. 5.13). However, it is difficult to understand the longitudinal information of anal canal. If the inspector is familiar with the normal anatomic structure of anus during ultrasonic examination, he or she can make up for this deficiency. During the examination, the ultrasonic probe inserted into the anus is moved up and down for several times to observe the anatomical relationship between the location of the primary lesion, the course of fistula, and the anal sphincter and anal levator ani muscles surrounding the fistula.

5.2.1.2 Examination Methods
According to the method of ultrasound echo display, there are two methods. (1) The two-dimensional section diagnostic method (abbreviated as B-mode ultrasound) is the most widely used ultrasound diagnostic method in clinics at present. In the anorectal department, it is often used for abdominal and perianal examinations. The real-time two-dimensional ultrasound tomography of human soft tissue organs is obtained by linear scanning. (2) Color Doppler flow imaging (CDFI) is a method of using autocorrelation technology on a two-dimensional ultrasound section to quickly obtain all echo information in a larger chamber or pipeline and then color coding and overlapping in the corresponding area of the same two-dimensional grayscale image. This can reflect the blood flow movement situation in local tissues. According to the path of examination, it can be divided into the body surface ultrasonography and the endoluminal ultrasound. Anal fistula is usually examined by endoluminal ultrasound. Because transanal ultrasound examination is specialized, it has great clinical significance for anal fistula and other diseases. This chapter mainly introduces the transanal ultrasound examination method.

Transanal ultrasonography
The enema should be given with 100 ml of glycerol in advance, and the left lateral position should be taken. The ultrasonic probe should be inserted through the anus, and the urethra should be firstly scanned to mark the position of 12 o'clock. Then move the ultrasonic probe up and down to confirm the internal sphincter, external

Fig. 5.13 Image of radiant ultrasound system

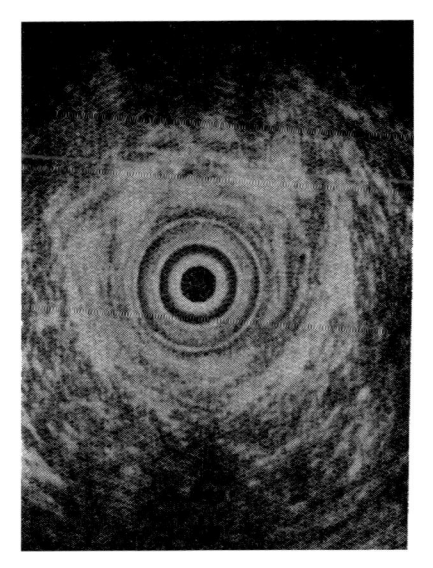

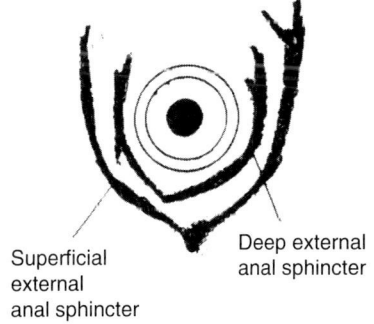

sphincter, and levator ani muscles as diagnostic targets and observe the presence of lesions and the direction of expansion. In order to locate the dentate line, a crypt hook can be placed in the dentate line when combined with high intersphincteric lesions.

When the ultrasound probe is inserted from the anus, the lower part of the external sphincter is located at the superficial part of the lower part of the anus and shows low echo and round around the anus. The sphincter muscle bundle is weaker in females than in males, especially in the front of the anus. According to the contraction of the anus, the voluntary contraction of the muscle can be observed, and this indicates that the muscle bundle is striated muscle.

The superficial part of the external sphincter and the subcutaneous part of the circular external sphincter have obvious shape differences and show low echo. The superficial part of the external sphincter is the largest, longest, and strongest muscle bundle in the external sphincter. It shows three forms on ultrasound, but all three of them fix the anus in the back from the left or right sphincters. When contracting the anus, random contraction of the muscle is observed, indicating that the muscle bundle is striated muscle. On the inner side of the superficial external sphincter, we can see that the deep external sphincter, which is described as a low echo, is circular around the deep anal sphincter as the subcutaneous part of the external sphincter. However, this muscle bundle is anatomically tightly attached to the posterior puborectalis muscle, and in many patients, it cannot be clearly scanned.

The levator ani muscle can be divided into three parts: puborectalis muscle, pubococcygeal muscle, and iliac coccygeal muscle according to its course. However, there is no clear demarcation between the three parts, so it is difficult to completely differentiate them in the ultrasonographic images. Because the internal sphincter is thin, in many patients it cannot be clearly described.

Endoscopic Ultrasonography

Endoscopic ultrasonography is simple, rapid, and easily accepted by patients. During operation, the patient takes the left lateral position or the prone position, the probe is gently inserted into the distal rectum, and the lens is retreated outward while the examination is performed.

There are three criteria for finding the internal opening under endoscopic ultrasonography: ① the internal sphincter is detected through the intersphincteric fistula (positive predictive value: 80%); ② obvious defect of internal sphincter (positive predictive value: 79%); and ③ clear subepithelial fistula with localized sphincter defect (positive predictive value: 94%). The overall sensitivity of these three signs in combination is 94% (specificity: 87%, positive predictive value: 81%).

5.2.1.3 Normal Anatomy of Transanal Ultrasound Examination

The images of internal sphincter, external sphincter, and levator ani muscle are recorded by preoperative ultrasonography. The muscles are exposed during the operation. Ultrasound examination is to be performed. If it is consistent with the preoperative findings, the muscles are identified as certain muscles. In addition, cases of internal hemorrhoids and anal fissure are also examined by ultrasound. Through the above efforts, the normal ultrasound anatomy of anal canal can be mastered.

1. Internal sphincter

    On ultrasound, it appears to be the innermost region, circular around the anus, and appears to be hypoechoic. Due to the thin layer, many cases cannot be scanned.

2. The subcutaneous part of the external sphincter

    Close to the outside of the internal sphincter, a clear circular hypoechoic image is easily found (Fig. 5.14).

3. Superficial external sphincter

    When the ultrasonic probe is moved upward from the trace to the subcutaneous part of the external sphincter, the image is the superficial part of the external sphincter, and its shape is significantly different from that of the subcutaneous part of the external sphincter (Fig. 5.15). The superficial appearance of

Fig. 5.14 Ultrasonic images of the subcutaneous and internal sphincter of the external sphincter

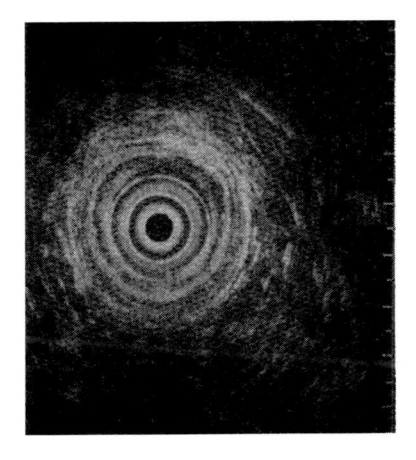

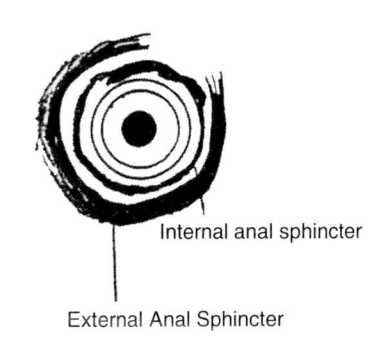

Fig. 5.15 Ultrasound images of the superficial and deep parts of the external anal sphincter

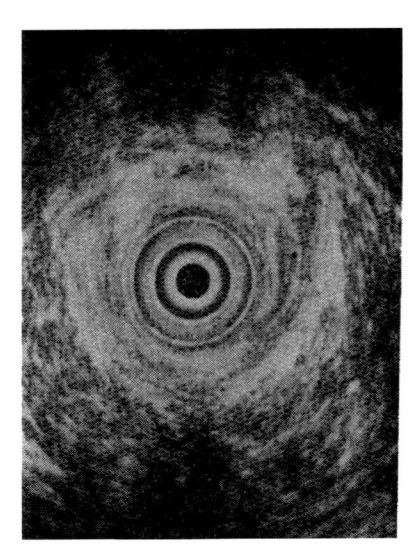

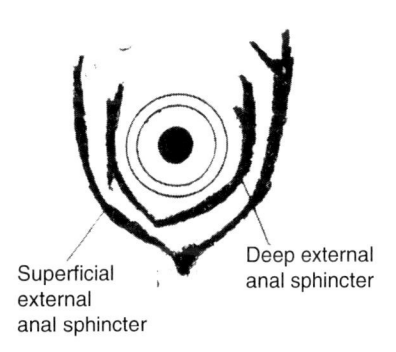

the external sphincter in the vast majority of cases is described as any of the three patterns shown in Fig. 5.16, a distinct low echo.

4. Deep external sphincter

    At the same height as the superficial part of the external sphincter, the inner part of the superficial part of the external sphincter is round around the anus and also presents as hypoechoic, but the deep image of the external sphincter in many cases is not clear.

5. Levator ani muscle

    At the height of the probe, it should be scanned from the superficial and deep parts of the external sphincter; moving the probe upward, there is a low muscle echo image that is U-shaped around the anus (Fig. 5.17).

6. Dentate line

    Under normal conditions, it is impossible to locate the dentate line by ultrasonic examination. Therefore, a liquid should be used to better characterize the characteristics of ultrasonic wave in the dentate line, i.e., with 0.5% serucaine E (0.5 ml) for local injection of about 5 places. This can accurately determine the position of the dentate line. It is also possible to position the dentate line by placing a crypt hook at the dentate line portion.

5.2.1.4 Ultrasonic Characteristics of Different Types of Perianal Abscesses and Anal Fistulas

When meeting specific cases in the clinic, doctors should compare the results of palpation

Fig. 5.16 Three forms of the superficial part of the external sphincter. The three pictures A/B/C on the left show the ultrasound images of the superficial part of the external sphincter muscle traced at different positions A/B/C in the right picture

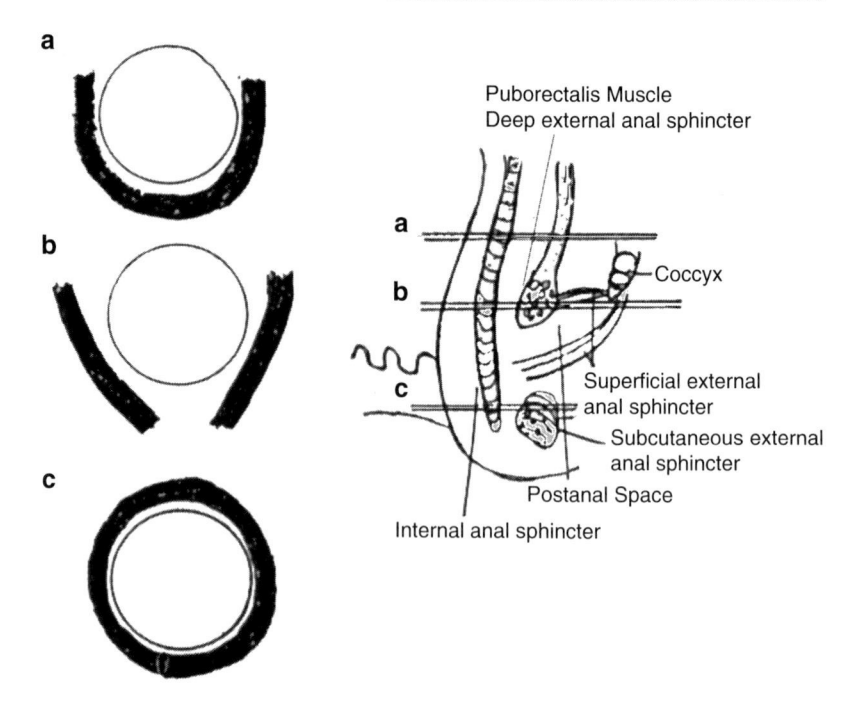

Fig. 5.17 Ultrasonic image of the levator ani muscle

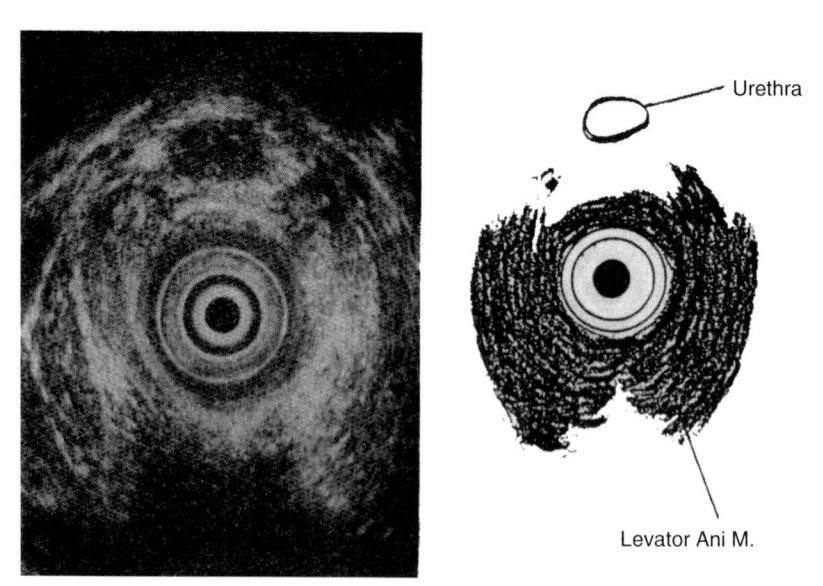

with the ultrasound images and the intraoperative findings so as to determine the ultrasound images of various types of perianal abscess and anal fistula and grasp the characteristics of the lesions.

Intersphincteric Abscess, Intersphincteric Fistula (II Type)

On the ultrasonographic images, the intersphincteric lesions present as a hypoechoic mass in the medial external sphincter. The abscess is cystic, and the anal fistula is a mass with approximately the same echo density as the sphincter. The high intersphincteric fistula (II H) or low intersphincteric fistula (II L) can be distinguished by locally injecting serucaine E into the dentate line to locate the dentate line.

Case 1: II HA, II LA (Figs. 5.18 and 5.19)
In Fig. 5.18, the superficial external sphincter appears as a U-shaped hypoechoic layer surrounding the anus. The intersphincteric lesion presents as a 6-point hypoechoic mass. Figure 5.19 is the image of the ultrasonic probe being pulled outward. The subcutaneous part of the external sphincter appears as a round hypoechoic layer around the anus. II LA and II HA also show the sphincter within 6-point inside the low echo. Therefore, a diagnosis of II HA II LA is made.

Case 2: II Hs (Fig. 5.20), **II Ls** (Fig. 5.21)
The circular hypoechoic layer surrounding the anus in Fig. 5.20 is the superficial part of the external sphincter. At six o'clock, the masses at the same level as the superficial part of the external sphincter can be seen, showing as II Hs. In

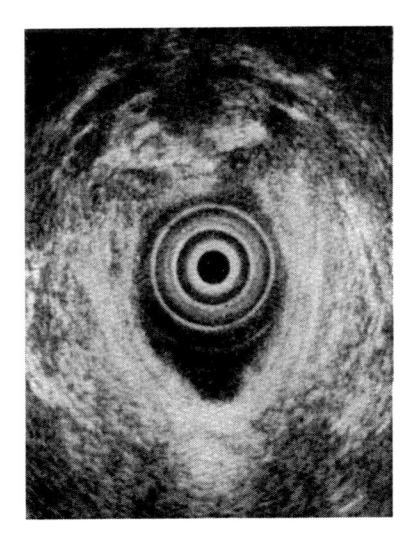

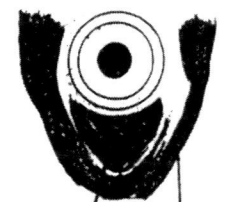

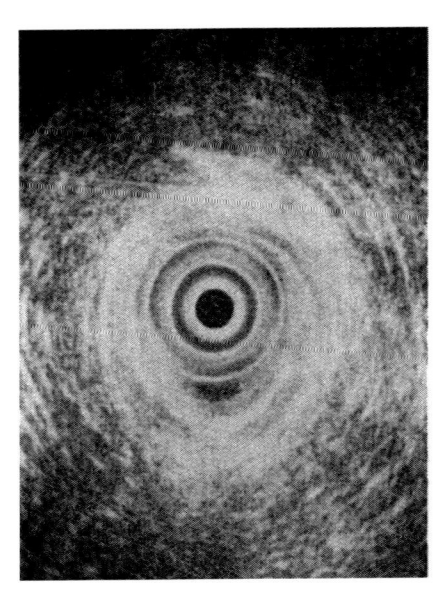

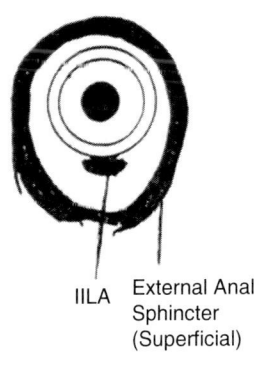

Fig. 5.18 Ultrasound image of high intermuscular abscess

Fig. 5.19 Ultrasound image of low intermuscular abscess

Fig. 5.20 Ultrasound image of high intermuscular fistula

External Anal Sphincter (Superficial) — IIHs

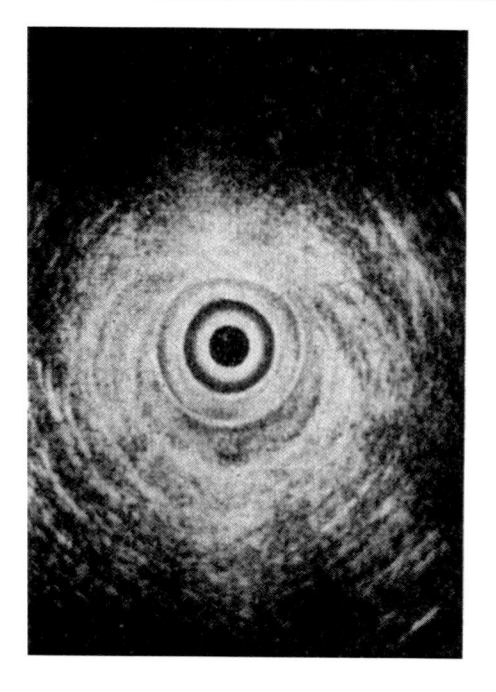

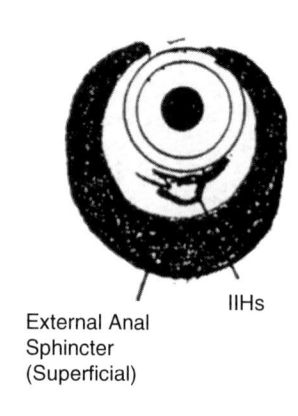

Fig. 5.21 Ultrasound image of low intermuscular fistula

External Anal Sphincter (Subcutaneous) — IILs

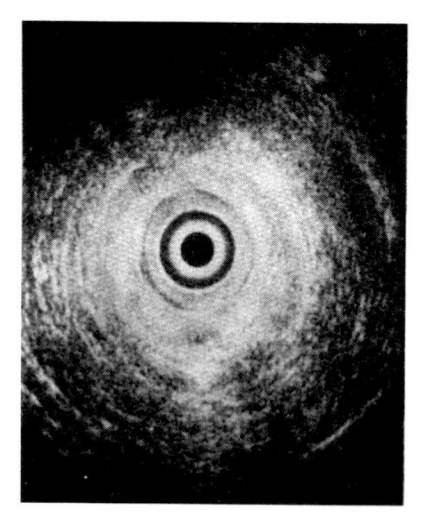

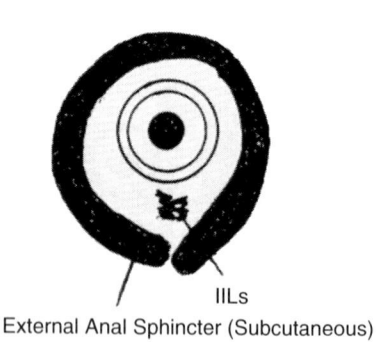

Fig. 5.21, the subcutaneous part of the circular external sphincter can be seen, and the lesion of II Ls can be seen at six o'clock. According to the above characteristics, the case is diagnosed as II Hs, II Ls.

Ischioanal Abscess, Ischioanal Fistula (Type III)

Because the gap behind the anus is full of pus, the ischioanal abscess shows a cystic shape in the gap behind the anus on ultrasonic examination, and the pus is discharged simultaneously when pressing on the superficial part of the external sphincter. Ischioanal abscess needs to be differentiated from intersphincteric abscess. It is very difficult to identify by palpation, but it can be easily identified by ultrasound.

In the case of ischioanal fistula, the purulent fluid in the posterior anal space decreases, and the inner cavity becomes smaller, presenting as a low-echo mass extending along the superficial part of the external sphincter to the horseshoe-shaped masses on both sides. Most cases of ischiorectal space lesions are associated with intersphincteric lesions (mostly II H).

When Takano Masahiro studied the formation pattern of ischioanal abscess by ultrasonic examination, he found something very interesting: in the production process of ischioanal abscess, an intersphincteric abscess was formed first, and then the intersphincteric abscess bursts through the external sphincter and extends deep into the posterior anal space, and then forms the ischioanal rectal abscess. When ultrasound examines the posterior anal space, there is no posterior anal space near the outside of the internal sphincter at the superficial height of the external sphincter. On the outside of the internal sphincter, there is a deep part of the external sphincter, and the outside of the deep part of the external sphincter has a deep postanal space. Therefore, the infection of the anal gland between the internal and external sphincter does not directly spread to the deep space but first forms the intersphincteric abscess. In some cases, the intersphincteric abscess ruptures the deep external sphincter and spreads to the deep space, forming ischiorectal abscess and ischiorectal fistula (Case 3).

When observing the lesions of the ischioanal abscesses with ultrasonic examination, the lesions in the deep space were first seen, the abscess is presented as a cystic shape, while the anal fistula presented as a mixed echo mass. Almost all cases are accompanied by low echo masses (intersphincteric lesions) on the inside of the external sphincter, and it is necessary to properly treat the lesions here during surgery (Case 3, Case 4).

Case 3: III BA (Fig. 5.22), **II HA, II LA** (Fig. 5.23)

In Fig. 5.22, II HA can be seen at six o'clock, and deep external sphincter can be seen behind it. The deep part of the external sphincter ruptured at six o'clock, and the lesion spread to the posterior anal space. In Fig. 5.23, we can see the subcutaneous part of the sphincter round around the anus, in which II LA can be seen. According to the above findings, the diagnosis of this case is III BA, II HA, and II LA.

Case 4: III Bs, II Hs (Fig. 5.24)

Unlike in the abscess stage, in the posterior anal space at 6 points, fibrin in the pus precipitates after a long period of development and becomes a horseshoe-shaped lesion with a mixture of strong echo and low echo, and is expressed as III Bs. The hypoechoic mass, II Hs, can be seen in the inner side of the internal sphincter at 6 points. Therefore, the disease is diagnosed as III Bs, II Hs.

Fig. 5.22 Ultrasonic images of ischiorectal fossa abscess and high intermuscular abscess

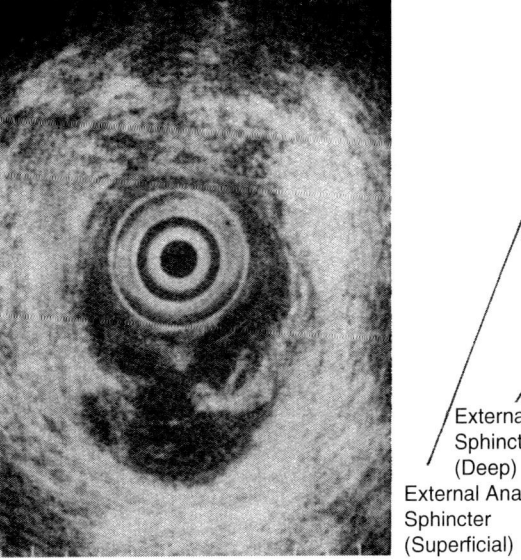

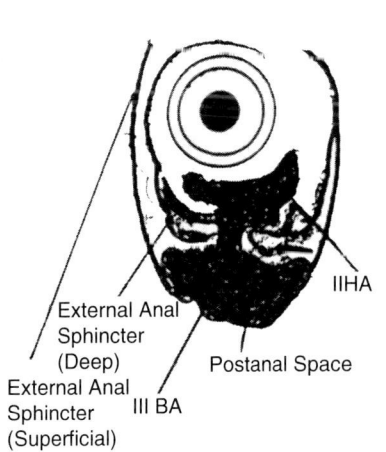

Fig. 5.23 Ultrasonic images of pus species and low intermuscular abscess in ischiorectal fossa

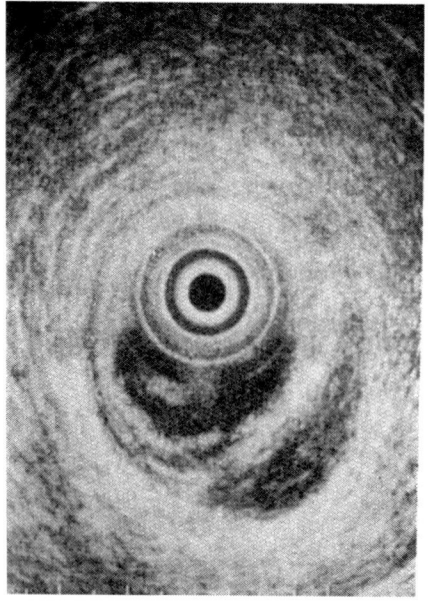

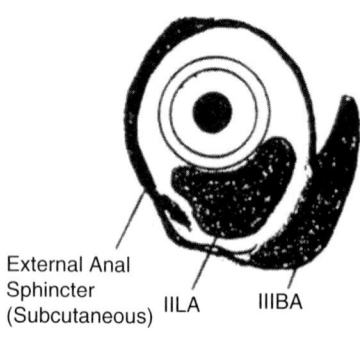

External Anal Sphincter (Subcutaneous) IILA IIIBA

Fig. 5.24 Ultrasonic images of ischiorectal fossa fistula and high intermuscular fistula

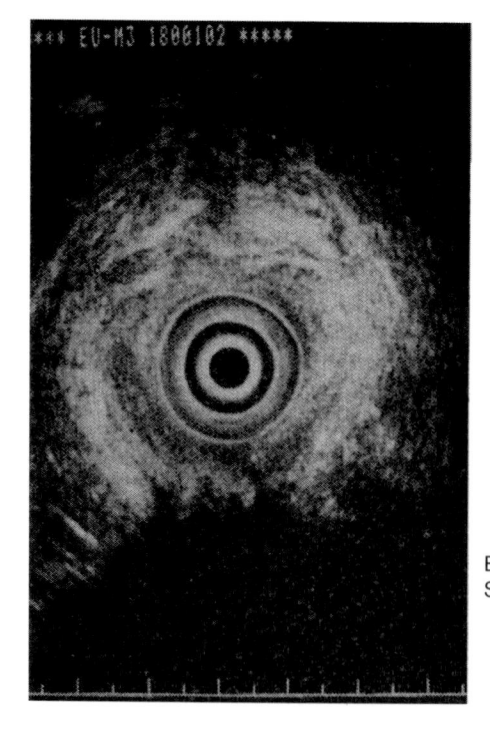

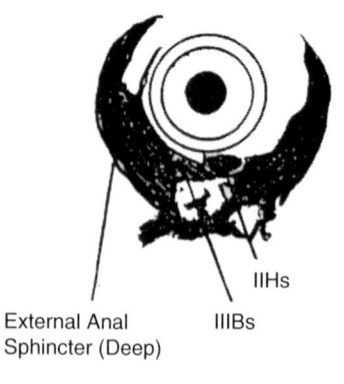

External Anal Sphincter (Deep) IIHs IIIBs

Pelvirectal Abscess, Pelvirectal Fistula (Type IV)

As with the ischiac rectum lesion, except for the result of Crohn's disease and foreign body, it is rare for individuals to have multiple intersphincteric lesions and ischiac rectum lesions.

It is believed that it is caused by the upward spread of the high intersphincteric lesions (II H) or the upward spread of the ulceration of levator ani muscle in ischiorectal fossa lesions (III). Therefore, pelvic rectal lesions are mostly associated with intersphincteric lesions and

Fig. 5.25 Ultrasound image of pelvic rectal fossa fistula

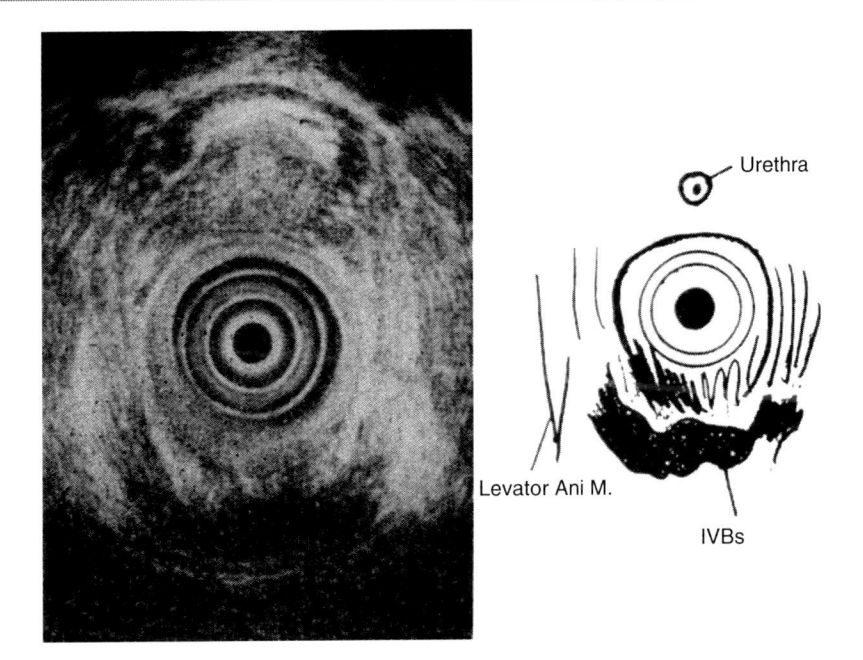

ischiorectal lesions. Ultrasound examination is characterized by low echo mass in pelvic rectal, which is easy to diagnose, especially in cases of IV B.

Case 5: IV Bs (Fig. 5.25), **III Bs, II Hs** (Fig. 5.26)

In Fig. 5.25, the levator ani muscle surrounds the anus, and bilateral lesions can be seen in the rear, represented by IV Bs. In Fig. 5.26, bilateral lesions can also be seen in the rear. Hypoechoic masses, expressed as III Bs and II Hs, are also recorded in the inner side of the external sphincter. According to the above findings, the diagnosis of this case is IV Bs, III Bs, and II Hs.

5.2.1.5 Accuracy of Transanal Ultrasonography

Lindsey et al. collected data from 38 consecutive patients with anal fistula before operation to evaluate the diagnostic value of anal ultrasonography in the diagnosis of anal fistula. The results indicated that in determining the presence and location of anal fistula, the consistency rate of ultrasonic examination of anal canal with anesthesia was up to 84%. The results showed that the coincidence rate of anal ultrasonography with anesthesia was 84% in determining the presence and location of anal fistula. In one patient, anal fistula was not found in the ultrasound examination of anal canal, and later he was diagnosed under anesthesia. Five patients, who were diagnosed with anal fistula by anal ultrasonography, had no fistula when examined under anesthesia. The results of anorectal ultrasound examination provided favorable information for the operation of nine patients (38%). Two cases of concealed sphincter defects were found. Three patients who were originally diagnosed with low anal fistula were corrected and diagnosed with high anal fistula. However, endoscopic ultrasonography has two obvious defects: (1) ultrasound is not enough to penetrate the external sphincter (especially the high-frequency transducer), so some fistulas may be missed through this method. (2) It is difficult to distinguish recurrent abscess from fibrous degeneration of the remaining fistula because both are infected and fibrotic tissues are hypoechoic under endoscopy.

Takano Masahiro et al. have performed transanal ultrasound examination on 200 cases of anal fistula and perianal abscess before operation and compared the diagnostic accuracy of finger examination and transanal ultrasound examination on anal fistula and perianal abscess according to different types of anal fistula and based on

Fig. 5.26 Ultrasonic images of ischiorectal fossa and intermuscular lesions of pelvic rectal fossa fistula

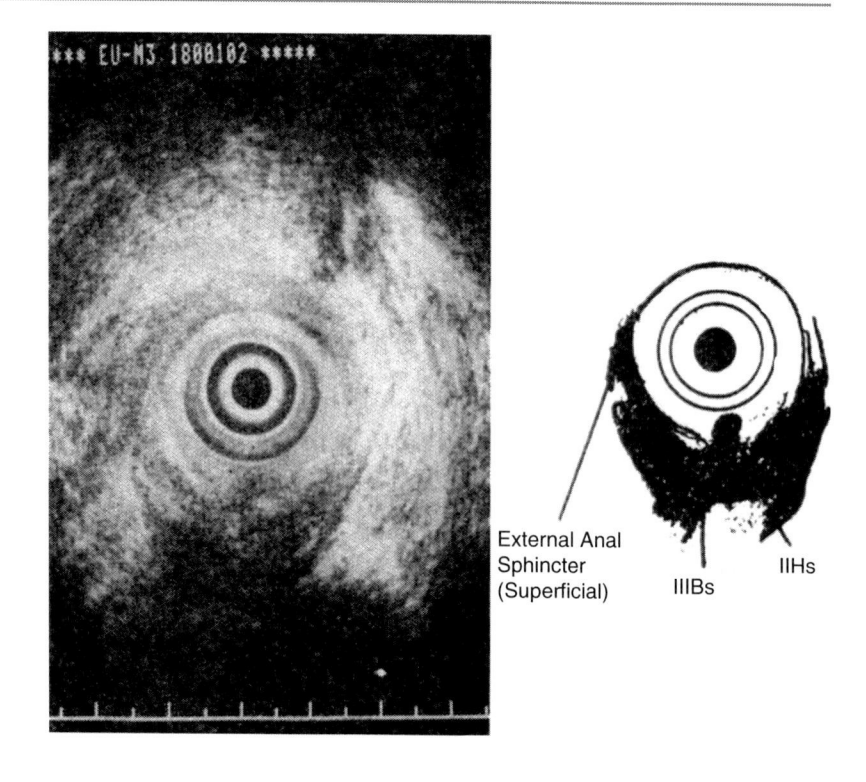

the operation results. In general, the correct diagnosis rate was 63.5% in finger diagnosis and only 58.5% in transanal ultrasonic examination, so finger diagnosis was better. The misdiagnosis rate of the basic correct part was 17.5% for finger diagnosis and 31.0% for transanal ultrasound examination. According to the different types, type I–III finger diagnosis is superior, while type IV finger diagnosis has the same accuracy. The misdiagnosis rate was 19.0% for finger diagnosis and 10.5% for transanal ultrasonography. Except for type I, the misdiagnosis rate of types II, III, and IV was high. Further analysis showed that 23 (65.5%) of the 35 misdiagnosed cases were missing partial fistula, and 12 of them were missing low intersphincteric fistula (IIL). That is to say, when there is deep anal fistula, it is easy to miss the superficial anal fistula, which may be caused by the negligence of others when people find large lesions, so it is necessary to cultivate the habit of comprehensive and careful examination. Nine cases (25.7%) were typing errors, of which seven cases were mistaken for simple (S) and complex (C), unilateral (U), and bilateral (B). Three cases (8.6%) had no anal fistula and were misdiagnosed as anal fistula, all of which were misdiagnosed as high intersphincteric fistula. Among 38 cases of complete misdiagnosis of finger diagnosis, 34 cases (89.5%) were misclassified, of which 25 cases (73.1%) were misclassified as the deeper type. Sebaceous cyst and scar after anal fistula operation were mistaken for anal fistula in three cases. Among 62 cases misdiagnosed by transanal ultrasound, 44 cases (71.0%) were misdiagnosed as anal fistula, which was significantly higher than that by finger examination. It is suggested that the technique of distinguishing anal fistula from sphincter needs to be improved, and the problem of high misdiagnosis rate needs to be solved by improving the techniques. Only nine cases (14.5%) were missed, which was less than that of finger diagnosis. There were six cases of typing errors, suggesting that transanal ultrasonography is difficult to diagnose distal branch end fistulas such as type I and type II, which should be remedied by finger diagnosis. Twenty-one cases were completely misdiagnosed by transanal ultrasonography, which was less than that by finger examination. Among them, 19 cases (90.5%) were mistyped, accounting for the overwhelming majority, 12 cases (63.2%) were diagnosed as the deep type, 7 cases (36.8%) were shallower than the actual type, and 2 cases (9.5%) were misdiagnosed as anal fistula.

Domestic doctors Ye Ling and Zheng Mingxiao reported that the location, size, distribution, and maturity of the abscess in perianal abscess were judged by ultrasonography. The location and direction of anal fistula, the number and distribution of branches, and the location and number of internal openings could provide qualitative and localized diagnosis for clinical operation. Clinical observation of 198 cases showed that the diagnostic accuracy of B-mode ultrasonography group was 100%, and the cure rate of one operation was 98%, which was significantly higher than that of the control group. It is believed that endorectal ultrasound can improve the diagnostic quality of perianal abscess and anal fistula and the cure rate of one operation.

However, Choen et al. thought that ultrasonic examination was actually no better than anal finger examination. They collected data from 38 anal fistula patients who visited the hospital continuously to compare the accuracy of anal finger examination and endoscopic ultrasonography in describing the anatomical structure of anal fistula. The results showed that 26 internal openings (33 in total), 29 main fistulas (34 in total), and 15 branches (21 in total) were accurately located in digital anal examination. Endoscopic ultrasonography accurately located 26 internal openings, 24 main fistulas, and 10 branches, and there was no statistically significant difference between the two.

Wang Zhenjun and Yang Bin performed endoscopic ultrasonography in 12 patients who failed to find the internal opening of anal fistula during routine operation. They were treated with endoscopic ultrasonography, and this was compared with other routine methods. Results showed that endoscopic ultrasonography revealed the exact location of healed internal openings in 12 patients, which was superior to the Goodsall rule, digital examination, sinus angiography, methylene blue injection, or sinus probe exploration. They found that saline injection through the external opening of the sinus could better show the location of the sinus and the internal opening during examination. It is recommended that blue dye be injected into the internal opening through endoscopy after the internal opening is found by endoscopy, which can greatly facilitate the surgeon to locate the internal opening quickly and shorten the operation time. It is believed that transanal endoscopic ultrasonography is an accurate, rapid, simple, and well-tolerated method for locating the anal internal opening of a healed anal fistula.

It is reported that hydrogen peroxide ultrasonography can significantly improve the accuracy in diagnosing fistulas and the internal opening. Kruskal and other scholars examined more than 60 cases of anal fistula patients with hydrogen peroxide ultrasound. They realized that this method is helpful to explore the existence, number, and structure of fistula and to select appropriate surgical methods for the surgeon. Buchanan and other scholars also believe that hydrogen peroxide ultrasonography is beneficial for finding the main fistula and internal opening in recurrent or complex cases of anal fistula. Nineteen patients with anal fistula had their data collected and observed with three-dimensional ultrasound reconstruction before and after injection of hydrogen peroxide. Two experienced radiologists independently analyzed the results of ultrasound diagnosis and compared them with the results of magnetic resonance imaging and surgical exploration. The results showed that most of the internal openings (19/21VS18/21), main tracts (17/21VS15/21), and branches (13/19VS12/19) were found by three-dimensional ultrasound and hydrogen peroxide three-dimensional ultrasound. Although the diagnostic significance of the two methods is comparable, the bubbles produced by hydrogen peroxide can make the fistula and the internal opening more obvious. Navarro-Luna conducted a prospective study of patients who underwent indirect enhanced endoanal ultrasound examination and surgery between 2001 and 2004. They contrasted the various features of anal fistula with the findings of the operation and classified the fistulas according to the ultrasound image. Results showed that in 94% of cases, the internal opening was identifiable. In only one case, the authors were unable to obtain sufficient information on the fistula and its course. In 95% of cases, endoanal ultrasound can correctly identify whether the fistula is straight or curved; in 85% of cases, the course of the fistula diagnosed by ultrasound is consistent with the findings of surgery; and 75% of chronic fistula is confirmed by surgery. Therefore, it is believed that the use of endoanal ultrasound, under the enhancement of hydrogen peroxide, can provide ideal results in the surgical pre-examination of anal fistula.

Through specialist examination methods such as ultrasonic examination and surgery on by examination of using touch, it was found that the reason why perianal sebaceous cyst is easily misdiagnosed as anal fistula or abscess was because the edge of the cyst is too close to the anus, so that suspicious hard nodules of the dental line could be easily found in the anal finger examination, but mistaken for the internal opening. Especially when the medial hard wall of the cyst is located just at the dental line height, it is difficult to distinguish the hard nodule of the internal opening from the hard wall of the mass.

Three-dimensional anorectal ultrasound developed on the basis of two-dimensional ultrasound can obtain three-dimensional modules of lesions from different angles at the same time. It can intuitively display the size of pus cavity, the course of fistula, and the relationship with the sphincter. The diagnostic accuracy of the internal cavity is higher than that of two-dimensional ultrasound. However, for high complex anal fistula with recurrence and fibrosis of the fistula wall and scarring, the inflammation process in the sphincter is a low echo area, which is difficult to distinguish from the low echo area caused by scarring. Therefore, there are omissions in the determination of the fistula, and there is no evaluation of fistula branches outside the anal margin.

5.2.1.6 The Role and Significance of Ultrasound Examination

Transanal ultrasound examination has obvious advantages in the diagnosis of anal fistula and perianal abscess. For example, ultrasound examination can accurately display the shape of the lesion and can save the image for comparative study before and after operation. In addition, the traditional examination method can only touch the size of the mass. The size of the abscess cavity mainly depends on experience. It is a blind area. The size of the abscess cavity can be more accurately understood by using transanal ultrasound examination. Therefore, transanal ultrasound examination has gradually become an important means of diagnosis of perianal abscess and anal fistula.

Transanal ultrasound can also find some internal openings that cannot be found through finger examination, can better grasp the direction of fistula and its branches, and make up for the shortcomings of traditional finger examination and anal endoscopy. Under endoscopic ultrasonography, the closed internal opening of anal fistula is characterized by defects such as the interruption and hypoechoic focus of submucosa or internal sphincter; some defects are connected with the defect of the external intestinal sphincter.

But there are still some limitations in ultrasonic examination. The limitations of ultrasonography are (1) limited penetrating ability, unable to reveal deep fistulas and small abscesses; (2) difficulty to display three-dimensional structure on a single plane; (3) if there is a probe squeezing, it may cause false closure and unnecessary pain of the fistula, and thus will reduce the accuracy of examination; and (4) diagnosis depends very much on the experience of the examiner. The accuracy of the results is related to the operator's experience, techniques, and the duration of illness. It is also related to the duration of fistula formation, the maturity of fiber duct, and the clarity of ultrasound image. (5) Some ultrasonic examination models are relatively expensive and not easy to promote in primary medical institutions.

5.2.2 Magnetic Resonance Imaging (MRI)

Nuclear magnetic resonance imaging (NMRI) is a new medical imaging technology based on the principle of nuclear magnetic resonance (NMR). Because of its good resolution of soft tissue, it is widely used in the examination of whole body organs; for substantive organs such as the brain, thyroid, liver, gallbladder, spleen, kidney, pancreas, adrenal gland, uterus, ovaries, prostate, and heart and great vessels, it has excellent diagnostic function. Compared with other auxiliary examination methods, MRI has many advantages such as more imaging parameters, faster scanning speed, higher tissue resolution, and a clearer image. At MRI examination has become a common imaging examination tool.

5.2.2.1 Examination Methods

Before conducting an MRI examination, all the metal objects on the body must be removed. Magnetic items such as watches, metal necklaces, dentures, metal buttons, and metal contraceptive rings should not be worn for the MRI examination. The upper abdomen (such as liver, pancreas, kidney, adrenal gland, etc.) must be empty for MRI examination, but sufficient water can be drunk before examination, which is conducive to clearer boundaries between the stomach and liver and spleen.

MRI examination of anal fistula can be achieved in two ways: through the rectal cavity coil and the surface phased array coil. The rectal cavity coils are expensive and have similar defects as ultrasound probes, with a reported accuracy of only 68%. Therefore, there is little use for the rectal cavity coil in clinical practice. Surface phased array coil is simple to operate, well-tolerated, has a large field of vision, and produces satisfactory images. It can also display the lesions above the levator ani muscle well.

During scanning, the positioning line should be vertical and parallel to the standard anal canal meridian, and the scanning layer thickness should be less than 4 mm.

Although MRI examination will not affect human health, six groups of people are not suitable for MRI: patients with a cardiac pacemaker, those with or suspected of having intraocular metal foreign bodies, patients with aneurysm clip ligation, those with retained metal foreign bodies or metal prostheses in vivo, critically ill patients with life-threatening conditions, and those with claustrophobia. It is not possible to bring monitoring instruments and rescue equipment into the nuclear magnetic resonance examination room. In addition, pregnant women less than three months along should best not to do magnetic resonance imaging.

5.2.2.2 Diagnostic Value

MRI has a high resolution for soft tissue, can directly produce multiplanar imaging, can collect high-quality images due to the low movement of pelvic organs, can clearly show fistulas without any drugs, and there is no radiation injury. For simple anal fistula, MRI can display abnormal signals of the intersphincteric space and the fistula downward to the skin. As for complex anal fistula, MRI can show whether the fistula passes through the anal canal or rectum wall through the pararectal space and can better show the anal sphincter and rectum of the surrounding structure of fistula (Fig. 5.27). Many scholars compared the MRI diagnosis results with the final surgical results, confirming the accuracy of the diagnosis of anal fistula. It is reported that the accuracy rate of anal fistula diagnosis in MRI is as high as 90%–93%.

Lunniss et al. conducted a prospective study in 1992 to assess the value of magnetic resonance imaging in the diagnosis of anal fistula. A total of

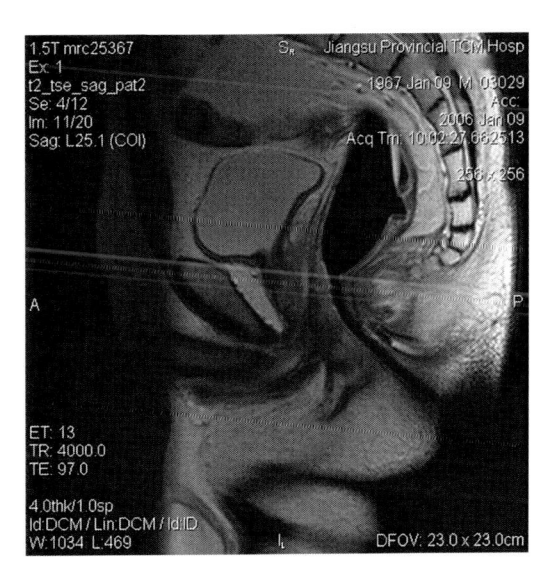

Fig. 5.27 MRI image of partial fistula of high complex anal fistula

16 patients with anal fistula (24–66 years old, average age 42 years old) underwent preoperative MRI, and 14 of them were found to have the same fistula course and location as those reported by MRI.

Scholefield and other scholars believe that patients with anal fistula do not need conventional magnetic resonance scanning before operation, but for patients with complex anal fistula, this method is particularly important. To assess the diagnostic value of MRI in patients with suspected anal fistula, they assigned an anorectal surgeon who did not know the results of the MRI to perform surgery under local anesthesia. The results showed that 33 patients with a clinical diagnosis of anal fistula were included in the experiment, and 27 patients were confirmed to have anal fistula through operation. MRI showed 42% of the fistulas, 63% of the internal openings, 13.33% of the external openings, and 50% of the perianal abscesses.

For recurrent anal fistula and Crohn's anal fistula, MRI is more important to diagnose complicated branches and residual abscess cavities. MRI has an irreplaceable diagnostic value in the diagnosis of complex anal fistula complicated by Crohn's disease. Beetstan and other scholars collected data on 56 patients with anal fistula. MRI was performed before surgery (24 patients with primary onset of anal fistula, 17 patients with recurrent anal fistula, and 15 patients with Crohn's disease complicated with anal fistula). The results confirmed that MRI provided important imperceptible additional information for 12 patients (Crohn's complicated anal fistula in six cases, recurrent anal fistula in four cases, and primary anal fistula in two cases). The sensitivity and specificity of magnetic resonance imaging for diagnosing fistula were 100% and 86%, respectively, the sensitivity and specificity for diagnosing perianal abscess were 96% and 97%, respectively, the sensitivity and specificity for diagnosing horseshoe fistula were 100%, and the sensitivity and specificity for diagnosing internal opening were 96% and 90%, respectively. MRI is of great significance in the diagnosis and treatment of the branches above the levator ani muscle. Under normal circumstances, these branches are not only difficult to find but also extremely difficult to handle.

MRI has been proved to affect the treatment of anal fistula patients. In a prospective study of 56 patients with anal fistula (15 of whom were patients with CD anal fistula), the preoperative MRI results were initially kept secret from the surgeon, then provided to the surgeon when the operation was completed, and the surgeon was allowed to perform further operations based on the information provided by MRI. Also, 21% of the patients underwent further operations due to the additional information provided by MRI, but if only CD patients were counted, the amount of further operations was increased to 40%.

With the development of MRI technology, MRI study of anal fistula has become more and more detailed. It has been reported in the literature that DWI can be used to evaluate anal fistula. ADC value can be quantified to reflect the inflammatory activity of the fistula and can replace enhanced scanning. Because dynamic contrast-enhanced scanning reflects the activity of the anal fistula and the response of the fistula to drug therapy, MRI can guide clinicians in the treatment and medication of CD anal fistula patients.

MRI examination also has some shortcomings: (1) the examination takes a long time, usually 20–30 min, and some patients with serious illnesses may not be able to finish it consistently; (2) some patients with active CD have fevers. It is risky to use 3.0T MR for examination, and when using 1.5T MR, doctors should also pay attention to the fever. (3) Compared with other examination methods, MRI examination has relatively more contraindications.

5.2.2.3 MRI Features of Anal Fistula

The basic sequence includes SE T1WI, FSE T2WI, T2-weighted fat suppression sequence, and T1WI enhanced scan sequence. On T1WI images, the fistula showed isotopic or slightly low signal, and also slightly high signal when combined with hemorrhage; the fistula and abscess could be clearly displayed on T2WI images, showing obvious high signal; T2-weighted fat suppression images could differentiate the fistula from perianal adipose tissue, which was not easily distinguishable on T2WI images; T1WI enhanced images showed relatively rich blood supply. The wall of the fistula was obviously enhanced, and the rate of enhancement could reflect the intensity of inflammatory activity in the fistula. However, the enhancement of fibrotic fistula is relatively weak or even has no enhancement at times.

The Internal Opening

The internal opening of the fistula presents tubular long T1 and long T2 signals in MRI images. One end is connected with the fistula, and the other end is facing the rectum. The transverse section shows a localized interruption of the intestinal wall near the dentate line of the rectum and a slight thickness of the adjacent rectal wall. Both superior sphincter fistula and lateral sphincter fistula may enter the pelvic floor through the puborectalis muscle. However, the location of the internal opening is completely different. Usually, the internal opening of the superior sphincter fistula is located in the anal canal, while the lateral sphincter fistula is located in the rectum. Sometimes the anal canal cannot be traced along the fistula on the MRI image. In this case, only the possible location of the internal opening can be inferred according to the shape of the fistula.

Main Tract of Fistula

The main active fistula was filled with pus and granulation tissue and showed a long high signal structure in T2-weighted or STIR sequence. In some patients with recurrent attacks, the fistula wall becomes thicker, showing that the active fistula is surrounded by a low-signal fibrous tissue wall. Sometimes this high signal can be seen because of tissue edema. If the high signal shadow appears outside the fistula wall, it indicates that there is inflammation in adjacent tissues. MRI shows that the external sphincter is a low signal structure in T2-weighted or STIR sequence, and the fat in the lateral ischiorectal is a high signal. Therefore, it is easy to analyze whether the fistula passed through the external sphincter or across the external sphincter. If the primary main tract is completely confined to the inside of the external sphincter, this should be an intersphincteric fistula. Conversely, any evidence of fistula in the ischiorectal suggests nonsphincter fistula.

Branch of Fistula

The branch tract is connected with the main tract at one end and the blind end at the other end. MRI findings of the existence of branch canal are of great significance for the diagnosis and treatment of anal fistula. MRI can accurately find and locate the branch canal and residual abscess cavity of the anal fistula. In T2-weighted and STIR sequences, the branches and residual cavities showed high signal structures around the primary main tract of fistula, and local signal enhancement was induced by intravenous administration of contrast agents. The most common form of branch canal is the intersphincteric anal fistula, where the main tract passes through the external sphincter into the anal canal and the branch enters the apex of the ischioanal rectum formosa.

5.2.3 CT Examination

Computed tomography (CT), that is, electronic computed tomography (CT), is the use of an accurate X-ray beam and extremely sensitive detector together around a part of the body for one after another cross-section scanning, with the characteristics of fast scanning time, clears image, etc., and can be used for the examination of a variety of diseases.

5.2.3.1 Examination Methods

Prior to examination, patients were asked to empty their stools and lie flat on the spiral CT machine. The routine scanning range was from the upper edge of the acetabulum to the entire lower edge of the hip. Multiplane reconstruction and volume reconstruction were used after scanning the images. It is also reported that for patients with anal fistula and perianal abscess, after the abscess is extracted from patients with perianal abscess, soft catheter is placed in the external opening of anal fistula or perianal abscess, and 20 ml of 5% diluent of meglumine diatrizoate is injected while scanning, with the injection speed of about 3.0 ml/s. Generally, the patient feels a little swelling and pain.

CT includes plain CT scan, contrast enhancement (CE), and contrast scan. Plain scan is a common scan without contrast enhancement or contrast. Enhanced scanning is a method of using 60 ml of intravenous injection of water-soluble organic iodine by high-pressure syringe, such as 60%–76% meglumine diatrizoate before scanning. With the increase of iodine concentration in blood, the concentration of iodine in organs and lesions can be different, resulting in a poor density, and can make the lesions more clearly developed. The main methods are group injection and intravenous drip.

5.2.3.2 Diagnostic Value

Since the advent of CT in the 1970s, it has been developed into multilayer spiral CT technology. Spiral CT combined with various reconstruction techniques can clearly display fistula morphology, length, the edge, and direction, help determine the extent of the structures near the fistula and the scope of the inflammation, and also can be observed from multiple directions. Multiple planar locations of the abscess, the space to be spread, and relationship with the anus levator ani muscle, pus and anus on the edge of the distance and the size of cavity, the presence of the opening, and the inlet position and quantity (with oral contrast agent can enter inside a straight bowel wall cavity) can also be displayed, and this allows surgeons to timely judge whether or not the patient has a fistula. Sometimes it can also judge whether the chronic anal fistula is cancerous. It can provide direct examination data for the clinician and has certain guiding functions for the clinical determination of the operation plan.

5.2.4 Fistula Angiography

Radiographic diagnosis of the fistula by fistula angiography (hereinafter referred to as fistula angiography) is a method of contrast imaging the fistula with a contrast agent. It is also the earliest examination method applied to anal fistula. When CT, MRI, and ultrasound were not popular, fistula angiography was an important examination method for anal fistula. It has been used for various kinds of anal fistula, especially for high complexity fistula. Although this method is still in clinical use, it has been gradually replaced by other examinations and has been relatively less used in clinical practice.

5.2.4.1 Examination Methods

Before fistula angiography, a metal marker (such as a paper clip) is placed at the anus to mark the position of the anal margin, and a thin catheter or silica gel tube is inserted into the fistula slowly from the outside of the anal fistula until there is resistance to mark the anal and rectum. The metal marker should also be disposed of outside. Then, a suitable amount of contrast agent is slowly injected into the external opening, and the external opening is blocked to prevent the leakage of the contrast agent. Then, positive and lateral films including anal canal, rectum, and sacrococcyx are taken to show the course, depth, branches, position of internal and external openings, the relationship between fistula and anal canal and rectum, and the relationship between fistula and surrounding organs.

The contrast agent used for fistula angiography used to be 40% iodized oil, but it is prone to allergic reactions. In severe cases, it can cause a shock. If the rescue is not timely, the patient will die. Therefore, an iodine allergy test should be performed before the test, and allergic reactions should be carefully watched out for during the test. The rescue medication after the occurrence requires the medical staff to accompany the whole inspection process. Therefore, at present, the contrast agent is generally changed to a safer agent that is less susceptible to causing allergic reactions such as iopromide.

5.2.4.2 Diagnostic Value

For relatively unobstructed fistulas, fistula angiography can effectively show the direction of the internal opening and the fistula and has a certain diagnostic value. Weisman et al. reported that 48% of anal fistula angiography could observe lesions not detected by routine examination.

However, fistula angiography has some obvious limitations: ① when there is no external opening in anal fistula, fistula angiography cannot be performed; ② when fistula branches adhere or the duct is narrow, the fistula and the internal opening often cannot be accurately visualized because of the difficulty of the contrast agent to pass through; ③ the contrast agent can flow from the internal opening and the external opening to the surrounding area, resulting in misdiagnosis; and ④ the angiography of the fistula does not show the sphincter, so it is impossible to judge the relationship between the fistula and the sphincter. The surgeon can only guess the relationship between the fistula and the sphincter, and the guiding significance for the operation is not enough. Therefore, fistula angiography may only be beneficial to patients in the case of combined magnetic resonance imaging and/or ultrasound endoscopy. In addition, fistula angiography can cause bacteremia due to the pressure injection or adverse reactions caused by the contrast agent. Compared with other examinations, fistula angiography still has the damage of ionizing radiation, which is not suitable for pregnant women and some other patients.

In order to evaluate the diagnostic value of fistula angiography in anal fistula, Kuijpers and other scholars compared and analyzed the fistula angiography results of 25 patients with anal fistula from the results of surgical exploration. They found that the accuracy rate of fistula angiography was only 16%, the false-positive rate was 10%, and the diagnostic rate of the internal opening was only 20%. They believed that fistula angiography examination has only limited effectiveness in surgical treatment.

5.2.5 Anal Fistula Endoscopy

Anal fistula endoscopy is a rigid endoscopy for the examination and treatment of anal fistula. Anal fistula mirror has an 8-degree angle eyepiece and light source channel and also an operation/flushing hole with a diameter of 3.3 × 4.7 mm and an operable length of 18 cm. It has a removable handle for easy operation. Anal fistula has two sub-interfaces, one of which can connect to 1% glycine mannitol solution (5000 ml bag).

5.2.5.1 Inspection Methods

Anal fistula endoscopy is usually performed under spinal anesthesia. Anal fistula endoscopy is usually performed before operation, and then the treatment of anal fistula is performed under anal fistula endoscopy.

During the examination, the anal fistula mirror should be inserted from the external opening. When there is very hard scar tissue around the external opening, the scar tissue must be removed to ensure that the anal fistula mirror can be inserted. Glycine is injected into the endoscope to fill the fistula for observation. By adjusting the anal mirror gently from top to bottom, the fistula channel can adapt to or accommodate the anal canal fistula mirror and then straighten the fistula. While observing, the anal fistula mirror is pushed forward. When there is obstruction of necrotic tissue in the fistula, appropriate scraping and removal are needed.

When performing anal fistula endoscopy, attention should be paid to finding the internal opening and fistula branches of anal fistula. When the anal fistula canal is narrow and the internal opening is closed, the internal opening of the anal fistula can be inferred by observing the translucent points of the anal fistula mirror displayed on the rectal mucosa.

5.2.5.2 Diagnostic Value

Anal fistula endoscopy, as a new type of inspection and treatment instrument, provides a video inspection method to see the internal condition and direction of the fistula, which can be recorded and saved. However, because of its high cost, the need for anesthesia, and its time-consuming and laborious nature, it has no obvious benefit as an examination method, so it is seldom used alone for the examination of anal fistula in China. It is generally used in the video-assisted surgical treatment of anal fistula.

5.2.6 Pathological Examination

In order to clarify the cause and nature of fistula, for suspicious cases or fistula history of more than five years, biopsy tissues should be taken before, during, or after surgery for pathological examinations to determine whether the anal fistula has cancer, tuberculosis, or anal fistula complicated by Crohn's disease. If a single test is negative or cannot be diagnosed, multiple live tissue tests can be taken. Attention should be paid to how to obtain the correct specimen, which should include the fistula wall and the tissue connected to the pipe wall or the tissue of the specific changed area.

5.2.7 Bacterial Culture

Bacterial culture and drug sensitivity tests of anal fistula secretions can assist in diagnosis and treatment. Bacterial culture and drug susceptibility tests are more important for those wounds that grow slowly and do not heal after a long time. Pathogenic bacteria examination and drug sensitivity during the abscess stage of anal fistula are also helpful to guide the rational use of antibiotics after operation.

In Japan in recent years, there were many reports of bacterial culture of abscesses. In Takano Hospital, bacteria were cultured in the abscess of 83 patients with perianal abscess, and 144 strains of bacteria were isolated. Among 82 patients, 30 (36.1%) were infected by one bacteria, 46 (55.4%) by two bacteria, 6 (7.2%) by three bacteria, and 1 (1.3%) by four bacteria. It was found that there was no correlation between the number of strains and the severity of the perianal abscess. Escherichia coli was the most common bacteria (56 strains, 38.4%), followed by *Bacteroides* (34 strains, 23.6%). If aerobic bacteria and magnetic anaerobes were separated, 95 strains of aerobic bacteria (66.0%) and 49 strains (34.0%) were anaerobes. Among the aerobic bacteria, *E. coli* was the most common (56 strains), followed by *Klebsiella* (17 strains). Among the anaerobic bacteria, *Bacteroides* were the most common (34 strains), followed by anaerobic gram-negative cocci (12 strains). There were 9 cases (10.8%) of anaerobic bacteria infection alone, 34 cases (40.0%) of aerobic bacteria infection alone, and 40 cases (49.2%) of mixed anaerobic bacteria and aerobic bacterial infection. In addition, Sinagawa reported that the infection rate of aerobic bacteria was 31.0%, that of anaerobic bacteria was 5.2%, and aerobic bacteria and anaerobic bacteria mixed infection rate of 62.8%. The results were basically consistent with those reported by Takano. But Okubo's report was different from that of Takano and Sinagawa. His reported rates of isolated infection of aerobic bacteria, anaerobic bacteria, and mixed aerobic and anaerobic bacteria were 56.3%, 1.9%, and 22.3%, respectively.

In recent years, the reports on pathogenic bacteria examination of perianal abscess in China have increased year by year and are different from those in Japan. According to Guan Ruijian et al., the positive rate of bacterial culture was 100% in 90 patients with perianal abscess, 63 cases (70%) had mixed infection, 14 cases (15.6%) had simple aerobic infection, and 13 cases (14.4%) had simple anaerobic infection. *Escherichia coli*, *Staphylococcus*, *Proteus*, and *Streptococcus* were the main aerobic bacteria, while anaerobic coccus, actinomycetes, and *Eubacterium* were the most common anaerobic bacteria.

According to the composition of intestinal bacteria, *Bacteroides* should be the most common bacteria, but the current results show that the most infectious bacteria are *Escherichia coli*. Takano believed that this may be related to the virulence of *Escherichia coli* and the anatomical characteristics of the anal canal and glands.

It is reported that intestinal bacterial infections are easy to become fistulas, while dermatological bacterial infections are relatively rare. Grace (1982) et al. analyzed 114 cases of enterogenous bacterial perianal abscess, 70 of which (61.4%) formed anal fistula. The detection rate of enterogenous bacteria in abscess with fistula was as high as 86%. Enterogenous bacteria included *Streptococcus*, *Bacteroides*, *Clostridium*,

Escherichia coli, and so on. Guan Ruijian et al. reported that five out of six cases of pure *E. coli* infection formed anal fistula, while none of the six cases of staphylococcal infection formed anal fistula. Anal fistula was found in 8 out of 13 patients with simple anaerobic bacterial infection (61.5%).

5.2.8 General X-Ray Examination

Pelvic radiography and X-ray angiography can be performed in patients with complex anal fistula, repeated operations, or suspected cystic anal fistula, or fistula after the rupture of presacral cyst or teratoma, or anal fistula or pelvic disease complicated by tuberculosis, Crohn's disease, or ulcerative colitis. Generally, the pelvis and sacrococcygeal region can be displayed by taking positive and lateral pelvic films. If it is bone tuberculosis or osteomyelitis, bone destruction can be seen, as well as pus cavity, dead bone, etc. If it is a teratoma, hair calcification, bone, and teeth can be seen, and rectal forward displacement often occurs.

5.2.9 Colonoscopy

With the advancement of colonoscopy technology and the popularization of instruments, colonoscopy has become a common examination item in the Department of Anorectology. Colonoscopy is not a necessary preoperative examination for patients with anal fistula, but it is better to perform colonoscopy before operation if conditions permit. Anal fistula patients have the following conditions: (1) abdominal pain, diarrhea, mucous stool, purulent stool, and other symptoms; (2) rough or thickened intestinal mucosa, rectal mucosa has obvious congestion and erosion; (3) too many fistula branches, too high a location, rectal ulceration, fistula wall tissue that is too hard or soft wall; (4) pus or wound secretion. Also, if the wound heals very slowly after operation, colonoscopy is necessary for these patients.

5.2.9.1 Preparation Before Colonoscopy

1. Inquire about the medical history of the patient, undertake necessary examinations such as electrocardiogram, blood biochemistry, etc., and understand if there are any contraindications for examination. Make the necessary explanations with the patient to eliminate their psychological concerns or fears.
2. Pay attention to eating a less or no dregs diet two days before the examination, and in the morning of enteroscopy, the patient should fast.
3. Make good preparation for intestinal cleansing. At present, the commonly used intestinal preparation schemes for colonoscopy are the following: (1) two packs of compound polyethylene glycol electrolyte powder, which is dissolved in 2 L cold boiled water or pure water, should be taken about four hours before the examination and be taken not less than within one hour. The method is simple, safe, with little adverse reactions, and does not affect the treatment of incision and cauterization when necessary. (2) 250 ml of 20% mannitol should be taken orally six hours before examination, and then 3000 ml of balanced solution or 5% saline should be taken intermittently within three hours. However, the intestinal preparation made by this method is not suitable for the treatment of enteroscopic cauterization and electrotomy. (3) Atropine 0.5 mg intramuscular injection can be used before enteroscopy if necessary to reduce the discomfort of intestinal spasm. For those with excessive mental stress, diazepam 5–10 mg can be injected intramuscularly or intravenously before the examination so as to stabilize the patient's mood.

5.2.9.2 Operating Methods

1. Check colonoscopy equipment and accessories; pay attention to check the light source, air and water suction device, and operation area.

2. The patient should be in the left lateral position with both legs bent toward the abdomen.
3. Before the examination, the operator gives the patient a digital rectal examination to find out whether there are tumors, strictures, hemorrhoids, anal fissures, etc. The assistant smears a proper amount of lubricant on the front end and surface of the colonoscopy. The patient should relax the anal sphincter, and the examiner should press the lens with his right index finger to slide the lens into the anus and let it slowly enter the anus.
4. Follow the cavity with the endoscope, slide the endoscope slowly, inject a small amount of air, pull properly, adopt a straight approach, and insert the endoscope in step by step with the avoid-loop, release-loop, and other insertion techniques. Pay attention to shortening suction and taking a straight line around the sigmoid colon and transverse colon, proper hooking and rotating mirror should be used at the spleen and liver curvature, and proper respiratory coordination and posture adjustment should be undertaken.
5. The assistant should press the abdomen with appropriate techniques to reduce intestinal curvature and knot loops.
6. When the front end of the lens reaches the ileocecal region, the signs are the crescent-shaped appendix hole and the ileocecal flap like fish mouth. At this point, adjust the angle of the lens end of the colonoscopy and insert it back into the blind valve to observe and examine the intestinal cavity and mucosa within a range of 15–30 cm of the terminal ileum.
7. During the withdrawal of the colonoscopy from the colon, observe the intestinal wall from left to right, and carefully observe the intestinal cavity size, intestinal wall, and pouch conditions step by step through a proper amount of air injection and extraction. Adjust the angle of the lens and the depth of entering for the turning part or the intestinal segment that is not seen around the colon.
8. Video, biopsy or biopsy of valuable parts for pathological examination.
9. At the end of the examination, the gas in the intestinal cavity should be removed as much as possible so as to reduce the discomfort to patients such as abdominal distension and abdominal pain. After the examination, observe the patient for 15–30 min. If there is no discomfort, and the patient agrees, the patient can leave.
10. For polyp removal and hemostasis treatment, patients should take a half-stream diet and rest for three to four days after treatment. Antibiotics should be applied appropriately according to the situation. If there is sudden abdominal pain, bleeding, and other discomforts, they should be treated promptly in hospital.

5.2.9.3 Diagnostic Value

One of the purposes of colonoscopy for anal fistula is to exclude surgical contraindications such as Crohn's disease and ulcerative colitis and perforation of intestines in anal fistula, which can be found during examination. Colonoscopy is very important for the diagnosis and treatment of some types of anal fistula. At present, the incidence of inflammatory bowel disease continues to increase, and more and more anal fistulas are caused by Crohn's disease. However, the anal fistulas of patients with inflammatory bowel disease can appear before intestinal symptoms. Many patients have long-term nonhealing wounds after surgery, and Crohn's disease and ulcerative colitis are found to be the cause after the examination.

The anal fistula of patients with Crohn's disease is mostly treated with conservative treatment or nonradical treatment. Surgical treatment should be avoided. Preoperative colonoscopy is helpful to avoid surgical treatment for patients with Crohn's disease and other patients not suited to surgery.

To sum up, there are various examination methods in the examination of anal fistula, such as finger diagnosis, fistula angiography, ultrasonic examination, MRI and CT examination, and anal fistula mirror, which all have their own indications and examination values, and their accuracy levels are also different.

Buchanan et al. performed fistula angiography, endoanal ultrasound, and MRI on 104 patients and compared them with the actual situation in the operation. The coincidence rate of anal fistula classification was 61% by fistula contrast, 81% by endoanal ultrasound, and 90% by MRI. For horseshoe anal fistula, the coincidence rate of endoanal ultrasound and MRI was 90% and 96%, respectively. It was considered that MRI was more suitable for the examination of anal fistula. Schwartz and others believe that MRI has absolute superiority and accuracy in the diagnosis of high complex anal fistula, horseshoe anal fistula, and other difficult clinical cases.

Schratter-Sehn et al. collected data on 25 patients with Crohn's disease to compare the advantages and disadvantages of transrectal (or transvaginal) endoscopic ultrasonography and CT in the diagnosis of anal fistula, perianal abscess, and low pelvic inflammation. Postoperative results showed that ① transrectal (or transvaginal) endoscopic ultrasonography was superior to CT in the diagnosis of anal fistula and low pelvic inflammatory infiltration (14 cases of anal fistula and 11 cases of low pelvic inflammation were correctly diagnosed by endoscopic ultrasonography; only 4 cases of anal fistula and 2 cases of low pelvic inflammation were correctly diagnosed by CT). ② The accuracy of the two examination methods in the diagnosis of perianal abscess is equal. ③ CT can accurately diagnose inflammatory infiltration of pararectal fascia and adipose tissue. Endoscopic ultrasonography has no such function.

Some scholars compared the accuracy of MRI and EUS in evaluating anal fistula in primary Crohn's disease, but the results reported by them were quite different. The reason may be related to different equipment used, patient selection criteria, and operator experience. Beckingham et al. believe that the sensitivity and specificity of dynamic enhanced MRI are better than AES.

At present, in the examination of anal fistula, there is no examination method with absolute superiority, and which can diagnose anal fistula 100% correctly. For the examination of anal fistula, different examination methods should be selected or comprehensively used according to the different types of anal fistula so as to improve the diagnostic accuracy and comprehensively grasp the morphological characteristics of the anal fistula. In the process of anal fistula diagnosis, flexible use of one to two or even a variety of methods is often needed to accurately and comprehensively diagnose anal fistula. The diagnosis of low anal fistula, intersphincteric fistula, and other simple anal fistulas can often be confirmed by conventional anal visual examination and finger examination. If necessary, endoanal ultrasound examination is performed, and MRI, CT, and other examinations are usually unnecessary. But for high complex anal fistulas such as extrasphincteric fistula or transsphinteric fistula, due to the fistula involving many surrounding tissues, the internal opening position is high, and there are more branches; ultrasound diagnosis and finger examination have limitations. It is difficult to fully understand the direction of the anal fistula and the relationship between the anal fistula and sphincter due to such limitations. MRI examination is necessary for high anal fistula because the deep tissue can be shown well.

5.3 Examination and Evaluation of Anal Function

Anal fistula is closely related to anal sphincter. It is easy to cause injury to the anal sphincter during operation and consequently lead to the damage of anal function. Therefore, it is necessary to undertake proper examination and evaluation of anal function before and after operation.

Anal finger examination is the most simple, noninvasive, and low-cost method for examining anal sphincter function. It is reported that the sensitivity and specificity of anal finger examination were 67% and 55% respectively. However, anal finger examination relies on experience and is difficult to be objective and quantified. At present, the methods of objectively detecting and evaluating the anal sphincter and its function include anorectal manometry, endoanal ultrasound, electromyography, rectal sensory function, and so on. These examinations not only can understand the function of the anus and rectum after operation but also help to analyze the causes from the angle of anatomy and pathophysiology to a certain extent, guide rehabilitation treatment, and help to judge the prognosis.

In addition, nerve conduction studies, electromyography, X-ray examination of fecal incontinence, determination of latency of pudendal nerve endings, mucosal inductance, and anal echo reflex are also methods to evaluate anal function, but few studies have been conducted.

It should be pointed out that there is no uniform and detailed standard for accurate and rigorous functional examination and evaluation, so it is often difficult to compare the results of different hospitals. How to improve the detection standard and standardize clinical operation is worth studying and looking into in order to find more appropriate solutions.

At present, the Anal Function Assessment Scale and QOL Questionnaire are mainly used to evaluate anal function, but the scale and QOL Questionnaire are subjective and have some limitations in evaluating anal function, so they cannot be used alone.

5.3.1 Anorectal Manometry

Anorectal manometry is measured by a physiological pressure tester to measure the pressure in the anus and the rectum and the physiological reflex between the anorectal areas to understand the functional status of the anorectal area and to evaluate the structural integrity of the muscles and nerves supporting the functional status.

Anorectal manometry is currently commonly used in the diagnosis of congenital megacolon, functional constipation, anal incontinence, anal flatulence, anorectal pain, as well as in the evaluation of the function and surgical injury of the anus and rectum, and the evaluation of the treatment of anorectal diseases. This examination has certain significance for the study of anorectal physiology, diagnosis, and treatment of anorectal diseases and evaluation of curative effects. It is the most important method in evaluating anal function at present. Anorectal manometry during anal fistula is helpful to judge the functional status of the anal sphincter before operation and the effect of operation on anal sphincter and its function. Anorectal manometry can also be used for biofeedback therapy of functional anorectal diseases. However, the anorectal manometry test still has some shortcomings such as the large fluctuation in test data, the translocation of receptors, the operation of different examiners, and so on. So far, even for the same brand of equipment, there is no standard value of indicators to refer to, and even the data of the same indicators vary greatly among different units.

5.3.1.1 Equipment

Anorectal manometry measuring device is composed of the baroreceptor, pressure conversion, and recording device. The baroreceptor is used to sense the change in anorectal pressure. The pressure conversion and recording device converts the pressure change signal sensed by the baroreceptor probe into electrical signals through the transducer, then transmits them to the amplification and recording device, and displays and records them in numerical and graphic form. At present, the baroreceptor part mainly has the air bag or water bag method, water perfusion method, and solid-state micro-converter method.

Different anorectal pressure testing equipment has different requirements and different operation methods. Surgeons need to be trained and certified before they can carry out testing.

5.3.1.2 Detection Indicators

There are four types of indicators for anorectal manometry.

Stress Indicators
1. **Anal Resting Pressure**
   The anal pressure is measured under the resting state of the anal canal; 80% of the resting pressure of the anal canal is caused by the contraction of the tension of the internal sphincter, while the tension of the external sphincter accounts for only 20% of the resting pressure of the anal canal. Generally speaking, the resting pressure of anal canal in

women after multiple births is lower than that in men, and that in the elderly is lower than that in the young.

Anal resting pressure decreases significantly in patients with anal incontinence, spinal anesthesia, and unilateral or bilateral sacral nerve resection. The resting pressure of anal canal in patients with anal fissure and some internal hemorrhoids is higher than normal, and it can return to normal after anal dilatation.

2. **Maximum Anal Systolic Pressure and Systolic Time**

   The maximum anal systolic pressure was generated when the subjects tried to contract the anus, and the systolic time was from the sudden rise of pressure to the return of pressure to the level of resting anal pressure. Anal systolic pressure is produced by the contraction of pelvic floor muscle and external sphincter. It can be used to judge the function of the external anal sphincter. The overall function of the anal sphincter can be understood by combining the maximum anal systolic pressure with the anal resting pressure.

3. **Anal Hypertensive Zone**

   After the probe is inserted into the rectum, the probe is pulled out of the anus with a uniform dragging speed. When the pressure suddenly rises, it is located at the proximal starting point of the high-pressure zone of the anus (the probe should be calibrated), and when the pressure of the anus sharply drops to the atmospheric pressure level, it is the distal end of the high-pressure zone of the anus (usually the anal margin).

   The anal hypertensive zone shows the distribution of internal and external sphincter function, which is caused by static tension contraction of internal and external sphincter. Anal sphincter injury can shorten the high-pressure zone of the anal canal.

4. **Active Systolic Pressure**

   The value of active anal systolic pressure is obtained by subtracting the maximum anal resting pressure from the maximum anal systolic pressure. It represents the net increase of active contraction of the external anal sphincter and pelvic floor muscle.

5. **Rectal Resting Pressure**

   Rectal resting pressure is the pressure in the resting state of the rectum. Normally, the resting pressure of the rectum is very low and can rise briefly during some physiological activities such as defecation and coughing.

Anorectal Reflex Activity

1. **Anal Reflex**

   Stimulating the skin around the anus can cause contraction of the external sphincter, which will lead to a sudden increase in anal pressure followed by a sudden decrease. It produces a high and narrow pressure wave, which is an anal reflex. Normal people have a normal reflex, but some elderly people need electrical stimulation to induce the reflex. If the nerve that controls the pelvic floor is seriously damaged, the reflection is reduced or destroyed.

2. **Rectoanal Inhibitory Reflex (RAIR)**

   When the rectum is dilated by intestinal contents or an artificial balloon, it can cause relaxation of the internal sphincter and a decrease in anal pressure. This reflex phenomenon is called the RAIR. The normal RAIR pressure map illustrates that the anal pressure decreased sharply from the resting level to original level after rectal dilatation and then slowly returned to the original level. Adults usually inflate at an incremental rate of 10 ml per test, and newborns can be as low as 3 ml. Abnormalities in or the disappearance of RAIR is mainly seen in patients with Hirschsprung's disease, after low rectal resection, and with neurogenic fecal incontinence. If the resting pressure of the anal canal is very low, RAIR can also disappear.

3. **Anal Relaxation Reflex**

   Pelvic floor muscle, puborectalis muscle, and external sphincter are striated muscles that can relax freely when simulating defecation, thus reducing the pressure of the anal canal. On the contrary, anal pressure increased in patients with pelvic floor striated muscle loses relaxation during defecation.

4. Anorectal Contractile Reflex

When the anorectal contractile reflex is injected into the rectum rapidly, the pressure of the anal canal rises suddenly and decreases after one to two seconds. Clinical significance: it indicates that the external sphincter responds to the stimulation of rectal dilatation and reflects the self-control function of the external sphincter to a certain extent. The reflex disappears when the nerve innervating the pelvic floor muscle is injured.

Wave Phase Activity of Anal Resting Pressure

When the resting pressure of anal canal is measured steadily and continuously, it can be found that the pressure of the anal sphincter in some people is not fixed but exhibits a rhythmic wave phase activity. According to the waveform, it can be divided into two categories: ultra-slow wave and slow wave. Waveform changes vary greatly among different age groups, and most of them are discontinuous and nonperiodic pressure changes. Ultra-slow waves usually have frequencies of 1–2 times/min and small amplitudes. Slow wave is easy to recognize. Its frequency is 10–20 times per minute in adults, 10–14 times per minute in children, and its amplitude is about 1.33–4 kPa. When the internal sphincter is diseased, normal wave phase activity can also be disrupted or disappeared.

Rectal Compliance

Rectal compliance is an important feature of rectal movement, reflecting the dilatancy of the rectum wall, that is, the volume change of rectum expansion when the pressure inside the rectum increases. Normally, when the rectum swells and its volume rises to 300 mL, the rectal pressure does not change, or can even decrease, in order to maintain anal self-control until the maximum capacity that the rectum can tolerate is reached and induces fecal urgency. At this point, the pressure increases significantly. This characteristic is called rectal compliance. It is a reflex adaptive response that enables the rectum to store a certain amount of feces before defecation and postpone defecation.

Rectal compliance = rectal pressure at the maximum tolerable capacity/maximum tolerable capacity of the rectum. Compliance reflects intestinal wall extensibility and rectal storage function, which is an important factor affecting fecal self-control. Rectal compliance is significantly decreased after proctitis, rectal resection, and colon or ileum anastomosis with anal canal or rectal radiotherapy, and the clinical manifestation is an increase in the number of stools per day. The rectal compliance of patients with megacolon, severe denervation of pelvic floor, and slow transit constipation is often increased.

5.3.2 Transanal Ultrasound Evaluation Method

Transanal ultrasound (endoanal ultrasound, EUS) can be used to observe the morphology of the anal rectum wall, internal sphincter, external sphincter, levator ani muscle, and female vaginal and rectal septum under dynamic and static conditions, respectively. Postoperative EUS imaging is helpful to evaluate postoperative anorectal function and guide rehabilitation. When EUS is performed, the patients usually take a left lateral position. During rest and maximum contraction of the anus, serial imaging of the anorectal junction and the three positions of the anal canal (upper, middle, and lower) is performed. The most prominent feature of this method is that it can display the anatomy of sphincter muscle and pelvic floor tissue directly. If the sphincter is damaged, in EUS examination, the hypoechoic sphincter ring may suddenly stop at a certain part, and a local hyperechoic region may occur instead. For anal and rectal postoperative incontinence in patients, EUS examination can find the site of sphincter injury and evaluate the severity of the injury, so as to provide necessary information for surgical repair. After repair, EUS can be used to observe the postoperative sphincter shape to evaluate the repair effect. Another feature of EUS is that it can be directly examine during the operation, which helps operators to timely understand the status of the sphincter, rectum, anus, and surrounding tissues during the operation so that the functions of anus and rectum can be retained as much as possible while the diseased parts are removed.

At present, 3D EUS has been widely accepted and used in the world, which improves the accuracy of diagnosis of anal sphincter injury and improves doctors' understanding of the pathological changes of anal sphincter injury. According to Bei Shaosheng and Li Huashan, 3D EUS is helpful to accurately evaluate the degree of anal sphincter complex injury in patients with high anal fistula.

Although EUS is widely used to determine the function of the anal sphincter complex, it has been reported that the related research methods of B-ultrasound are different at present, and there is heterogeneity in the research object, so it needs to be further studied and improved on.

It is worth noting that sphincter injury after anal and rectal surgery is more common, but a considerable number of patients do not show related symptoms. Stamatiadis et al. found that 75% of patients with IAS injury and 62% of patients with sonographic evidence of EAS injury did not show corresponding clinical symptoms. If not treated in a timely manner, these patients may end up with incontinence due to long-term complications, neuromuscular degeneration, or further improper surgery. Therefore, it is important to evaluate the sphincter status by EUS after operation in order to understand anal function.

5.3.3 Nuclear Magnetic Resonance Imaging Assessment Method

MRI can clearly show the structure of the pelvic floor muscle and whether there is muscular atrophy. MRI is superior to EUS in diagnosing EAS injuries. In terms of IAS testing, EUS has a better effect. EUS can provide anatomical explanations of IAS and EAS injuries intuitively and can be examined intraoperatively. For all kinds of patients after anal and rectal surgery, routine EUS examination is recommended to understand the status of the sphincter and guide further treatment. According to a foreign study, EUS can be the first choice for anal and rectal function evaluation in patients with sphincter injury, and MRI and EUS can be used together to evaluate the anal and rectal functions of patients.

5.3.4 Pelvic Floor EMG Examination

Electromyography (EMG) is a scientific method that detects and studies the bioelectrical activity of muscles to determine the functional changes of the neuromuscular system. The object of EMG is the motion unit potential (MUP), which refers to the comprehensive reflection of the myoelectric activity produced by a group of muscle fibers dominated by a lower motor neuron. The number of muscle fibers dominated by each motor neuron axon is different. A lower motor neuron, together with the muscle fibers it dominates, forms a functional unit called a motor unit.

The muscle fibers of different motor units are interlaced to some extent (one muscle fiber can be dominated by several motor units). Therefore, 10 to 20 motor units can be induced by an electromyographic examination with the same core needle electrode.

The commonly used EMG is to insert a core-needle electrode into the muscle and collect the EMG activity of the surrounding muscle fibers for analysis. In addition, there are single-fiber EMG, giant EMG, and scanning EMG. EMG examination is mainly used to (1) judge the functional activity state of pelvic floor muscle, such as abnormal electrical activity of pelvic floor muscle in pelvic floor achalasia syndrome; (2) assess the causes of pelvic floor dysfunction—if congenital or traumatic pelvic floor muscle defect, EMG activity is weakened or disappeared, or pathological electrical activity; and (3) provide biofeedback treatment of chronic functional constipation and anal incontinence. This examination is mainly used to evaluate the functional status of anorectal and pelvic floor muscle groups in patients with anal fistula so as to determine the status of surgical injury.

5.3.4.1 Inspection Methods
The patient should take the right recumbent position, the right leg is slightly flexed, the left leg is

pulled forward to fully expose the examination area, the examiner wears gloves on the left hand, the paraffin oil lubricated index finger is inserted into the rectal cavity, and the palmar side of finger touches the anal and rectal ring. The needle insertion area should be sterilized. The needle should be inserted from the appropriate position on the line between the posterior median line of the anus and the coccyx tip in the right hand with the needle electrode. Through the guidance of the left index finger, it advances toward the rear free edge of the anal straight ring. Adjust the position of the needle tip until a very clear electromyographic sound of machine gun firing is obtained. Rest for three minutes after positioning and then start the inspection.

The external sphincter is generally tested for its shallow part, the needle should retreat to the subcutaneous, and the finger abdomen should point to the sphincter sulcus and between the straight anal ring so that the tip of the needle is located in the appropriate position of the external sphincter.

5.3.4.2 Testing Indicators

Electromyographic Activity in Resting State

The needle is inserted into the measured muscle, and the observation starts after the electromyographic activity is stable. First observe whether there is a pathological wave. Because the pelvic floor striated muscle is showing low frequency continuous electric activity in quiet, the reason fibrillation potential, bundle fibrillation potential are hard to distinguish, but a positive acute wave can be recorded sometimes. A positive sharp wave is a positive phase, then from the pointed peak goes downward to a two-phase wave, first for a low amplitude positive phase peak wave, and then for an extended, minimal amplitude of negative post-potential, and most do not return to the baseline. The final shape is like the letter "V," with waveform stability. The parameters are a large amplitude difference, mostly low amplitude wave (generally 50–100 μv). The time limit is generally 4–8 ms, and it can be as long as 30–100 ms. The waveform is a two-phase wave, first positive phase, then negative phase. The frequency is usually 1–10 times/S, up to 100 times/S. Positive acute waves occur only in muscles that lose nerve control.

The average amplitude of the puborectalis and external sphincter in the resting state was recorded. The sensitivity of the amplifier was 0.2 mv/cm, and the scanning speed was 100 ms/cm. The amplitude is generally between 150 and 300 μv.

Simulated EMG Activity During Defecation

If the patient was to perform defecation, observe whether the EMG activity was reduced and record it. This process is sometimes difficult to do in the limited window of opportunity; when necessary, repeat this several times to determine the true status of EMG changes during defecation.

When normal people simulated defecation, the electromyoelectric activity of the pelvic floor decreased significantly compared with the resting state, and the amplitude decreased to between 50 and 100 μV, or presented electric resting. When simulating defecation, EMG activity does not decrease but increases, which is called abnormal electrical activity. When abnormal electrical activity is detected, false positives due to an inappropriate environment are shown. Mental tension, needle electrode stimulation, and pain should be excluded.

Mild Contraction of the Myoelectric Activity

When the pelvic floor muscle is slightly contracted, a separate single unit potential can appear. A single unit of motion reflects the synthetic potential of muscle fibers dominated by a single spinal cord anterior horn cell or the synthetic potential of a subunit of motion, which can be used for the analysis of the unit of motion potential. Motion unit potential analysis includes amplitude, duration, waveform, and discharge frequency. Because of the large time range variation, it is generally necessary to take an average of 20 motion unit potential times.

Strong Contraction of the Muscle Activity

When the skeletal muscles undergo the maximum contraction, almost all the sports units participate in the contraction. As the number of sports units involved in the discharge increases by each movement unit, the frequency of discharge also increases. Different potentials interfere with each other and overlap, and it is impossible to distinguish a single movement unit potential, called the interference phase. Its voltage is generally 600–1000 μV. The maximum contraction can only produce a single unit potential, which is termed a reduction in the number of unit potentials. It is found in anterior angular cell disease or peripheral nerve incompleteness damage.

5.3.5 Anorectal Sensory Function Examination

The anus can maintain normal abstinence function, which is closely related to the sensory function of the anus and rectum. The anal canal is dominated by the free nerve endings and sensory organs. The anal crypt, mucosa on the head side of the crypt, and anal canal transition zone are the most intensive place of free nerve endings distribution. The distal anal canal epithelium is sensitive to pain, temperature, and touch, and there is no pain-sensing fiber at the proximal end, but there are many Golgi-Mazzoni bodies and Pacinian corpuscles that are sensitive to pressure changes such as intestinal lumen expansion and a sense of fullness. Since the mucosa has almost no nerve fibers, it is speculated that this feeling is not caused by the mucosa but by the stimulation of receptors in the pelvic floor muscles and surrounding structures.

The exact role of sensation in controlling bowel movements is unclear. The sampling reflex plays an important role in distinguishing whether the anus needs to exhaust or defecate or produce solid stool. Sample reflexes disappear after ileal anal anastomosis or colon anal anastomosis. However, these patients are often able to maintain a controlled bowel function. Moreover, there was no difference in anal function after resection or preservation of the anal transitional area. In addition, normal human anal topical application of lignocaine gel does not cause incontinence.

Anorectal sensory function examination in anal fistula is mainly used to evaluate the anorectal function and surgical injury.

5.3.5.1 Observation Indicators

Mucosal Electrical Sensitivity Test
This method requires a special probe that is lubricated with a conductive gel and placed in the upper portion of the anal canal. A DC generator capable of generating a square wave stimulus of 5-Hz frequency is used to generate the voltage required for the electrode. The stimulation increases gradually at a rate of 1 mA until the patient feels tingling pain. The measurement results are recorded digitally, and the mean value of the data obtained is considered as the sensory threshold. Then, place the probe in the middle of the anal canal and finally in the lower portion, and repeat the procedure.

Currently, this test is mainly used to examine patients with idiopathic and iatrogenic constipation. It was once thought that these patients had decreased rectal sensation, but recently this idea has been challenged. Meagher and her colleagues reported decreased rectal sensation due to damage to the sensory nerves in the surrounding muscles and fecal influence on the probe's full contact with the mucosa.

5.3.5.2 Temperature Sense Detection
There is evidence that temperature sensing plays a role in distinguishing between gaseous, liquid, and solid waste. Miller and colleagues used water-infused thermal electrodes to detect anorectal temperature sensitivity. The method is to use three thermostatic water tanks to supply water to the hot electrode so that the temperature can be maintained at 37 °C, or rapidly rise or fall by 4.5 °C. A thermocouple is used to measure the temperature of the contact surface between the thermal electrode and the mucous membrane. The thermocouple temperature was recorded as the patient felt the temperature change. The temperature sensitivity of patients was measured

from four temperature ranges from normal sensation to heat sensation, from heat sensation to normal sensation, from normal sensation to cold sensation, and from cold sensation to normal sensation. The average of the four temperature ranges was recorded to show how temperature-sensitive the patient was. The temperature ranges of the upper, middle, and lower parts of the anal canal were measured, respectively.

5.3.5.3 Rectal Volume Sensory Function

Air or liquid is injected into the balloon in the rectal cavity at a constant speed to detect the sensory threshold of the subject when the rectum is filled to varying degrees, including the rectal sensory threshold, the initial rectal sensory volume, and the maximum rectal tolerance.

Rectal Sensation Threshold

This is the volume at which the subject first injects air or liquid when there is an object in the rectum. At this time, if the injection is stopped, the subject's feeling of having an object in the rectum will disappear after a moment of rest. The rectal sensory threshold of a normal person is 10 to 40 ml.

Rectal Initial Intentional Capacity

This is the volume when the subject has a sense of defecation after the rectum continues to be injected with gas or liquid. The results vary widely from individual to individual and depend on the subject. The initial intentional capacity is usually 50 to 80 ml.

Rectal Maximum Tolerance Capacity

This is the maximum volume of gas or fluid injected into the rectal cavity that the subject can tolerate. It is about 100 to 320 ml.

There are two common methods for gas injection when rectal volume sensory function is measured: ① continuous injection method: continuously inject air into the rectal bulb at a certain speed, and inquire about the feeling of the subject while injecting, and make corresponding record of this. ② Intermittent injection method: inject air into the rectal cavity according to a certain volume intermittently. The volume to be injected is generally increased in the following amounts: 10 ml, 20 ml, 30 ml, 40 ml, 50 ml, 80 ml, 110 ml, 140 ml, 170 ml, 200 ml, 230 ml, 260 ml, 290 ml, 320 ml, and 350 ml. Leave one minute after each injection to ask for the patient's feelings. After emptying the balloon, rest for one minute, inject again, and complete the examination in turn.

It should be noted that the faster the infusion rate is, the easier it is to induce the sense of gas or liquid in the rectum, and the lower the sensory threshold. Therefore, air or gas should be injected at the same rate during the inspection to make the results comparable. In addition, due to the test relying on the patient's ability to explain the different feelings, care should be taken to explain these to the patient before undergoing the test in order for him or her to fully and correctly understand and cooperate well. As far as possible, try to reduce the error caused by patient's lack of understanding.

5.3.6 Anal Function Evaluation Scale

There are many scales to evaluate anal function, including Kirwan scale, Williams standard, Jorge/Wexner scale, and score of severity of fecal incontinence. The anal function evaluation scale is subjective and has its own advantages and disadvantages. This kind of scale is divided into two categories: the rating scale and the total score rating scale.

5.3.6.1 Rating Scale

Parks, Broden, Keighley, Hiltunen, Kirwan, Corman, Williams, Rainey, and Womack all designed their own rating scales. At present, there are many anal functional rating scales in China, such as those of Parks, Womack, Kirwan, and Williams.

Parks Anal Function Classification: Grade 1: completely normal; Grade 2: gas and diarrhea cannot be completely controlled; Grade 3: total inability to control diarrhea; Grade 4: unable to control solid bowel movements.

Womack anus function grading: Grade A: can control any form of defecation; Grade B: unable to control gas; Grade C: unable to control liquid defecation and gas; Grade D: no control over gases, liquids, or solids.

Kirwan anal function classification: Level I: anal function well; Level II: unable to control exhaust; Level III: accidental waste; Level IV:, often waste; Level V: anal incontinence. Williams standard: Grade A: good control of solids, liquids, and gases; Grade B: good solid and liquid control, gas incontinence; Grade C: occasionally a small amount of contaminated clothing, good solid control, occasionally liquid incontinence; Grade D: contaminated clothing, frequent fluid incontinence; Grade E: frequent solid and liquid incontinence. A and B grades are considered functional.

The rating scale is often regarded as too simple and only roughly evaluates the function of anus. It has some shortcomings such as inconsistency, incompleteness, and inaccuracy, so it is generally not recommended to use alone.

5.3.6.2 Total Score Evaluation Scale

The total score scale quantifies the anal function more objectively, specifically, and effectively. It can make up for the deficiency of grade evaluation and is more widely used. The current total score evaluation includes nine different evaluation methods. Rockwood, Hull, Wexner, Pescatori, Vaizey, Skinner, Bai, Rothenberger, and Lunniss all designed the total scores of their respective teams. Nancy et al. systematically summarized this. The score with the lowest total score is 0–6, and the highest is 0–120.

The anal function scoring method of Wexner (Table 5.1) is a widely used anal function evaluation method in China.

There are four types of fecal incontinence: gas incontinence, mucus incontinence, liquid incontinence, and solid incontinence. The severity and frequency of fecal incontinence are different. Therefore, the weight of different types of fecal incontinence should be taken into account in the total score evaluation. There are many ways to allocate weights. At present, there are three main ways to allocate weights: ① no weights are allocated; ② weight distribution; and ③ assign weights according to the widely used objective weight classification method.

The Jorge/Wexner Scale, Hull Scale, Valzey Scale, and Lunniss Scale are not weighted, and all types of fecal incontinence are considered to have the same severity. The Jorge/Wexner Scale is currently the most widely used scale without weight assignment because of its simplicity, reliability, and sensitivity. However, since no weight is assigned, the frequency of bowel movement was significantly affected by the subjective feelings of the subjects. Therefore, the Jorge/Wexner Scale, while proving useful, does not reflect the true feelings of patients and thus limits its application to some extent.

Self-allocation of weights is better than no allocation of weights, but it is not recommended because the calculation method is cumbersome and unscientific.

The Fecal Incontinence Severity Index (FISI) designed by Rockwood et al. used an objective weight allocation method. FISI consists of four components: gas, mucus, liquid, and solid. It contains six different frequency categories: two or more times per day, once a day, twice a week or more, once a week, one to three times a month, and never. The total score is 0–61. While this study helps us understand the importance of weighting different types of fecal incontinence, it will need to be replicated in other groups before it can be widely used because of the small number of participants. However, FISI is recommended when fecal incontinence occurs frequently. In addition, some scholars believe that any method to evaluate anal function should include tenesmus, as tenesmus is a common clinical symptom and has a great impact on patients' quality of life. According to Lika et al.'s study, the evaluation results of Wexner Scale, Vaizey Scale, Pescatori Scale, and AMS Scale were consistent in the postoperative anal function measurement of patients with different anal preservation methods and TNM stages, suggesting that the combined evaluation of the four scales had a good consistency effect.

Table 5.1 Wexner anal function scoring method

Incontinence	Frequency				
	Never	Rarely	Sometimes	Usually	Always
Dry stool	0	1	2	3	4
Loose stools	0	1	2	3	4
Gases	0	1	2	3	4
Need to pack	0	1	2	3	4
Lifestyle change	0	1	2	3	4

NB: never: 0; rarely: less than once a month; sometimes: more than once a month and less than once a week; often: more than once a week but less than once a day; always: more than once a day. 0 is considered normal and 20 is considered complete anal incontinence, with a low to high score representing the severity of anal incontinence

5.3.7 Questionnaire Survey on Patients' Quality of Life

The quality of life questionnaire survey of patients can also indirectly reflect the anal sphincter function; the disadvantage is that it is highly subjective, so it is difficult to evaluate the anal function objectively.

Quality of life questionnaire (FIQL) of fecal incontinence was developed by the American Society of Colon and Rectal Surgeons. ① It is a specific quality of life questionnaire related to defecation function. ② It deals with psychological coping/behavior (nine provisions). ③ It deals with depression/self-perception (seven provisions). ④ It deals with embarrassment (three provisions). Feedback on each specific item has a specific value, ranging from the ideal to worst quality of life, and then the total score is calculated to indirectly assess changes in anal function. At present, FIQL is widely studied and has certain practical value and certain validity and sensitivity, so it is recommended for use.

Suggested Reading

1. Masahino Takano. Compiled by Shi Renjie. Essential Diagnosis and Treatment of Anorectal Disease. Beijing: Biomedical Branch of Chemical Press, 2009, 107–166.
2. Cao Jixun. Chinese Hemorrhoids and Fistula Science. Chengdu: Sichuan Science and Technology Press, 2015, 37–64.
3. Huang Naijian. Anorectal Diseases in China. Jinan: Shandong Science and Technology Publishing House, 1996, 735–742.
4. Zhu Rui, Zhang Pingsheng, Shen Lin, et al. Advances in the diagnosis and treatment of anal fistula. Integrated Chinese and Western Medicine, 2011, 03 (3): 156–161, 166.
5. Shi Renjie, Gu Yunfei, Li Guonian, et al. 20 cases of anal fistula and perianal abscess examined by transanal ultrasound. Chinese Journal of Anorectal Disease. 2004, 24 (12). 28
6. Zhao Zehua, Li Ming, Wang Weizhong, et al. Preoperative diagnostic value of body surface coil magnetic resonance imaging for anal fistula. Chinese Journal of Medical Computer Imaging, 2007, 13 (6): 440–443.
7. Yang Bolin, Gu Yunfei, Zhuxin et al. Application of magnetic resonance imaging in the diagnosis of complex anal fistula. Chinese Journal of Gastrointestinal Surgery, 2008,11(4): 339–342
8. Zhang Dewang, Li Xin, Tang Guangjian, et al. A comparative study of preoperative MRI findings and surgical pathological findings of anal fistula. Chinese Journal of Medical Imaging, 2014, 22 (6): 441–445.
9. Cao Liang, Yang Bolin. Progress in the application of imaging examination in the diagnosis of anal fistula. Journal of Nanjing University of Traditional Chinese Medicine, 2012, 28 (2): 198–200.
10. Wu Yanlan, Wang Yehuang. Research progress of imaging examination in the diagnosis of anal fistula. Hebei Medicine, 2015, 37 (11): 1715–1717.
11. Feng Qunhu, Feng Guicheng, Lin Hongcheng et al. Diagnostic value of multi-slice spiral CT in perianal abscess and anal fistula. Shanxi Medical Journal, 2014, (3): 346–347.
12. Ma Haifeng, Wang Song, Wang Xifu et al. A new method for preoperative evaluation of anal fistula: clinical application of three-dimensional reconstruction technique of multi-slice spiral CT rectal tamponade fistula angiography. Journal of Clinical Radiology, 2007, 26 (6): 605–608.
13. Li Wenru, Yuan Fen, Zhou Zhiyang and others. Imaging diagnosis of anal fistula in Crohn's disease. Chinese Journal of Gastrointestinal Surgery, 2014, 17 (3): 215–218
14. Guan Ruijian, Yuan Hanxiong, Ren Donglin. Bacterial factors of perianal abscess and the relationship between abscess and anal fistula. Chinese Journal of Integrated Traditional Chinese and Western Medicine Surgery, 1996, 2 (6): 437–438.

15. Wan Xingyang, Lin Xiaosong, Hubang et al. Clinical significance of preoperative colonoscopy for benign anorectal diseases.Chinese Journal of Digestive Surgery, 2014, 13(1): 47–50.
16. Zhang Bo, Wang Fan, Chen Wenping. Diagnostic value of pelvic floor electromyography in outlet obstructive constipation. Colorectal and Anal Surgery, 2007, 13 (2): 68–70.
17. Chen Jinping, Liu Baohua, Luo Donglin, et al. Evaluation of electromyography in the diagnosis of puborectalis syndrome. Journal of Chongqing Medical University, 2007, 32 (11): 1185–1188, 1192.
18. Anorectal Surgery Group, Pediatric Surgery Branch, Chinese Medical Association. Recommendation of objective methods for the detection of anorectal function. Chinese Journal of Pediatric Surgery, 2011, 32 (8): 633–634
19. Wang Zhifeng, Ke Meiyun, Sun Xiaohong et al. Anorectal Dynamics and Sensory Function in Patients with Functional Constipation and Their Clinical Significance. Chinese Journal of Digestion, 2004, 24 (9): 526–529.
20. Huang Yan, Jin Xianqing, Li Xiaoqing, et al. Significance of endoanal ultrasound and anorectal manometry in the evaluation of anal function after anorectal atresia surgery. Chongqing Medical College, 2014, (28): 3704–3707, 3712
21. Gong Xiaoyong, Jin Zhiming, Zheng Qi, et al. Progress in the evaluation of anal and rectal function after low rectal cancer surgery. Shanghai Medical College, 2010, 33 (11): 1057–1061.
22. Yin Wanbin, Zhao Xiaotang, Dai Lei, et al. Progress in the study of anal sphincter function determination methods. International Journal of Surgery, 2015, 42 (8): 567–570

Classification and Diagnosis of Anal Fistula

6

Renjie Shi and JinHui Gu

Abstract

In ancient China, anal fistulas were classified by the location, shape, and characteristics. According to the current classification method, the anal fistulas above the deep external anal sphincter are defined as high anal fistulas, while those below the deep external anal sphincter are defined as low anal fistulas. The anal fistulas with relatively straight pipelines and fewer than one inner opening/outer opening/pipelines are defined as simple, while those with curved, more branches pipelines and multiple external openings/internal openings/pipelines are defined as complex. Parks' classification of anal fistula and Yuyuko's classification of anal fistula (Japan) are also widely used in China. The diagnosis of the anal fistula is based on the symptoms, signs, and various auxiliary examinations. It is important to make good use of all kinds of examination methods and to complete the colonoscopy and anal function evaluation before operation. Hidradenitis suppurativa, presacral cyst, and other diseases are easy to be misdiagnosed as anal fistula, and attention should be paid to prevent the errors.

Keywords

Anal fistula · Diagnosis · Differential diagnosis · Classification of diseases · Parks Yukio Sumikoshi

6.1 Classification of Anal Fistula

6.1.1 Classification of Anal Fistula in Traditional Chinese Medicine

The classification of anal fistula is complex. Ancient Chinese physicians classified the fistula according to its location, shape, and characteristics.

6.1.2 Classification of Anal Fistula in Western Medicine

6.1.2.1 Classification of Anal Fistula by the National Conference on Anorectal Surgery (1975)

Anal fistula classification has been commonly used in China since 1975. In July 2012, the Guidelines for the Diagnosis and Treatment of

R. Shi (✉)
Department of Anorectal Surgery, Affiliated Hospital of Nanjing University of Traditional Chinese Medicine, Nanjing, Jiangsu, China

J. Gu
Suzhou Hospital of Traditional Chinese Medicine, Affiliated to Nanjing University of Chinese Medicine, Suzhou, Jiangsu, China

© Chemical Industry Press 2021
R. Shi, L. Zheng (eds.), *Diagnosis and Treatment of Anal Fistula*,
https://doi.org/10.1007/978-981-16-5804-4_6

Common Diseases in Anorectal Department of Traditional Chinese Medicine was published by the National Administration of Traditional Chinese Medicine and still adopted mostly the same classification methods. Although there were slight differences in expression, the contents were basically the same.

The distinction is marked by the deep line of the external sphincter, the fistula passing above this line is deemed high, and the fistula below this line is deemed low. If there is only a single internal orifice, the fistula and external orifice are called simple. It is called complexed when there are two or more internal orifices, fistulas, and external orifices. This classification is still widely used in China.

Low Simple Anal Fistula

The internal orifice is in the anal recess with only one fistula passing through the subcutaneous or superficial part of the external sphincter, which communicates with the skin.

Low Complex Anal Fistula

There are more than two internal or external orifices, and the fistula is located in the subcutaneous or superficial part of the external sphincter.

High Simple Anal Fistula

The internal orifice is in the anal recess, with only one fistula, which runs above the deep layer of the external sphincter.

High Complex Anal Fistula

There are more than two external orifices connected with the internal orifice through the fistula or with a branch cavity. The main fistula passes through the deep layer of the external sphincter.

6.1.2.2 Parks 4 Class Method (1976)

According to the relationship between the fistula and sphincter, anal fistula can be divided into four categories (Fig. 6.1). This is the main anal fistula classification method most commonly used abroad.

Intersphincter Fistula (Low Anal Fistula)

This is most common, accounting for about 70% of cases, and is the result of perianal abscess. The fistula passes only through the internal sphincter. There is usually only one external orifice, which is close to the anal margin, about 3–5 cm. A few fistulas go upward, forming a blind end between the rectal circular muscle and the longitudinal muscle or penetrating the rectum to form a high sphincter fistula.

Transsphincter Anal Fistula (Low or High Anal Fistula)

Accounting for about 25% of cases, it is the result of abscess in the ischiorectal fossa. The fistula passes through the superficial and deep parts of the internal and external sphincters. There are often several external orifices and branches communicating with each other. The external orifice is about 5 cm away from the anal margin. A few fistulas pass upward through the levator ani muscle to rectal connective tissue, forming a pelvic-rectal fistula.

Superior Sphincter Anal Fistula (High Anal Fistula)

This is rare, accounting for about 5% of cases. The fistula goes up through the levator ani muscle, then down to the ischiorectal fossa and penetrates the skin. Because this type of fistula often involves the anal and rectal rings, it is difficult to treat, and it often requires staging an operation.

External Anal Fistula of Sphincter (High Anal Fistula)

This is rarest, accounting for only about 1% of cases, and is the result of pelvic and rectal space abscess combined with ischiorectal fossa abscess. The fistula passes through the levator ani muscle and connects directly to the rectum. This type of anal fistula is often caused by Crohn's disease, intestinal cancer, or trauma. Treatment should therefore pay attention to the primary focus.

Marks and Ritchie (1977) pointed out that the clinical manifestations of sphincter fistula were simple, while the last three types of anal fistula had a long history, more rounds of operation and

6 Classification and Diagnosis of Anal Fistula

Fig. 6.1 Classification of fistula-in-ano (Parks)

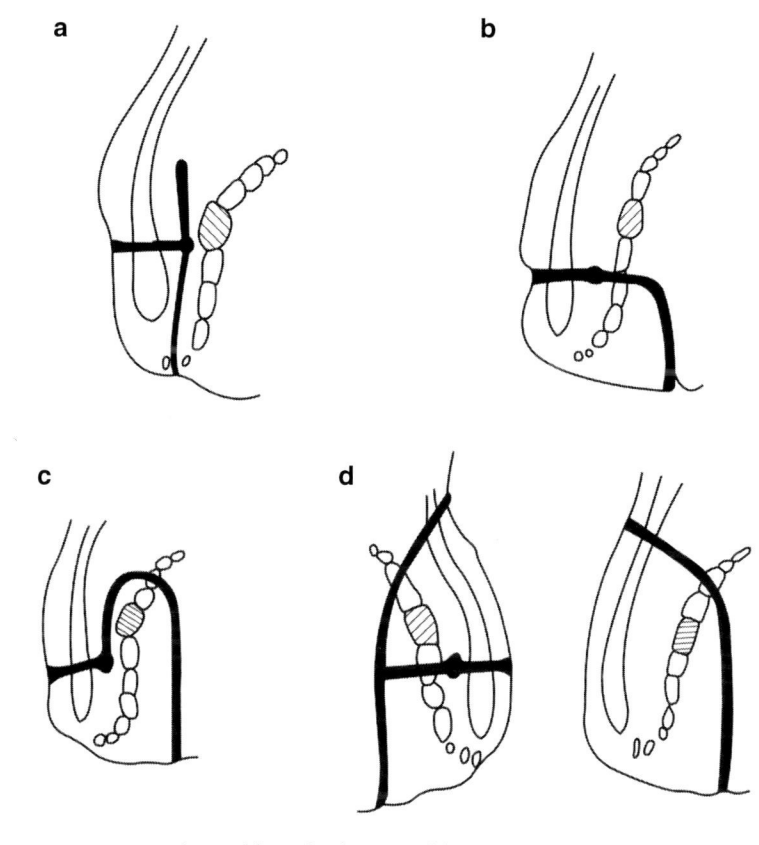

a. Intersphincteric   b. transsphincteric
c. Suprasphincteric   d. extrasphincteric

abscess drainage, more horseshoe type or spread, and more lateral and multiple external orifices.

6.1.2.3 Yukio Sumikoshi's Classification of Anal Fistula

In 1972, Japanese scholar Yukio Sumikoshi put forward the anal fistula classification method based on the relationship between anal fistula and sphincters (Fig. 6.2). This method is widely respected and applied in Japan and is basically the national anal fistula classification method in Japan. Japan's renowned anorectologist Masahino Takano said that, except for a few special cases of mutation, the method is based on anatomical formulation, strong theories, clinical practice, and very practical classification. Taka Utui also commented that "among all the classification methods, only Yukio Sumikoshi's classification can

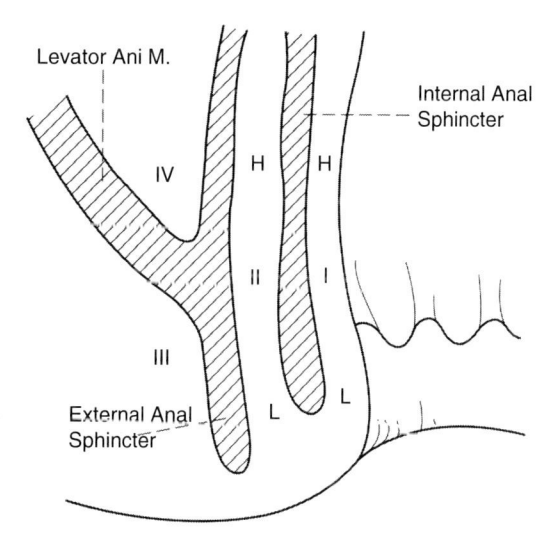

Fig. 6.2 Classification of fistula-in-ano (Yukio Sumikoshi)

fully display the three-dimensional shape and straightforwardly show the location, direction and complexity of anal fistula."

The anal fistula was classified into four categories in Yukio Sumikoshi's classification method and then divided into 11 subcategories, which were shown by marks and easy to remember. Based on the internal and external sphincters and levator ani muscles, the gap between the mucosa or anal epithelium and the internal sphincter is marked as I, the gap between the internal and external sphincters is marked as II, the gap under the levator ani is marked as III, and the gap above the levator ani is marked as IV. Traveling below the dental line is marked as L, and traveling above the dental line is marked as H. Those that walk on one side are represented by U (unilateral), while those that walk on both sides are represented by B (bilateral). Simple fistula and complicated fistula are called S (simple) and C (complicated) (Table 6.1).

According to the relationship between the abscess and sphincter and according to the Yukio Sumikoshi's classification of anal fistula (Fig. 6.3), Masahiro Takano divided perianal abscesses into six categories: subcutaneous abscess, submucosal abscess, low intermuscular abscess, high intermuscular abscess, sciatorectal fossa abscess, and pelvic and rectal fossa abscess. The forms I LA, II HA, II LA, III A, and IVA were used, respectively. A is an abbreviation for abscess.

Table 6.1 Yukio Sumikoshi's classification of anal fistula

I. Subcutaneous or submucosal fistula	Mark
L subcutaneous fistula	I L
H submucosal fistula	I H
II. Intersphincteric fistula	
L low intersphincteric.........S simple	II Ls
.................C complicated	II Lc
H high intersphincteric.........S simple	III Us
.................C complicated	III Uc
III. Infralevator fistula	
U unilateral.........S simple	III Us
.................C complicated	III Uc
B bilateral.........S simple	III Bs
....................C complicated	III Bc
IV. Supralevator fistula	IV

6.1.2.4 Other Taxonomies

Classification of Fistulas Based on Internal and External Characteristics
1. **Single-Orifice Internal Fistula**
   This is also known as internal blind fistula, where only the internal orifice communicates with the fistula, and there is no external orifice.
2. **Internal and External Fistula**
   This is the most common type of anal fistula. The fistula has both internal and external orifices. The external orifice is on the surface, and the internal orifice is usually in the anal sinus. The internal and external orifices are connected by the fistula.
3. **Single-Orifice External Fistula**
   This is also known as the external blind fistula. Only the external orifice is connected to the fistula, but there is no internal orifice. This type of anal fistula is rarely seen clinically.
4. **Total External Fistula**
   The fistula has more than two external openings, which are connected to each other by pipelines without an internal orifice. This kind of anal fistula is also rare in the clinic.

Classification of Fistulas Based on the Shape of Anal Fistulas
1. **Straight Fistula**
   The fistula is straight, and the internal and external orifices are in the same direction. It is more common in the clinic, accounting for more than 1/3 of cases.
2. **Curved Fistula**
   The fistula is curved in path, and the internal and external orifices are mostly not in the same direction.
3. **Posterior Horseshoe-Shaped Anal Fistula**
   The fistula is curved and shoe-shaped, in the posterior position of the anus, with the inner orifice in the middle of the posterior.
4. **Anterior Horseshoe-Shaped Anal Fistula**
   The fistula is curved and shoe-shaped, which is relatively rare, and is in front of the anus.

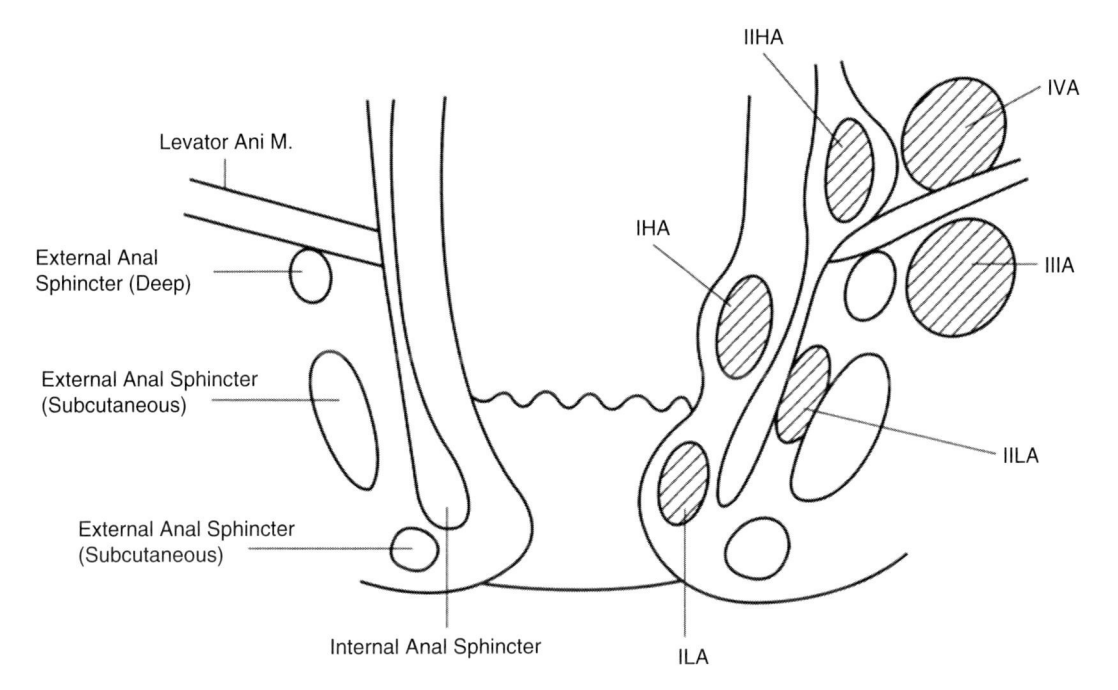

Fig. 6.3 Classification of perianal abscess. According to the classification of anal fistula, it is divided into subcutaneous abscess (ILA), submucosal abscess (IHA), low intermuscular abscess (III LA), high intermuscular abscess (IIHA), ischiorectal fossa abscess (IIIA), pelvic rectum Abscess (IVA) type 6. A is the abbreviation of Abscess

5. **Circumferential Fistula**
    The fistula surrounds the anal canal or rectum, and operation on it is difficult and complicated.

Classification of Fistulas Based on the Relationship Between the Fistula and the Sphincter

1. **Subcutaneous Fistula**
    In the anal subcutaneous layer, shallow, low position.
2. **Submucosal Fistula**
    Under the rectal mucosa, not on the surface of the body.
3. **Fistula Between Superficial External Sphincter and Subcutaneous Part**
4. **Fistula Between Deep and Superficial External Sphincter**
5. **Deep Fistula Between the Levator Ani and External Sphincter**
6. **Superior Levator Anal Fistula**

Classification of Fistulas Based on the Number of Internal and External Orifices and Fistulas

1. **Simple Anal Fistula**
    There is only one internal orifice, one external orifice, and only one fistula connecting the internal and external orifices.
2. **Complex Anal Fistula**
    There are two or more internal orifices or external orifices, more than two fistulas, or branches and blind canals.

Classification of Fistulas Based on the Etiology and Pathological Nature of Anal Fistulas

1. **Nonspecific Anal Fistula**
    The mixed infection of *Escherichia coli*, *Staphylococcus*, *Streptococcus*, and so on usually causes anorectal abscess and forms anal fistula after ulceration. This is most common in the clinic.

2. **Specific Anal Fistula**

    This includes tuberculous anal fistula, Crohn's disease anal fistula, and so on.

Eisenhammer: Three Categories and Five Types Method (1966)

Eisenhammer divided anal fistulas into the internal group, external group, and internal and external combined group according to the theory of intramuscular fistula abscess.

1. **Internal Group**

    Refers to the intramuscular fistula abscess and submucosal fistula originating from the anal recess inside the anal canal. There are three types of fistulas here: high internal and external sphincter fistula, low internal and external sphincter fistula, and submucosal fistula.
2. **Outside Group**

    Refers to infectious fistula abscess of non-anal recess gland originating from outside the anal canal, such as ischiorectal fossa abscess caused by hemorrhagic infection, trauma, etc. The outside group can be further divided into two types: (1) ischiorectal fossa fistula and (2) subcutaneous fistula.
3. **Internal and External Merger Group**

    Refers to the irregular type of infection originating from both sides of the anal canal, and this happens in many cases.

Goligher's Classification (1975)

The Goligher taxonomy was developed on the basis of the Milligan–Morgan taxonomy. It is divided into the following:

1. **Subcutaneous Anal Fistula**

    This accounts for 10%–15% of cases. The fistula is located in the lower part of the perianal skin, and the internal orifice is at the dental line. Sometimes it can be presented as blind subcutaneous external fistula (sinus tract).
2. **Low Anal Fistula**

    This is most common, accounting for 60%–70% of cases. The fistula passes through the subcutaneous part of the external sphincter or the inferior edge of the internal sphincter. The internal orifice is often near the dental line; sometimes it can be a blind external fistula (sinus tract).
3. **High Anal Fistula**

    This accounts for 15% of cases, and the fistula location is higher, close to the anal rectal ring, but not over this ring. The internal orifice is often near the dental line. The fistula can pass through the internal and external sphincters and become oblique. Sometimes there is no internal orifice, showing a high blind external fistula.
4. **Anorectal Fistula**

    Clinically relatively rare, this accounts for about 5% of cases, and there are two types. One is the ischiorectal fossa type. The fistula is under the levator ani muscle. Because the levator ani muscle is oblique, the fistula begins above the anorectal ring. The internal orifice can be single or multiple, often under the anorectal ring. The other is pelvic-rectal type with fistula above the levator ani muscle. The internal orifice may be under or above the anorectal ring, or it may be an external fistula of the blind end. The fistula is not connected with the rectum. Goligher believes that the internal orifice above the anal and rectal ring is often caused by artificial causes, such as inappropriate probe examination, artificial internal orifice, or by incorrect incision of pelvic and rectal space abscess or ischiorectal fossa abscess.
5. **High Intermuscular Anal Fistula**

    This is rare in the clinic. It is usually the blind sinus tract, extending upward from the dental line. The fistula is between the circular and longitudinal muscles. Sometimes it can be under the mucosa, and the skin has no external orifice. Sometimes it appears as an internal fistula.

6.2 Diagnosis of Anal Fistula

6.2.1 Diagnostic Methods of Anal Fistula

Diagnosis of anal fistula is not difficult. According to the history of intermittent onset of anal swelling and pain and purulence, combined with the symptoms of swelling and pain, purulence and other characteristics, and then according to an anorectal specialist examination, such as the detection of an external orifice, fistula, internal orifice, or other characteristic changes, anal fistula can be diagnosed. After the diagnosis of anal fistula, it is necessary to further clarify the location of the internal orifice of the anal fistula, whether the anal fistula is simple or complex, whether it is high or low, and the shape of the fistula, the relationship between the fistula and the sphincter, etc.

Generally, simple anal fistula has only one external orifice, one internal orifice, and one fistula, while complex anal fistula can form multiple branches, which connect to the external orifice and the internal orifice. However, some people believe that complex anal fistula should not be divided into the number of external orifices because sometimes the anal fistula has multiple external orifices but treatment is not difficult. The main pipeline affects anorectal ring or above anorectal ring. Although there may be only one external mouth and one internal mouth, it is difficult to treat, so it should be a complex anal fistula.

As for the classification of high and low anal fistulas, Parks's method (1967) has been widely used in clinical practice to classify high and low anal fistulas based on whether the fistula crosses the highest self-control muscular layer. He defined high anal fistula as "an anal fistula in which a fistula passes over the top of the highest self-control muscle." If the fistula passes through the levator ani muscle (mainly the puborectal muscle), it is a high anal fistula, and the lower anal fistula is the anal fistula below the levator ani muscle. Milligan–Morgan (1934) referred to fistula as high anal fistula if it is above the dental line level and as low anal fistula if it is below the dental line level.

The shape of the fistula can be a straight fistula, curved fistula, and horseshoe fistula. The external and internal orifices of the straight fistula are in corresponding positions, and the pipes are straight or slightly curved, often shorter. Straight fistulas can be low or high. Straight fistulas also have more than one line, or near one line, which is relatively easy to treat. The external and internal orifices of the curved fistula are often not in the same direction, and the curved condition can be quite different. Some have a very small curvature, whereas some have a very large curvature. Horseshoe-shaped anal fistula is mostly posterior horseshoe-shaped. Generally, the internal orifice is in the posterior, and the fistula is shoe-shaped behind the anus. Occasionally, there are anterior horseshoe anal fistulas and even whole horseshoe anal fistulas.

The nature of anal fistula should also be clarified in the diagnosis of anal fistula. General anal fistula refers to the anal fistula caused by common intestinal or dermatogenic bacterial infections and accompanied by noninflammatory bowel diseases. Specific anal fistula refers to tuberculous anal fistula and anal fistula complicated by Crohn's disease.

In the diagnosis of anal fistula, a comprehensive examination should be carried out on the basis of a detailed collection of medical history in order to determine the general situation and know whether the patient has diabetes, leukemia, Crohn's disease, ulcerative colitis, or other diseases and whether there are any surgical contraindications. This is important for treatment decision-making and the choice of treatment methods.

In addition, according to the clinical symptoms and signs, the duration of anal fistula should be determined as static, chronic active, or acute inflammation. These are also closely related to the choice of appropriate treatment methods.

6.2.2 The Importance of Preoperative Diagnosis of Anal Fistula

Preliminary diagnosis of anal fistula is not difficult, but for some high complex anal fistulas, it is still difficult to accurately know the number of fistulas, distribution, direction, and location of the internal orifice before operation. Precise preoperative diagnosis is of great significance in making an operative plan, reducing variability and randomness during operation, improving the cure rate of the anal fistula, and reducing postoperative complications and sequelae. In order to improve the accuracy of diagnosis, we must pay attention to the following aspects.

6.2.2.1 Make Good Use of Various Inspection Means and Techniques

At present, all kinds of methods used in the diagnosis of anal fistula have their respective advantages and limitations. It is helpful for the accurate diagnosis of anal fistula to use a comprehensive application of digital rectal examination, transanal ultrasonography, and rectal and pelvic floor magnetic resonance imaging. From the three-dimensional location and morphology of the anal fistula, we can have a comprehensive and accurate understanding of the internal orifice, direction, shape, and relationship with the sphincter of anal fistula. With the improvement in the examination technology of anal fistula such as MRI, it seems that the accurate location of complex anal fistula, from its shape and course, can be on the whole achieved at present. However, not all clinicians can understand the information reflected by the MRI images or accurately understand the morphological structure of anal fistula and its relationship with the sphincter, etc. Therefore, colorectal and anal surgeons should learn and master anal MRI film reading in order to help further improve their expertise in diagnosis and treatment.

6.2.2.2 Colonoscopy Before Anal Fistula Operation Should Be Done as Much as Possible

At present, the incidence of Crohn's disease and ulcerative colitis tends to increase, and the concept of colonoscopy before complex anal fistula to exclude perianal Crohn's disease has become more widely supported. It has been reported that more than 10% of complex anal fistula is actually a perianal fistula change of inflammatory bowel disease, which means that preoperative colonoscopy can help about one-tenth of complex anal fistula patients avoid inappropriate surgery and get more suitable treatment. Although the current guidelines for the treatment of anal fistula (including Crohn's disease and anal fistula) do not include colonoscopy as recommended, we recommend that preoperative colonoscopy be performed for all patients with anal fistula, especially for those with high complex anal fistula. Colonoscopy before an operation on anal fistula can exclude perianal Crohn's disease, intestinal malignant tumors, intestinal tuberculosis, and so on. It does not increase the additional risk of diagnosis and treatment.

6.2.2.3 Preoperative Evaluation of Anal Function Is Helpful to Formulate Individualized Treatment Plans

Preoperative decline of anal defecation control function is a risk factor for postoperative anal incontinence. Anorectal finger examination and other examinations can be used to understand the situation of anorectal defect, the integrity of the anorectal ring, and the diastolic and contractile function of the anorectal muscles; an appropriate scoring scale can be used to evaluate the preoperative anorectal function; MR examination and anorectal color Doppler ultrasound are used to determine whether there are any minor injuries to the anal sphincter; and anorectal manometry is used to assess the contraction and sensory function of anal muscles. Then, according to the different conditions of each patient, doctors should develop targeted surgical methods for improving the one-time cure rate of anal fistula, better protection of patients' anal function, and even prevention of doctor–patient disputes.

Anorectal manometry is one of the most commonly used methods for preoperative evaluation of anal function. Although there are many reports in the literature and the examination is considered to be of great significance, the data obtained by the examination are not stable, so there is no accepted standard value. Because of the influence of translocation, examiner, and even patient's cooperation and other inherent defects, the examination results may not truly reflect the most realistic functional state of a patient's anus before operation. Therefore, the author believes that anorectal manometry can only be used as a reference in the evaluation of anal function. In the preoperative functional evaluation of anal fistula, the patient's complaint, anal function score, anorectal digital examination, and MRI examination are arguably more useful than anorectal manometry. We should learn to use all kinds of possible means of examination and functional evaluation in order to formulate a treatment plan more comprehensively and pertinently.

6.2.2.4 Preoperative Pathological Examination and Diagnosis If Necessary

Pathological examination is necessary for those patients who are clinically highly suspected of carcinogenesis, tuberculosis, and Crohn's disease complicated with anal fistula, seemingly simple cases that not cured after multiple operations, delayed wound healing, or difficulties in wound healing. In principle, specimens should be taken for pathological examination in all kinds of anal fistula operations.

6.3 Differential Diagnosis of the Third Anal Fistula

There are other diseases around the anus and sacrococcygeal region, such as ulceration and secretion, which are easily confused with anal fistula, and these need to be differentiated.

6.3.1 Hidradenitis Suppurativa

Hidradenitis suppurativa is a chronic suppurative disease of the skin and subcutaneous tissue. The lesions are often widespread, diffuse, or flaky, with many ulcers, pus, or particular odor. The skin in the lesion area is often blackened by pigmentation. Hidradenitis suppurativa is more superficial, generally only in the skin and subcutaneous tissue, mostly not connected with the anal canal. But sometimes it can communicate with the anal canal and rectum to form complex anal fistula or multiple anal fistulas, which needs attention.

6.3.2 Perianal Folliculitis and Furuncle

In perianal folliculitis and furuncle, small red, swollen, and painful nodules are found locally, which then gradually swell and protrude. Several days later, the central tissue of the nodule becomes soft and necrotic, and yellow-white pus will appear. The range of redness, swelling, and pain will also be enlarged. The pus drops off, and pus is discharged. The inflammation gradually disappears and recovers. Occasionally, the infection of boils spreads, causing lymphangitis and lymphadenitis. If multiple boils occur simultaneously or repeatedly, they are called furunculosis.

Perianal folliculitis or furuncle lesions are small, shallow, and limited, not connected with the anal canal. It is easy to know the limitations and superficial features of perianal folliculitis or furuncle when making sliding palpation, and therefore it is easy to differentiate from anal fistula.

6.3.3 Perianal Sinus Tract

Anal trauma or infection can form a sinus tract because it is not connected with the anus, and generally after a dressing change can be cured. If there is foreign body in the sinus tract, it is difficult to heal though drainage is smooth, so clinical attention must be paid to it. History is an important basis for differential diagnosis. Combined with the clinical features that are not connected with the anal canal, it is generally easy to differentiate from anal fistula.

6.3.4 Sacrococcygeal Cyst

Sacrococcygeal cyst is a congenital disease that is generally believed to be caused by abnormal embryonic development. Epidermal cysts and dermoid cysts are common, located in the anterior and posterior sacral space. Cysts can be monocystic, bicystic, or polycystic, as large as eggs, as small as yolk, and with gelatinous mucus in the cavity. The age of onset is mostly about 20–30 years old. There is no infection, often asymptomatic, or a slight sacrococcygeal pain. If the cyst grows in size or secondary infection occurs, fever, local swelling, pain, and other symptoms can occur. After ulceration or incision and drainage, a fistula might be formed, but there is no internal orifice. The main points of differentiation are the following: cysts often have sacrococcygeal swelling and pain; most of the fistulas are located in or near the middle hip suture, far from the anal margin and near the tip of the coccyx; epithelial tissue extends into the fistula; and the fistula is depressed, which is not easy to close. If the cyst is large, the presacral swelling can be found in digital rectal examination, and the cystic mass can be touched. The surface is smooth, and the boundary is clear. CT or MRI examination will show sacrococcygeal cystic lesions, often with obvious cystic wall and outer membrane.

6.3.5 Perineal Urethral Fistula

This kind of fistula is the urethral bulb connected with the skin. The orificium fistulae are often located in the perineal urogenital triangle. When urinating, there is urine flowing out of the external orifice. Most of them are congenital anomalies, but some are also caused by trauma, tumors, and so on. The diagnosis and differential diagnosis can only be made by a local specialist examination combined with CT and MRI.

6.3.6 Sacrococcygeal Osteomyelitis

Sacral osteomyelitis can cause an abscess between the sacrum and the rectum. The abscess is perforated near the coccyx to form a fistula. The fistula is usually on both sides of the coccyx tip and is even with the tip of the coccyx. Sometimes there are two symmetrical fistulas with equal distances. The probe can penetrate several centimeters. The fistula is parallel to the rectum. It is located in the anterior sacral fossa. There is no stiffening tissue between the fistula and the anal canal, and it is not connected to the rectum. Pelvic floor MRI is an important basis for differential diagnosis.

6.3.7 Sacroiliac Bone Tuberculosis

Sacral, iliac, hip, and pubic tuberculosis can form abscesses, pus in the buttocks or perineum, or inguinal perforation. The formation of fistula needs to be identified with anal fistula. The onset of bone tuberculosis is slow, mostly without acute inflammation. After the break, the purulent fluid flows away, the wound is not closed for a long time, the wound mouth is depressed, and the orificium fistulae are far from the anus, which is not connected with the rectum. Bone tuberculosis is often manifested as low fever, night sweat, poor appetite, and other tuberculosis. CT or X-ray examination of the sacrococcygeal bone can detect bone tuberculosis manifestations such as sacrococcygeal bone destruction.

6.3.8 Rupture of Anterior Sacral Space Teratoma

Presacral space teratoma is a congenital disease associated with abnormal embryonic development. Most of them occur in the young and middle-aged period and have no obvious symptoms in the initial stage. If the tumor enlarges and compresses the rectum, symptoms such as anal distension or difficulty in defecation may occur. Anal finger examination can often touch the sacral anterior cystic mass sensation but generally cannot find the internal orifice. Presacral space teratoma can sometimes burst from the back of the anus when it is secondary to infection. Imaging examination is an important means in differential diagnosis. It is often found that there are teeth and bones in the tumors during imaging examination or surgery. Hair, teeth, and other tissues are often seen in cysts removed during surgery.

6.3.9 Carcinoma of Anal Canal and Rectum

Anal fistula can also occur after canceration of anal or low rectal cancer. It can be found that there are hard masses in the anus and rectum with more fixed basement and less abscess. Sometimes it can be seen that the surface of the tumors has cauliflower-like changes, with pus, blood, mucus, and other secretions. Although it is easy to differentiate according to clinical features, definite diagnosis still depends on pathological examination.

Suggested Reading

1. Masahiro Takano. Compilation by Shi Renjie. The essence of treatment of anorectal diseases. Beijing: Chemical Press Biomedical Branch, 2009, 107–166.
2. Cao Jixun. Chinese Hemorrhoidology. Chengdu: Sichuan Science and Technology Press, 2015, 37–64.
3. Huang Naijian. Chinese anorectal pathology. Jinan: Shandong Science and Technology Publishing House, 1996, 731–734.
4. Wang F, Gong XC, Alimas et al. A collection of studies on the causes, classification and diagnostic methods of anal fistula. Xinjiang Medicine,2007,37(5):271–274.
5. Qian Qun. Diagnosis of anal fistula. Journal of Clinical Surgery, 2011, 19(4): 224–225.
6. Xu Mengting, Chen Fujun. Diagnostic status of anal fistula. Journal of Modern Traditional Chinese and Western Medicine,2009,18(8):936–938

The Therapeutic Principle of Fistula-in-Ano

Renjie Shi and Lihua Zheng

Abstract

The purpose of anal fistula treatment is to relieve the pain caused by anal fistula and improve the life quality of patients. Besides the cure rate, the protection of anal function should be taken into account in anal fistula surgery to the maximum extent possible. The basic requirement of curing anal fistula is a thorough treatment of the internal opening and the primary lesions in the sphincter. The sphincter involved in the surgery should be protected as much as possible, and the minimum requirement is to avoid direct incision of the deep external anal sphincter and levator ani muscle. Excision and drainage of the external opening are sufficient. It is important to ensure that the drainage of each wound is kept open so that the healing of the fistula is not influenced. The treatment should be individualized according to the type of fistula and the patient's physical condition. The surgical method should protect the anal sphincter as much as possible. Drainage or nonsurgical treatment could be used for those who are difficult to cure and for whom surgery can easily lead to anal incontinence.

Keywords

Anal fistula · Treatment · Principle
Operation · Seton therapy · Anal sphincter
Primary lesion · Drainage · Crohn's disease with anal fistula

It is impossible to accomplish autotherapy once fistula-in-ano or anal fistula has appeared. Put frankly, fistula-in-ano must undergo surgery. In the treatment of fistula-in-ano, some principles must be followed, and with reasonable techniques, an ideal clinical curative effect can be achieved. The basic principles of fistula-in-ano surgery are as follows.

7.1 Both Healing Fistula-in-Ano and Protecting Anal Function Are Equally Important

The purpose of fistula-in-ano surgery is to relieve the pain caused by an anal fistula and improve the patient's quality of life. Surgery is the necessary means for the treatment of fistula-in-ano; however, in healing anal fistula, surgery is bound to

R. Shi (✉)
Department of Anorectal Surgery, Affiliated Hospital of Nanjing University of Traditional Chinese Medicine, Nanjing, Jiangsu, China

L. Zheng
Department of Proctology, China-Japan Friendship Hospital, Beijing, China

cause some damage due to its disruptions. How to protect anal function to a maximum is always a problem in the operation of anal fistula. The so-called equal importance of curing anal fistula and protecting anal function is to cure anal fistula while at the same time maximally protect anal function by taking necessary measures in the operation.

It is the most basic and important principle that must be strictly grasped in anal fistula surgery: paying equal attention to curing the anal fistula and protecting anal function. Otherwise, even if the anal fistula is cured, if anal function is seriously damaged or there is even fecal incontinence, the quality of life of patients is greatly reduced after the procedure. In this case, the benefits of anal fistula surgery are offset, and the postoperative pain might even be greater than before surgery, so it will not be worth it.

Anal fistula surgery has many serious complications and sequelae of anal incontinence such as anal incontinence, anal stenosis, anal malformation, etc. In order to avoid the occurrence of these complications and sequelae and to maximize the protection of the anus function, doctors need to choose the appropriate surgical methods and measures. They should maximally protect the internal and external anal sphincters and anorectal tissue during surgery so as to minimize and avoid incontinence and anal malformation and improve patients' quality of life after surgery.

There has been a long-standing debate on the damage and retention of the anal sphincter in the domestic and foreign anorectal communities. Modern research shows that important factors affecting the function of anal continence include anal external sphincter integrity, integrity of internal sphincter reflex, anal local epithelial electrophysiological sensation, anal canal coloboma, etc. We need to point out that anal sphincter preservation is not a complete procedure that does not destroy the sphincter at all. It also causes some damage to anal sphincter but will try to protect the anal sphincter in terms of ideas and measures.

For high complexity anal fistula, Crohn's disease accompanied with anal fistula, anal fistula that recurs after multiple operations and whose cause of recurrence is unknown, when there is no cure or a low cure rate, or when anal function cannot be effectively protected, the operation may not be performed both temporarily or even permanently so as to avoid failure. For those difficult miscellaneous cases, drained by widening the wound, drained with medicated strip, traditional Chinese medicine for oral or external use, etc. can be used to reduce the scope of inflammation and the probability of repeated infection, protect the anal control function, reduce local symptoms, and improve the quality of life of patients. This "survival with fistula" method is also a reasonable choice or method in the treatment of fistula-in-ano. This practice is widely recognized at home and abroad, widely used in the treatment of anal fistula caused by Crohn's disease and anal fistula that is highly complexed.

7.2 The Treatment of the Internal or Primary Opening and the Primary Lesion Should Be Clean and Thorough

Most anal fistulas are caused by infection of anal glands; therefore, for the vast majority of anal fistulas, the thorough treatment of the internal opening and the primary intersphincteric abscess is the most basic and necessary condition for the healing of the anal fistula. Otherwise, it will easily relapse. Most recidivation of anal fistula correlates with inappropriate or halfway treatment of the internal opening or primary abscess.

Accurately finding the internal opening is the premise of handling the internal opening. Treatment for the internal orifice is usually incision, or excision, or ligation.

The primary abscess is the initial lesion caused by an infection of the anal gland. It includes the anal duct and intersphincteric anal abscess. The primary abscess is a submucosal induration of the internal opening during digital examination. During the operation, it is a tubal wall or an abscess wall that turns hard between the sphincters. These necrotic tissues cannot be left behind and need to be completely removed during surgery.

7.3 Protect the Anal Sphincter as Much as Possible

Because the anal fistula passes through the internal and external anal sphincters or the tract passes within the intersphincteric space, when dealing with the fistula, the anal sphincter will be damaged more or less a bit. Therefore, the anal sphincter must be protected as much as possible during the operation of anal fistula.

Protecting the anal sphincter as much as possible includes measures such as not letting the anal sphincter divide during surgery, or dividing it as little as possible. This requires certain principles to be followed and certain measures to be adopted during the surgery.

In an anal fistula surgery, the range of sphincters allowed to be cut is 1–2 pots in the lower half of the internal sphincter, 1–3 places in the subcutaneous parts of the external sphincter, 1–2 places in the superficial part of the external sphincter, and 1 place in the posterior deep part of external sphincter. According to this principle, it generally does not cause severe anal incontinence.

In anal surgery, the scope in which the sphincter cannot be incised is all of the internal sphincter, more than three places in the superficial part of the external sphincter, the deep part of external sphincter (except behind the anus), and all the levator ani muscles.

When cutting the internal sphincter deep or incising the internal sphincter in two or three places at the same time, the continuous occlusion of the internal sphincter will be lost; thus, the anus cannot remain completely closed. Although the external sphincter has a compensatory function, but because the external sphincter is prone to fatigue, it is worn out, and it tends to cause loose stools and gas leakage. This is the main cause of anus dampness, discharge, and underwear dirt after an anal fistula operation.

Cutting the external sphincter has less effect on anal function than it has on the levator ani muscle. But cutting too deeply or multiple incisions can also cause anal incontinence. In addition, a lateral incision of the sphincter can easily cause anal deformation.

The levator ani muscle is located in the deepest part of the anus and has the function of continuously and powerfully closing the anus from the back. As long as the levator ani muscle is retained, the basic constriction function of the anus can be preserved, and at the very least, function of control over solid feces can be maintained. Therefore, in general, cutting the levator ani muscle will cause anal incontinence except for very rare cases such as where the anorectal ring is already stiff. So in principle, unless the anorectal ring is already stiff, the levator ani muscle cannot be divided in one go.

At present, some scholars have different views on whether the levator ani muscle can be incised in one go. Hill reports three cases of incisions of all anal sphincter muscles including the levator ani muscle where after the operation, solid stools can still be controlled. The three patients he reported on had all their sphincters cut off, but there were no diarrhea or soft stools, and they had bowel movement once a day only. On the other hand, in patients with only mild to moderate incision of the sphincter, there are also cases of severe anal incontinence. The investigation found that these patients have nonanal local factors such as psychological factors, functional or organic intestinal diseases, etc. Therefore, it is necessary to know the psychological and defecation situations of patients before operating on anal fistula, as well as the functional or organic lesions of the large intestine anus.

On the other hand, the integrity of anal function is related not only to the anal sphincter but also to the soft tissue of the anus. When the anal soft group defect caused by anal fistula surgery is too large, the anus cannot be completely closed. Therefore, attention should be paid to protecting the soft tissue of the perianal rectum as much as possible during the anal fistula operations.

7.4 The External Opening and Wound Should Be Properly Managed in Fistulas

Fistulas and external openings of the anal fistulas need to be properly treated in order to ensure the smooth healing of the raw surface. If the intraoperative treatment is not in place, it is difficult for anal fistulas to heal smoothly. Clinically, even if the treatment of the primary lesion is correct, inadequate intraoperative treatment of the fistula, having an external opening or raw surface, can all lead to recurrence or partial recurrence of the anal fistula.

The septic tissue in the fistula must be scratched and scraped clean, and hard and thick tube walls must be completely or properly ectomized. Fistulas superficial to and below the external sphincter are usually incised or excised. However, care should be taken when opening anterior and lateral fistulas, especially in female patients and patients with particularly weak anterior sphincters. It is generally recommended to adopt the cutting seton method. A fistula in the intersphincter and which tracts upward above the depth of the external setonsphincter can be treated by cutting seton or drain seton or catheter drainage.

Drainage of the wound should be adequate and appropriate. The anal fistula wound in most cases treated with the method of open drainage, but because the wound surface in the anus is often contaminated by stool, mucus, exudation, etc., and also constricted by the sphincter, sometimes the wounds are difficult to heal. In order to drain the wound, it is necessary to extend the wound outwardly to the anus, a form that allows dirt on the surface of the wound to easily flow out. The size of the drainage wound depends on the size and depth of the lesion and the route of the lesion in the anus. Generally, the deeper and longer the fistula is, the larger and longer the drainage wound must be.

If the superficial fistula along the perianal circumference is longer, in order to ensure the smooth drainage of the lumen, it is necessary to make a cut at intervals of 2–3 cm in the middle of the fistula. Loose drainage should be undertaken between two adjacent incisions.

At present, pocket stitching is often used in the treatment of anal fistulas, and the edge of the wound is often clipped. All of these methods are not only beneficial to the wound drainage, but also in deflating the raw surface, which may speed up the duration of healing.

Usually, regardless of the number of external openings, in principle, all of them should be ectomized to form an open raw surface so as to facilitate drainage.

7.5 The Selection and Individualization of Treatment Program for Fistula-in-Ano

There is no technique available for treating all fistulas; therefore, the anal fistula treatment plan must be determined according to the etiology, anatomy, severity of the disease, whether there are any complications, and the surgeon's treatment experience. The pros and cons between sphincter cutoff range, cure rate, and anal function impairment should be traded off so as to develop a reasonable treatment plan. Meanwhile, for specific cases of anal fistula, the situation of anal fistula patients, combined with their physical state, mental state, etc., should also be taken into account. In order to develop targeted treatment plans, the choice of specific case treatment plans should both follow general principles and also meet the individual's particular circumstances.

7.5.1 Simple Anal Fistulas

7.5.1.1 Anal Fistulotomy
The cure rate of anal fistulotomy can reach 92–97% among particular patients. Recurrence is often associated with the following reasons: complicated anal fistulas, unclear position of the internal opening, and Crohn's disease.

At present, there is no consensus on how many anal sphincters can be cut without significantly affecting anal function. The rate of anal incontinence after anal fistulotomy is 0–73%. The large differences in incontinence rates are related to the definition of anal incontinence, the time of follow-up, and the degree of sphincter injury. Preoperative anal incontinence, recurrent anal fistula, complex anal fistula, previous history of anal fistula surgery, and even female anterior anal fistula are all risk factors for incontinence after surgery, so care must be taken when performing anal fistulotomy in such cases.

When performing anal fistulotomy, pocket stitching can reduce postoperative bleeding and shorten the duration of healing (4 weeks). The healing rates of anal fistulectomy and anal fistulotomy are similar; however, wound healing time of the former is longer because the wound is larger and the rate of incontinence is higher.

7.5.1.2 First-Stage Incision and Drainage with Anal Fistulotomy

When the anal fistula is associated with a perianal abscess, patients with clear internal openings can perform first-stage incision and drainage and anal fistulotomy. That way, they can avoid two surgeries. A meta-analysis of 405 patients enrolled in five studies indicated that the recurrence rate can be significantly reduced by abscising the sphincter muscle (anal fistulotomy or anal fistulectomy) during incision and drainage.

However, there is still controversy over performing anal fistulotomy while incising and draining the perianal abscess. Some people think that this one-stage operation increases the rate of anal incontinence. Also, although some patients can be cured by incision and drainage and may not need to undergo another operation, there might still be recurrence after the operation for others. Therefore, physicians should weigh the pros and cons of reduced recurrence rates against increased rates of anal incontinence before making a decision.

7.5.1.3 Fistula Debridement and Fibrin Glue Injection

Fibrin glue injection for anal fistula has the advantages of a simple method and good repeatability and avoids sphincter injury. Fibrin glue injection therapy is more suitable for the high-risk population prone to anal incontinence. However, the recurrence rate after fibrin injection is very high, and there are more failures.

Retrospective and prospective studies have shown that the healing rate of simple anal fistula treated with fibrin glue is 40–78%. Some control studies show that the healing rate of fibrin glue in treating simple low anal fistula is 50% (3/6), but the cure rate of anal fistulotomy is 100% (7/7). The incidence of anal incontinence was lower in both groups. It is suggested that fibrin glue injection therapy for simple anal fistula has no obvious advantages.

7.5.2 Complicated Anal Fistulas

7.5.2.1 Fistula Debridement and Fibrin Glue Injection

In a randomized controlled study published by Lindsey et al., 29 patients with complicated anal fistula were randomized to receive a mucosal advancement flap transfer or fibrin glue injection after seton and drainage. The healing rate of the fibrin glue group was higher (69% (9/13) vs. 13% (2/16), $P = 0.003$), and the rates of anal incontinence were similar in both groups (0/13 vs. 2/16). In nonrandomized controlled studies, the healing rate of fibrin glue in the treatment of complex anal fistula was 10–67%. Although the healing rate of fibrin glue in the treatment of complex anal fistula is relatively low, it can be considered as the initial treatment due to fewer complications.

7.5.2.2 Anal Fistula Plug

An anal fistula plug made of biological materials can suture internal openings and fill in the fistula. Some studies report that the healing rate of anal fistula plug in treating low anal fistula can reach 70–100%; however, its efficacy in complex anal fistula is poor. Early literature reported that the healing rate of anal fistula plug in the treatment of fistula in Crohn's disease was up to 80%. Patients in the same group that included all types of complicated anal fistula had an average cure rate of 83% after 12 months of follow-up.

However, most of the research reports failed to repeat the above results, and the cure rate of most of the studies on the treatment of anal fistula with anal fistula plug is less than 50%. The reduced cure rate may be related to the longer follow-up time. Due to fewer complications, good repeatability, and the lack of other ideal treatment methods, the fistula plug can be considered a good treatment for complicated anal fistula.

7.5.2.3 Rectal Mucosa Advancement Flap

Rectal mucosa advancement flap is a technique that can protect the sphincter muscle. Its specific operations include fistulous tract scraping and the normal proximal mucosal flap freeing (including anorectal mucosa, submucosa, and muscle layer) to cover the sutured fistula internal opening. The postoperative recurrence rate of this surgery is 13–56%. Combining fibrin glue failed to improve the cure rate. The associated factors for treatment failure were radiotherapy, Crohn's disease, active proctitis, rectovaginal fistula, malignancy, and the number of previous repair operations. Although the operation does not cut the anal sphincter, the rate of mild and moderate anal incontinence was still 7–38%. Postoperative anal pressure measurement indicated that both resting pressure and systolic pressure were reduced.

7.5.2.4 Seton and Fistulotomy in Stages

The goal of seton is to pass through the fistula, transforming the inflammatory process into a foreign body reaction that causes fibrosis around the sphincter. Seton is divided into cutting seton, slack seton, and virtual and real combination seton. The cutting seton is gradually tightened, and the fistula is cut down gradually within several weeks, thus resulting in part scar and healing. Loose seton acts as a drainage and reduces recurrence, which can be retained for a long duration or removed in the next treatment. The virtual and real combination seton is the combination of the cutting and slack seton: cutting seton in the first week, gradually cut a part of the high fistula; in the second to third week, the loose seton will play the role of drainage, and the stitches will be removed in 20 days and until the wound has healed. There are only four randomized controlled studies, but the results vary.

Seton for complicated anal fistula is usually performed in stages. Seton to control infection in the first stage, a few weeks later, secondary procedures (such as mucous advancement flap, fibrin glue injection, and anal plug tamping) will be performed. This can avoid cutting the sphincter. Due to the different techniques of the second phase operation, the cure rate of the threaded treatment is 62–100%. The rate of anal incontinence treated by staging and cutting seton is 0–54%. When anal incontinence occurs, the control of gas function is significantly worse than that of liquid or solid feces.

7.5.2.5 Ligation of Intersphincteric Fistula (LIFT)

LIFT is an operative procedure that ligates and cuts the fistula between the anal canal sphincters. The classic description includes drain seton for more than 8 weeks to promote fibrosis of the fistula; intersphincter incisions will be performed to separate the fistulas, ligate both ends, and remove; close the internal opening as much as possible and expand the external opening to facilitate drainage.

The technique does not theoretically cut the sphincter and does not impair anal sphincter function. Reported in the literature, the mean follow-up time was 3.8 months, and the cure rate was 57–94%. The recurrence rate was 6–18%. There is still some controversy about LIFT. Although it is recommended in foreign guides, the recurrence rate of this operation is higher, and there are certain requirements for indications.

7.5.3 Treatment of Anal Fistula in Crohn's Disease

The incidence of perianal disease in Crohn's disease ranges from 40 to 80%. Drug treatment of anal fistula in Crohn's disease is the first choice. Surgical treatment is used to control infection and is occasionally chosen as a treatment.

Antibiotic treatment is especially effective: 90% of patients respond to the treatment of arilin plus quinolone antibiotics (at least temporarily). Limited data have shown that azathioprine, 6-mercaptopurine, ciclosporin, and tacrolimus can also cure fistula in Crohn's disease. Infliximab is a human and mouse chimerical antibody that specifically blocks tumor necrosis factor α (TNF-α) and has been shown to improve the healing rate of anal fistula to 46%.

Surgical treatment of anal fistula in Crohn's disease must follow the principle of individualization, and decisions must be based on the degree of illness and severity of symptoms. Despite various treatment options, patients with severe fistula in Crohn's disease may still need to undergo rectal resection or permanent enterostomy.

7.5.3.1 Asymptomatic Crohn's Disease Anal Fistula Does Not Require Surgical Treatment

Fistula in Crohn's disease may be secondary to Crohn's disease or crypt infection. Regardless of the etiology, anal fistulas with no symptoms and local signs of infection can remain in a static state for a long time without requiring surgical treatment.

7.5.3.2 Symptomatic Simple Low Anal Fistula in Crohn's Disease Can Undergo Fistulotomy

All simple lower fistula in Crohn's disease involving or rarely involving the external sphincter can safely and effectively receive an anal fistulotomy. In view of the chronic course and high recurrence rate of that disease, sphincter function should be preserved as much as possible. All risk factors, especially the severity of anorectal disease, sphincter function, rectal compliance, presence of active proctitis, history of anorectal surgery, and defecate concordancy, should be considered before incision. The appropriate surgical cure rate for patients is 56–100%, the rate of mild anal incontinence is 6–12%, and the duration of healing requires 3–6 months. Anal incontinence may be associated with a previous history of anal fistula surgery.

7.5.3.3 The Complicated Anal Fistula of Crohn's Disease Can Be Treated Palliatively with Long-Term Drain Seton

In patients with complicated anal fistula in Crohn's disease, long-term (usually more than 6 weeks) seton is aimed at continuous drainage and preventing closure of the external opening of the anal fistula in order to smooth the drainage and control the development of inflammation. Even so, the repeated infection rate of patients with anal fistula is still 20–40%, and 8–13% of patients have different degrees of leakage. Recent data have shown a healing rate of 24–78% after induction therapy with drain seton combined with infliximab and 25–100% of patients responding effectively to infliximab maintenance therapy.

7.5.3.4 If the Rectal Mucosa Is Generally Normal, Complex Anal Fistula of Crohn's Disease Can Undergo Mucous Advancement Flap Metastasis

The complicated anal fistula of Crohn's disease without active proctitis can be treated by mucous advancement flap metastasis, the short-term cure rate is 64–75%, and the recurrence rate is positively correlated with the follow-up time. The short-term cure rate of Crohn's disease complicated by rectovaginal fistula is 40–50%. Patients with active proctitis can be treated by biologics first, and then with surgery after the disease is in remission.

7.5.3.5 Complex Anal Fistula of Crohn's Disease That Cannot Be Controlled May Require Permanent Neostomy or Rectum Resection

In a few cases of extensively crescendo complicated anal fistulas of Crohn's disease and in cases that are ineffective with medications and thread drainage, in order to control perianal infection, patients need to undergo enterostomy or rectectomy. Enterostomy is required in 31–49% of patients with complicated perianal Crohn's disease. Risk factors for permanent enterostomy and rectectomy include accompanied by colonic disease, persistent perianal infection, previous temporary neostomy, fecal incontinence, and stricture of the anus. Despite appropriate medication and minimally invasive treatments, 8–40% of patients require rectectomy to control persistent symptoms.

7.6 Nonradical Drainage or Drug Treatment Should Be Used in Some Patients

Not all patients are suitable for radical surgery. Sometimes nonradical treatment or expectant treatment to remiss symptoms and control the development of the disease may be more beneficial to patients. Expectant treatment is suitable for the following patients:

1. Those who have important organ diseases such as heart, brain, lung, liver, and kidney disease or have other surgical contraindications.
2. Those who have anal fistula associated with Crohn's disease and ulcerative colitis.
3. Those who have anal fistula with high position, too complex tendency, and the failure rate of operation greater than the success rate.
4. Those in whom anal fistula has not been cured by multiple operations, but there was mild or moderate incontinence of the anus, and reoperation may lead to further low anal function or even severe incontinence.
5. Patients who require expectant treatment.

Suggested Reading

1. Masahino Takano. Shi renjie compilation. Essence of anorectal diseases diagnosis and treatment. Beijing: biological medicine branch of chemical industry press, 2009, 137–166.
2. Cao Jixun. Hemorrhoidology of China. Chengdu: sichuan science and technology press, 2015, 165–170.
3. Huang Naijian. Chinese Proctology. Jinan: shandong science and technology press, 1996, 745–766.
4. American Society of Colorectal Surgeons. 2011 American guidelines for treatment of perianal abscess and anal fistula [J]. Chinese journal of gastrointestinal surgery, 2012, 15(6):640–643.
5. Cao Yongqing. Several ideas on the study of the standardization of anal fistula diagnosis and treatment [J]. Journal of traditional Chinese medicine, 2003, 44(z1):85–86.
6. Ren Donglin, Zhang Heng. Several key problems needing attention in the diagnosis and treatment of complicated anal fistula [J]. Chinese journal of gastrointestinal surgery, 2015, 18(12):1186–1192.
7. Cao Yongqing, Pan Yibin, Guo Xiutian et al. Clinical treatment strategies for anal fistula [J]. World journal of traditional Chinese medicine, 2010, 05(4):275–277.

Surgical Treatment of Anal Fistula

Renjie Shi and Lihua Zheng

Abstract

The anal fistula surgeon should be experienced in the necessary skills, including correctly finding and managing the internal opening and primary lesions, handling the anal sphincter, working with the complex fistula, making the smooth drainage wound, handling the soft tissue around the fistula, handling the coexisting lesions, handling the perforation of rectum, etc. There are many treatment methods for anal fistula, which can be divided into three categories: incision, seton therapy, and sphincter preserving, each of which has its own indications and limitations. In China, seton therapy has been widely used in the treatment of anal fistula since the Ming Dynasty and has undergone six major changes. The function of anal fistula thread is to cut the anal sphincter chronically so that the broken end of anal sphincter remains continuous through the scar while acting as the drainage at the same time. Methods of seton therapy include low incision and high thread-ligating therapy, low incision and high virtual seton therapy, combination of virtual and real seton, tunnel thread drawing, traditional medicine seton therapy, catheter drainage therapy, long-term drainage seton therapy, etc. There are still some controversies about seton therapy. Sphincter preserving surgery is the development direction of anal fistula treatment, which is carried out earlier and has rich experience in Japan. LIFT and mucosal flap advancement are the most popular sphincter preserving methods.

Keywords

Anal fistula · Operation · Handcraft Operation method · Seton therapy · Sphincter preserving surgery · LIFT · Mucosal flap advancement

R. Shi (✉)
Department of Anorectal Surgery, Affiliated Hospital of Nanjing University of Traditional Chinese Medicine, Nanjing, Jiangsu, China

L. Zheng
Department of Proctology, China-Japan Friendship Hospital, Beijing, China

In principle, anal fistula needs surgery to achieve a radical cure. The efficacy of anal fistula surgery and the incidence of complications are related to the operative method and depend on the operative skills and experience of the surgeon.

8.1 Basic Techniques of Anal Fistula Surgery

8.1.1 Intraoperative Techniques for Finding and Handling the Internal Orifice

8.1.1.1 Intraoperative Techniques for Finding the Internal Orifice

Accurate finding of the inner opening is one of the prerequisites for radical treatment of anal fistula. If the positioning of the internal orifice is not correct, the internal orifice treatment will not be in place, leading to the complete failure of anal fistula surgery. The ability to search for an internal orifice during surgery is largely dependent on the skill and experience of the surgeon.

The internal orifice is mostly located in the anal sinus on the dentate line, the internal orifice of horseshoe-shaped anal fistula is mostly located in the dentate line behind the anus, and the internal orifice of simple anal fistula is mostly located in the dentate line of the same position as the external orifice of the fistula. Although it is possible to infer the approximate orientation of the interior orifice from the position of the outside orifice according to Goethe's Rule or Solomon's Law, this is not accurate. So Goethe's Rule is often used to guide preoperative examination and rarely intraoperative examination. During the operation, palpation, methylene blue, and probe examination are the main methods to examine the internal orifice.

During digital examination, the typical anal fistula opening presents a small induration that can be touched under the mucous membrane of the dentine line during palpation. The anal recess with a deep depression can be seen when the anus is examined by anoscope. If the recess is deep, it is likely to be the internal opening.

However, sometimes the characteristics of the internal opening of patients with anal fistula are not obvious, and the typical characteristics of the internal orifice cannot be found before and during the operation. In the intraoperative exploration of such patients, the fistula can be extracted from the outer orifice, and a segment of the fistula can be extracted and pulled outward by holding the outer mouth, and there will be an obvious depression at the corresponding inner mouth so that the location of the inner mouth can be inferred. In the operation, the primary abscess can be found by cutting open the internal and external sphincter muscle and then through the anal duct to find the internal orifice connected with the primary abscess.

8.1.1.2 Tips for Handling the Internal Orifice

The treatment of the internal orifice depends on the surgical procedure. Most of the existing anal fistula surgical methods need to cut and remove the internal opening and separate the internal opening to create both edges and the adjacent anal sinus ligation, which can improve the thoroughness of the internal orifice treatment and at the same time prevent postoperative bleeding of the wound mucosa, which is conducive to wound drainage.

When there is a large scleroma or obvious inflammation in the internal orifice, it is necessary to remove the scleroma and severely inflamed tissues. However, excision of these tissues can easily lead to large defects in the inner mouth and prolong the healing time. In this regard, some surgical methods advocate suturing the wound surface of the inner orifice or covering it with a mucous flap. It is very important to eliminate tension when suturing the wound surface and moving the flap. The transferred flap must maintain good blood supply and prevent the formation of hematoma.

If the internal orifice treatment is not in place, it can easily lead to anal fistula recurrence. In the anal fistula sphincter retention operation, the treatment method of cutting out the fistula at the inner opening is often adopted. If the treatment is not good, it will easily lead to partial fistula residue, which is the main reason why the recurrence rate of anal fistula retention sphincter operation is higher than that of open surgery.

8.1.2 Techniques for Dealing with Primary Lesions Between the Internal and External Sphincters

Improper treatment of the primary abscess is the most common cause of anal fistula recurrence, and good treatment of the primary abscess and primary fistula is the second most important requirement for the healing of anal fistula.

8.1.2.1 Techniques for Finding Primary Lesions

The primary intermuscular lesion can be found from the inner or outer opening. The method to search for the primary lesion from the external opening is as follows: fistula is cut around the external opening, fistula at the external opening is clamped, and then the fistula is exfoliated along the outer wall of the fistula until the exfoliation reaches the internal and external sphincter muscle, and then the primary abscess lesion is found between the muscles. The way to find the primary lesion from the inner opening is that after treating the inner opening, the primary abscess can be exposed by separating it outward along the primary fistula and separating the internal and external sphincter muscle. The above two methods can also be used to find primary lesions.

8.1.2.2 Management Skills of the Primary Abscess

The basic principle for treating primary lesions is to remove the primary abscess as thoroughly as possible. It is recommended to remove the hard intermuscular tissue until the hard tissue cannot be touched. However, it is necessary to prevent excessive excision of tissue from causing unnecessary damage and leading to excessive tissue loss between the internal and external sphincters. If the lacunae that are produced between the internal and external sphincter muscles after excising the primary hair abscess are bigger, the surgeon can break the end with the external sphincter muscle, external sphincter muscle subcutaneous ministry or gluteus maximus, and find a tissue to make the pedicle muscle flap filling after creating a cavity again. The suture should then be fixed.

In anal fistula that is newly formed, when the tissue does not have apparent hardness between muscles, the surgeon should only scratch the local purulent area and clean the tissue, and next open drainage of wound cavity should take place. If the fistula is small and the primary abscess is small, the fistula can be cut open or removed, and the wound surface can be opened for drainage without special treatment for the primary abscess.

8.1.3 Anal Sphincter Management Skills

Most anal fistula operations involve the management of the anal sphincter. Moderation and necessity should be taken into account when dealing with the anal sphincter. Improper incision or resection of the anal sphincter muscle will increase anal function damage. However, if the surgeon is too worried about injury to the anal sphincter muscle and does not make the correct incision, it may affect the treatment of the focal point. Because of this, or because of the impact of drainage, this might also lead to anal fistula recurrence or delayed healing.

Grasping the skills of anal sphincter degree in anal fistula surgery: (1) since the subcutaneous fistula does not involve an anal sphincter, it can be directly cut. (2) External sphincter muscle subcutaneous and superficial can be cut directly, but the anterior anal fistula and sphincter muscle are particularly weak. Even if only opening the external sphincter muscle subcutaneous or superficial, the surgeon should be cautious. (3) In principle, deep external sphincter muscle and puborectalis muscle cannot be cut directly. If necessary, the method of thread hanging is usually used for the incision to maintain the integrity of the anorectal ring. (4) When incisions are made on the front and side of the anus, the incisions on the back of the anus are more likely to lead to postoperative anal deformation and loose closure, thus requiring attention. Especially in women, care should be taken to avoid as much as possible cutting too far in the front of the anus or the side when directly opening the anal sphincter. It is recommended to use the method of strangle cut slowly. (5) The anal sphincter cannot be cut in more than three places at the same time. Because the anal sphincter has the effect of continuous closure of the anus, it is easy for this function to deteriorate if it is cut off, and some patients will have sequelae such as anal moisture and overflow.

The number and necessity of incisions to the sphincter muscle are related to the operative style and the surgeon's concept and clinical experience. Even for the same anal fistula, the degree of sphincter injury often varies greatly with different procedures or by different operators. As surgeons, we should improve theoretical and clinical literacy, accumulate more experience and skills, fully weigh the pros and cons while ensuring the cure when facing specific cases, ensure anal function as far as possible, and pay attention to protecting the anal sphincter during the operation.

8.1.4 Management Techniques of Fistulas

When dealing with fistulas, the management of the main canal is critical. The main tract should be treated thoroughly, and the drainage of the wound should be maintained unobstructed. Small branch ducts can be scratched after the use of elastic bands, such as loose wire drainage. Superficial and obvious fistulas are easy to follow up on, but deep fistulas depend on the surgeon's touch and experience.

In general, when the canal cavity is small or the wall tissue is soft, only incision or partial resection of the fistula is performed in the anofistulectomy. However, when the fistula is complex, the tube is large or deep, the contents of the lumen are dirty, and the inflammation of surrounding tissues is severe, it is necessary to remove the purulent and rotting tissue in the fistula cavity and remove the fistula wall as far as possible.

When necessary, the wound surface after total resection of the main tract or branch canal can also be sutured. The key is to ensure that the lesion is completely removed and tightly sutured without leaving a cavity.

Fistula under the rectal mucosa or between the upper muscles may lead to rectal stenosis, which is difficult to remove completely. If the treatment of the inner orifice and primary lesions is thoroughly advanced, as long as the lumen is scraped clean, the fistula can be cut off longitudinally in one or two places. The rectal stenosis should also be relieved after cutting.

8.1.5 Wound Management Skills

The anal wound is easy to be contaminated by feces, secretions, poor exposure, and poor drainage. Effective countermeasures for these conditions are to make the anal wound drainage unobstructed. Smooth drainage is a necessary condition for the smooth healing of anal wounds.

In order to ensure smooth drainage of the anal wound, it is very important to take the following steps. In wound drainage, we should extend and expand the anal wound appropriately. The size of the drainage site should be determined according to the size, depth, and length of the anal wound. In general, the deeper the anal fistula is and the longer it is, the deeper, wider, and longer the drainage wound should be. Our experience is that the width and depth of the drainage wound are closely related to the healing time of the wound, and the deeper and wider the wound, the longer the healing time. However, the length of the wound does not affect the healing time, so we usually use the method of extending the drainage wound and not increasing the width of the wound as far as possible when making the drainage wound, which can not only effectively improve the drainage but also facilitate the early healing of the wound.

In general, if the fistula extends outside the anus for a long time, the length of incision of the fistula and the drainage wound surface is enough. However, if the fistula is short and deep, the wound needs to be extended and expanded outward, making the whole wound appear like a water drop. In the case of horseshoe-shaped fistula, the wound surface is often made into an arrow shape when it is extended outward for drainage due to the influence of the tailbone. Although the drainage wound outside the anus looks large, because the drainage is unobstructed, the healing is much faster than the wound inside the anus. Therefore, under normal circumstances, the drainage wound must be made small inside the anus and a large outside of the anus. This is expected to achieve the goal of healing the wound gradually from the inside out or at the same time.

The surface of drainage wound must be smooth without depression to ensure smooth drainage. If the wound has a depression, secretion will be easily retained and will affect the smooth healing of the wound. Therefore, the bottom and edge of the wound should be trimmed in order to ensure the smooth drainage of the wound.

8.1.6 Soft Tissue Management Techniques

The complete function of the anus is not only related to the anal sphincter but also to the soft tissue inside and outside the anal canal. When there is soft tissue defect inside the anal canal, even though the anal sphincter muscle is retained very well, it can also decrease anal function and the anus can easily become wet or leak liquid. Therefore, in anal fistula surgery, injury to the soft tissues around the anal fistula should be reduced as much as possible, and the soft tissues of the anus should be retained as much as possible.

8.1.7 Management Skills of Coexisting Other Anal Diseases

Anal fistula is often combined with internal hemorrhoids and external hemorrhoids, anal nipple hypertrophy, anal fissure, etc. Some of these concurrent lesions sometimes have symptoms, and some have no symptoms all the time. These coexisting lesions cannot be treated at the same time during anal fistula surgery, and these lesions are prone to postoperative swelling and enlargement, pain, bleeding, and other symptoms. External hemorrhoids and hypertrophic anal nipples at the wound edge can also affect the drainage of the anal fistula wound surface or directly put pressure on the wound surface to make wound healing difficult. Therefore, in anal fistula surgery, we also advocate simultaneous treatment of these wound edge lesions, even if there are no symptoms, so as to eliminate the impact on wound drainage and healing and prevent them from happening in the first place.

In the treatment of coexisting lesions, internal or external hemorrhoids can be excised or ligated. Anal papillary hypertrophy can be removed by ligation or direct resection. Anal fissure can be treated by excising redundant skin and anal papillary hypertrophy with excising the hard fissure and changed tissue. However, there is no need to cut off the anal sphincter muscle because this will decrease anal function.

8.1.8 Management Techniques for Rectal Perforation

Rectal perforation mainly occurs in cases of high intermuscular fistula and pelvic rectal fossa fistula. For rectal perforation, in principle, the internal orifice and the primary abscess should be treated well, the perforation part is well drained, and if necessary, the drainage line should be temporarily suspended. After the perforated part has subsided, the drainage line can be removed. It can also be treated through fasting and using central venous nutrition to control defecation. Generally, there is no need to create a temporary artificial anus.

8.2 Classification and Surgical Methods of Anal Fistula

Radical operation of anal fistula is basically based on the theory of the "infection of anal recess gland." The key aspects of operation include three aspects: first, the treatment of the inner mouth and primary lesions; second, the treatment of the sphincter; and third, wound drainage.

With regard to the treatment of the internal orifice and primary lesion, most surgical methods adopt the method of incision or excision. Only the coring-out operation of Takao Moriya, the submucosal primary lesion resection of Yasuo Yamamoto, the subcutaneous primary lesion resection of Shoji Sumie, and the intersphincter fistula ligation (LIFT) of Arun are special in the treatment of the inner opening (detailed discussion is given in the following corresponding surgical procedures).

Regarding the treatment of the sphincter, the main difference lies in the method of incision and treatment. In the author's opinion, according to the different treatment methods of the sphincter, the radical operation of anal fistula can be divided into three categories: anal fistulectomy, anal fistula thread-drawing and incision seton therapy, and the anal fistula retained sphincter method. As for intraoperative wound healing techniques, such as open suture, partial suture, full suture, bag suture, flap or mucous flap coverage, biomaterial filling, anal fistula endoscopic video auxiliary treatment, etc., the target is basically to provide the best condition for wound healing. The author believes that these techniques are not the core techniques for the treatment of anal fistula, but in essence, they are auxiliary methods in the treatment of anal fistula. Therefore, according to the different treatment methods of anal sphincter in this book, the author divides anal fistula surgery into three categories: incisional surgery, thread-drawing incision seton surgery, and sphincter retention surgery.

Operation points: routine disinfection, local anesthesia, or Yaoshu anesthesia. If there is an external orifice, a small amount of methylene blue can be injected from the external orifice to check whether there is staining and the staining position of the preset gauze in the anal canal so as to confirm whether the fistula is perforated and the position of the internal orifice. The probe should be inserted from the outer opening and gently probed along the pipeline. Under the guidance of finger touch, it should be pierced through the inner mouth and then tightened. All fistulas should be cut along the probe (Fig. 8.1). If the tube is bent, or the lumen is small, it can be cut at the same time as exploration and forward to the inner orifice until all fistulas are cut.

If there is no external opening or closure of the external opening, a small incision can be made at the top of the external end of the pipe or at the closed external opening to open the fistula, and the probe can be put into the pipe through this. Then, all the fistulas can be cut out after the probe is out of the internal opening.

If there is no outside mouth, but there is purulent in the inside mouth, one end of the probe can be bent into a hook. Under the guidance of the crypt hook, the probe can be probed into the inside mouth and tube, and all fistulas can be cut along the probe or from inside out.

After incision of the fistula, the tube wall should be scraped and trimmed to scrape away the necrotic tissue and cut off the very rough tube wall and uneven tissue (Fig. 8.2). Generally, it is not neces-

8.2.1 Anofistulectomy

8.2.1.1 Anal Fistula Incision (Excision)

It is mainly applicable to low simple anal fistula and high anal fistula where some anorectal rings have become stiff. However, for anal fistula in the front and anal fistula with weak sphincter muscle, especially those of female patients, special caution should be taken in the operation of anal fistulectomy, and it is recommended to adopt the surgical method of resecting and hanging the line or retaining the sphincter.

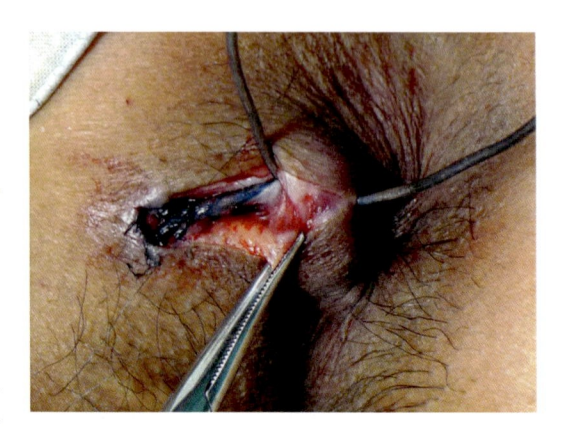

Fig. 8.1 Anal fistula incision

sary to remove all the tube walls in order to reduce tissue defects and shorten the course of treatment. During operation, the branch should be carefully explored. If there is a branch tube, the branch tube can be cut if the branch tube is relatively short. If the branch tube is long or bent, it can be treated with anal fistula incision and drainage.

After fistula incision, the wall of the tube should be scratched and repaired to remove corrupt tissue, and the thick and hard wall and uneven tissue should be cut off (Fig. 8.3). In general, it is not necessary to remove all tube walls to reduce tissue defects and shorten the course of treatment. The branch canal should be carefully explored during the operation. If there is a branch tube, it can be cut short. If the branch tube is longer or bent, it can be treated as an anal fistula incision and drainage should take place.

Hemostatic treatment of the wound should be performed before the operation is completed, and the edge and bottom of the wound should be repaired. The cross section of the wound should be shaped like a "V" with a large inner and outer side, so as to make the wound smooth and facilitate drainage and create favorable conditions for the smooth healing of the wound.

8.2.1.2 Anal Fistula Incision and Drainage

It is also known as open anal fistula surgery. It is mainly suitable for the treatment of low position, long pipeline, or curved anal fistula.

Operation points: the treatment of the main pipeline and internal orifice is equivalent to low anal fistulectomy. In order to reduce injury to the sphincter, it is not suitable to open the fistula obliquely. The main part of the sphincter is radially cut, and the drainage is extended outward.

The branches are carefully explored, and all fistulas are managed one by one. If the fistula is long but no more than 3 cm, a radial incision can be made at the end of the tube to loosen ligation between the incision and the main incision to facilitate drainage. If the length of the pipelines exceeds 3 cm, all openings can be made every 2–3 cm in the pipelines, and the rubber bands or skin sheets are relaxed with respect to drainage between all adjacent incisions (Fig. 8.4).

8.2.1.3 Anal Fistula Resection and Suture

Anal fistula resection is mainly used for the treatment of straight low simple anal fistula without obvious signs of infection.

Operating instructions: make the wound fresh and soft after incision of the fistula and excision of all the wall tissue. Then stop the bleeding completely, rinse the wound, and suture the wound with a full layer. Do not leave dead cavity when suturing and try to be tension-free. Defecation should be able to be controlled within 3–5 days after surgery, and stitches are removed 1 week later.

Anal fistula resection and suture can easily lead to anal fistula recurrence and operation failure due to postoperative infection, which may complicate the condition and prolong the course of treatment. Therefore, it is necessary to strictly adhere to the

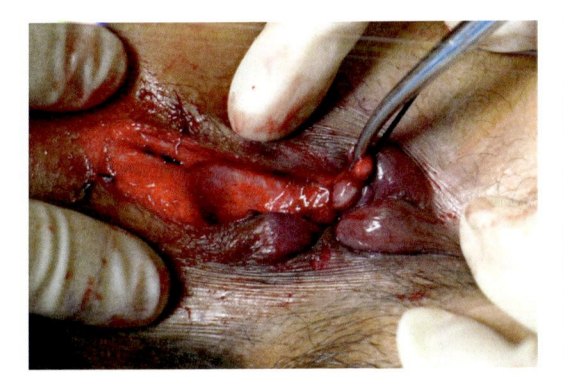

Fig. 8.2 Anal fistula incision to ligate the wound on both sides of the inner opening

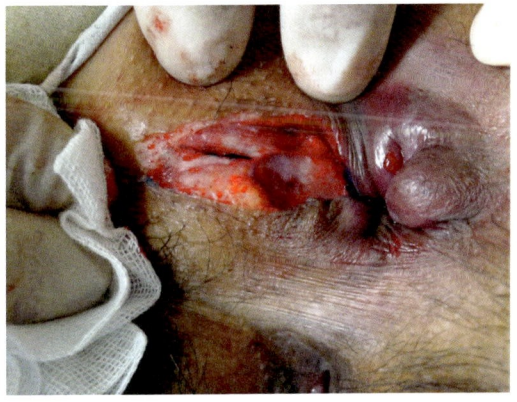

Fig. 8.3 After anal fistula incision has removed part of the wall

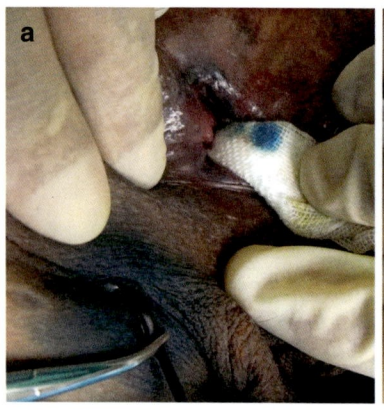

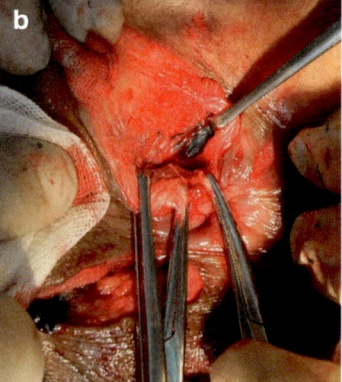

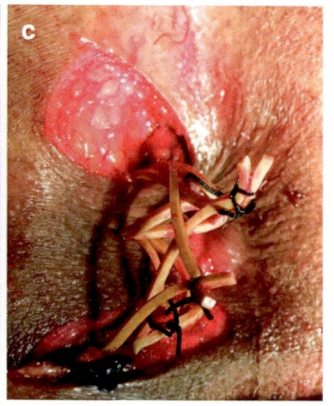

Fig. 8.4 Anal fistula incision and drainage. (**a**) After injecting methylene blue from the left front outer port, there is methylene blue overflow at the posterior tooth line. (**b**) The main incision is made on the posterior side. After opening the posterior fistula, a stained fistula is seen. (**c**) A rubber band is placed between the front and rear incisions drainage

indications and conduct adequate doctor–patient communication. In order to prevent postoperative infection, the intestinal tract should be prepared before the operation, and appropriate antibiotics should be used between 3 and 5 days after the operation to prevent incision infection.

8.2.1.4 Anal Fistula Resection and Semi-suture

It is suitable for the treatment of low anal fistula that is longer or has more branches.

Operation method: the main canal should be opened for drainage after the treatment of anal fistulectomy, and the fistulas or branches outside the main canal should be treated with resection and suture to reduce the wound surface and shorten the wound healing time. The wound treated in this way is half open and half stitched. Semi-suture of anal fistula resection is suitable for the treatment of low anal fistula that is longer or has more branches.

8.2.1.5 Hanley Method

Also known as the open orifice drainage method, mainly applied to the internal orifice in the anus behind the sciatic rectal socket fistula or posterior horseshoe fistula. The Hanley operation is suitable for anal fistula with small bilateral branches but not for those with large bilateral branches.

Operation points: after excision of the inner mouth, the wound should be made to extend outward, part of the internal sphincter and external sphincter are cut open, and the posterior anal space is exposed to deal with the primary lesion. After scratching and trimming the scar tissue, the wound is extended outward to make its drainage smooth. The necrotic tissue in the fistula extending to both sides is usually not treated by incision, but a small incision drainage can be made at the end of fistulas if necessary (Fig. 8.5).

8.2.1.6 Goligher-UI Method

It is also referred to as the open drainage of anal fistula. In 1970, Goligher designed this method for horseshoe anal fistula, and in 1982, UI improved the Goligher method, so it is called the Goligher-UI method in Japan. It is suitable for the treatment of complex anal fistula such as ischiorectal fossa fistula.

Operation points: the treatment of the internal orifice, the treatment of the primary intermuscular lesion, and the treatment of the drainage wound are the same as the Hanley method. A wide and narrow open wound is made behind the anus to remove infected and necrotic tissue, remove scar tissue, and scratch clean the wound. For the branches on both sides, Goligher adopts the method of cutting open fistulas that extend to both sides. The improvement of the Goligher method is to make triangular cutting and cutting in the middle sections of the fistulas that extend to both sides so as to reduce injuries. The fistulas

8 Surgical Treatment of Anal Fistula

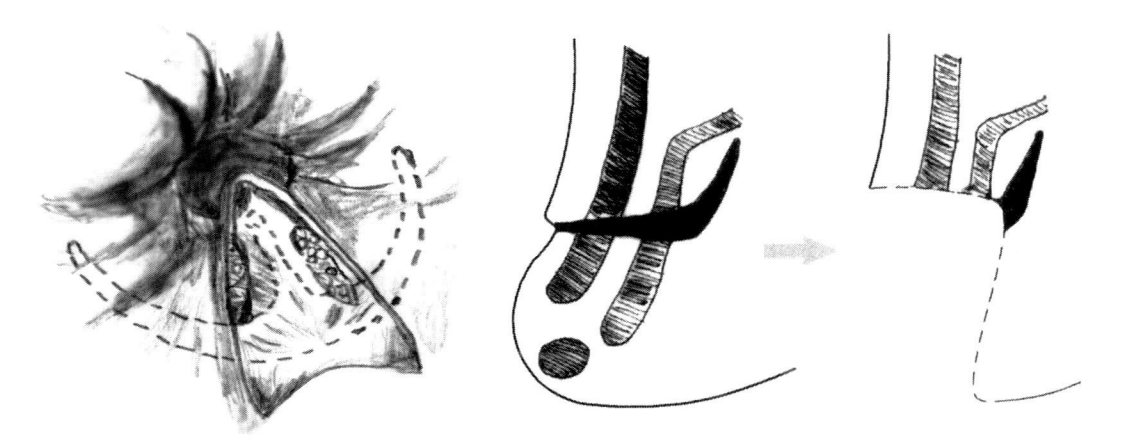

Fig. 8.5 Hanley's technique. When the ends of the branch pipes extending to both sides are thin, only the internal mouth and the original abscess are removed, the wound is open and drained, and the ends of the branch pipes on both sides remain

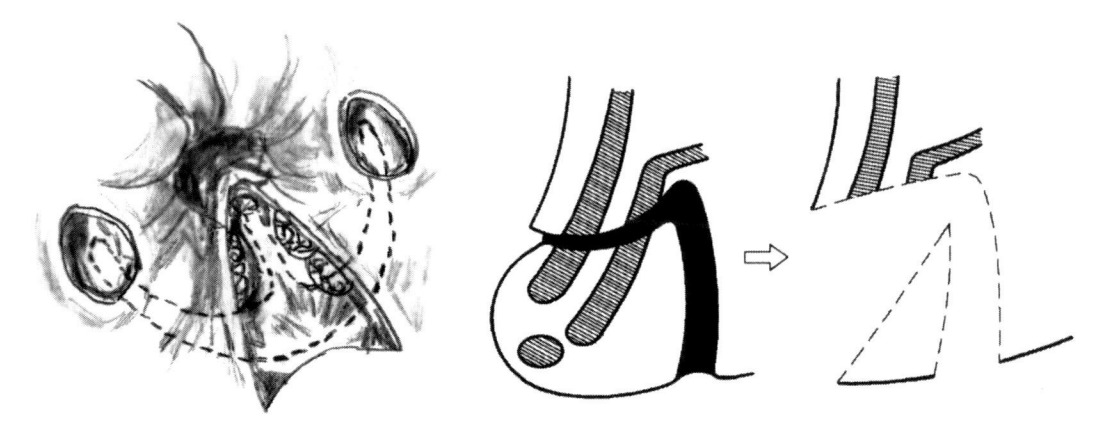

Fig. 8.6 Goligher's procedure for ischiorectal fossa surgery. When the branches extending to both sides are thick, only the internal mouth and the primary abscess are removed and the wound is open for drainage, and both sides open for drainage

are scratched clean, and wound drainage is conducted (Figs. 8.6 and 8.7).

8.2.2 Anal Fistula Thread-Drawing

8.2.2.1 The Origins

Thread-Drawing Was First Recorded in the Ming Dynasty

The thread-hanging therapy in China was first recorded in Gujin Yitong written by Xu Chunfu, a doctor in the Ming dynasty (1556 AD). The book records: "Chunfu's method of treating anal fistula, ... The far-reaching influence must be the thread-hanging therapy in "Yonglei Qian Fang," which can cure anal fistula thoroughly." Therefore, the term "seton" was first put forward in the "Yonglei Qian Fang," which is probably the earliest record of thread-drawing in China.

Previously, in almost all works of traditional Chinese medicine on anorectal diseases, it was believed that "Yonglei Qian Fang" had been lost. In fact, the book was not lost. At present, there are two editions printed by the People's Health Publishing House and Medical Science and Technology Publishing House, respectively. The author checked the two versions of the book and

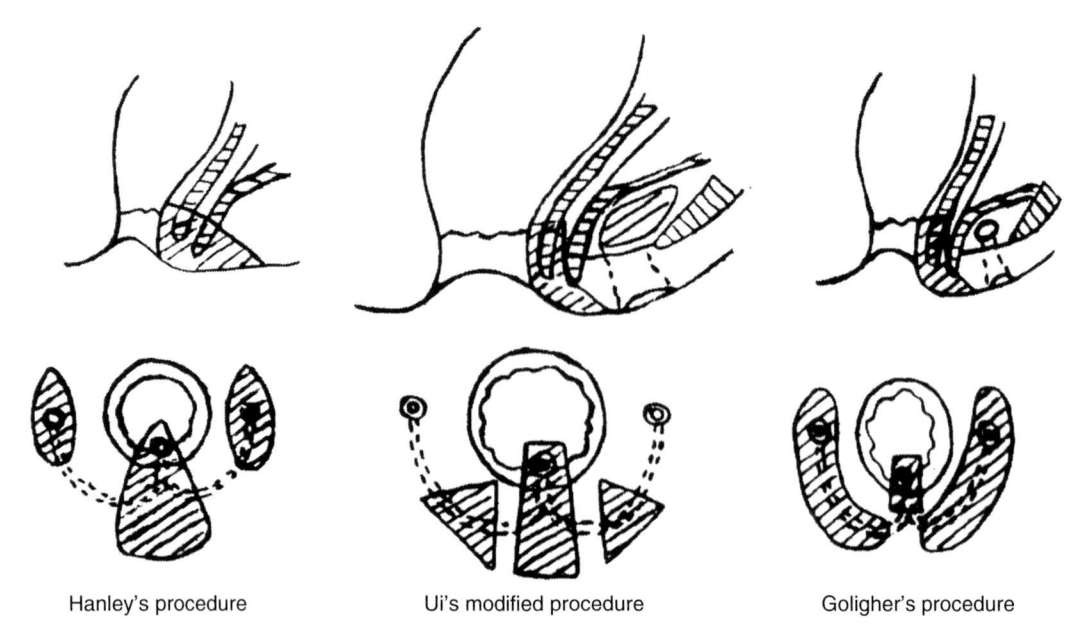

Fig. 8.7 Comparison of Hanley's procedure, Goligher's procedure, and UI's modified procedure

found that the contents are basically the same. However, the author could not find the relevant contents on the hanging line of anal fistula in "Yonglei Qian Fang" in these two editions, only the content of ligating of hemorrhoids by boiling the thread of Daphne genkwa root. Are the relevant pages or contents of the original book lost? This needs further research.

Anal Fistula Thread-Drawing Therapy in the Ming Dynasty Was Quite Mature

In "Gujin Yitong," the origin of thread-hanging therapy, the method of making the medicine line, the method of thread-hanging operation, the indication of thread-hanging therapy, the change of condition after thread hanging, the course of treatment, the curative effect, and even the mechanism of treatment were introduced comprehensively. The method of making the medicine line introduced in this book is "[to treat] external hemorrhoids and anal fistula, scrotal abscess, acute pyogenic infection of perineum, gluteal abscess. Roots of Daphne genkwa (no matter how much, pound the juice in the Tong Tiao, slow fire boil into an ointment, put raw silk thread into the ointment and boil for a long time until the ointment becomes thicker. Let the line dry in shade, and the ointment is retained for later use)." Indications are as follows: "when the anal fistula has more branches and a longer course of disease, although the San Pin Ding Zi is used to eliminate necrotic tissues and promote granulation, it is only for the treatment of low anal fistula. For high anal fistula, hanging thread therapy in "Yonglei Qian Fang" can almost always cure it". The hanging operation method is: "regardless of the number of sores, use grass to explore a hole, lead the line out of the intestinal, drop the plumb, and let hanging to take quick effect." The expected course of treatment was: "10 days or half a month, and no more than 20 days." Curative effect is: "The thread passes through the anus, if the hammer falls off, it cures a hundred times without perforating the sore, the goose tube disappears, and the skin returns to normal after 7 days." The treatment mechanism is as follows: "the medicine thread dips, the enteric muscle grows with time, the spot is replenished. Water flows down the line, like the dike, and the water has returned to being submersible. After all flows away with the flood, is there still a flood?"

At the same time, the book details the clinical application of how to hang the line, how to tie the knot after hanging the line, what to do when encountering an area difficult to pierce through, etc. Details include: "a fistula with three carbuncles, regardless of how many dozen sores, the choice to cure the anus is with the Irisensata Thunb. If there is a hole through the bowel, first bend the silver bar, dig into the valley road and hook out the straw. Thread six or seven inches of one end into a flexible buckle. Do not pull the head of the grass lead through the large intestine, the thread untangling head is one inch long inside the buckle, tie three, four or five cents onto the end to hang down, when sitting and sleeping keep clothes from sticking, quick results are desirable. Wash the line early every day for about five minutes long, leave one inch, the thread lasts 7 days and is more than three inches below the line. If the source is blocked, with no perforation and no abscess, the goose tube is changed, first remove it all. The sore is close to the anus for 10 days, then the semilunar line comes down through the anus, and it will drop after 20 days. If 7 days after the fall, the paracubic sores are still wet, the line must be hung again. If it cannot be pierced, dip the needle into the paper instead of sticking it until it hurts. That is, at the zigzag point, thrice pass the threading. When the line falls, use Shengji powder." The details of the relevant content are so clear, it would have been difficult to achieve this amount of detail without skilled and frequent practice. Therefore, it must have been put in practice many times, indicating that the therapy was already quite mature in clinical use at the time.

"Gu Jin Yi Tong"'s record of string therapy was so detailed mainly because the author himself was a patient of anal fistula and a beneficiary of string therapy. It is written in the book: "to have suffered from this disease for 17 years, I have read a lot of books, learned the ancient ways, received useless treatments, exposed myself to poison and worried about intaking food and sleep. After meeting Li Chunshan of Jiang You, he cooked the string of common turnip only and hung the large intestine. In more than 70 days only he achieved full success." From this, we can know that Xu Chunfu's thread-hanging therapy was learned from Li Chunshan, and he had personal experience of its application.

The Contents of Thread-Drawing Have Been Enriched Since Ancient Times with Modern Medicine, But There Has Been No Breakthrough

"Surgery Dacheng": "if you use thread hanging, if there are many holes, treat one hole first, and then every few days treat another hole." It detailed the thread-hanging treatment method of multiple external openings or multiple fistulas.

"Yi Men Bu Yao" pointed out that "if the patient is a virtual person, hanging the line method cannot be used and it is easy for the task to turn into an incurable labor." "Virtual people" are those that were found to be contraindications to hanging the line method. This is still of great significance. Currently, for patients with abnormal wound healing of Crohn's anal fistula and tuberculous anal fistula, it is forbidden in principle to use tight thread treatment.

"Surgery Illustrated" contained the atlas of "anal tube probes," "anal needles," "sickle knives," and so on, enabling later generations to have an intuitive understanding of the instruments used by doctors at the time for anorectal surgery.

The Real Reform of Thread Therapy Came After the Founding of New China

Since the founding of the People's Republic of China, thread-linked therapy has been continuously reformed and innovated by specialists in anorectal surgery in China, and its treatment pool has expanded from single anal fistula to perianal abscess, rectal stenosis, constipation, anal fissure, and other diseases, and its treatment mechanism has been further recognized. In its usage, continuous improvement has been made, from the initial drug line gravity hanging through the rubber band hanging line, to low incision high hanging line, virtual hanging line, virtual and real hanging line together with a series of changes. It has now become one of the most common traditional methods in the clinical application of anorectal treatment.

8.2.2.2 The Evolution of Thread Hanging

Since it was recorded in the Ming dynasty, thread-hanging therapy has been applied in clinics and recorded in the medical books of past dynasties. However, the thread-hanging therapy now in use is very different from the one Xu Chunfu talked about. In my opinion, there have been at least six major changes in the current thread-hanging therapy compared with Xu's original method.

The Change from Gravity Hanging Line to Daily Tightening Line

Because there is no textual research on thread-hanging therapy in "Yonglei Qian Fang" at present, it can only be analyzed by comparing the thread-hanging therapy in "Gu Jin Yi Tong." The "YiMen BuYao" recorded, "use a thin copper needle to create the medicine line, the right hand holds the needle to be inserted into the fistula, the left hand holds the thick spicule to be inserted into the anus, hook out the needle and medicine line, tie a knot, gradually tighten, add buttons to the end of the medicine line to pull it down, the pipe is open for 7 days, mix medicine into the raw muscle, the wound should be closed in a month." This shows that its method is a daily tight hanging line therapy and is different from "Gu Jin Yi Tong"'s gravity hanging line method, so it can be regarded as the earliest alteration to the hanging line therapy.

The Change from Using a Drug Wire to a Rubber Band

The traditional thread-hanging therapy (Fig. 8.8) uses medicinal thread, which is a raw silk thread boiled and soaked with the root of Daphne. In the process of use or in the drug line, it is sprinkled with Jiuyi Dan and other drugs. The thread itself contains the drug or can have characteristics of the drug.

When hanging the drug wire, insert the thread into the fistula through the outer opening and tie a movable knot to make a ring after piercing the inner opening. Because the thread itself does not have the force of contraction, copper or iron and other weights should be hung on the thread ring

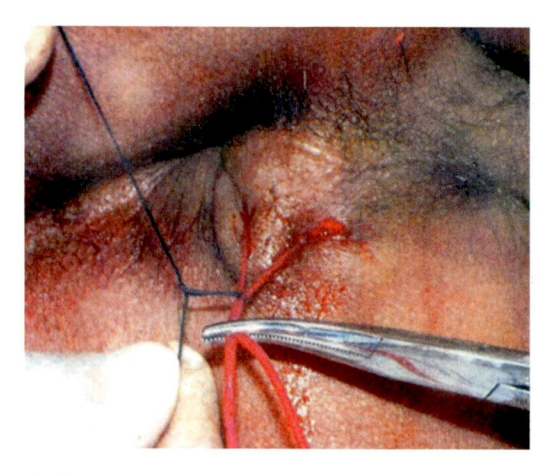

Fig. 8.8 Anal fistula's traditional medicine thread hanging therapy

after hanging to slowly open the fistula. As the fistula is gradually opened from the inside out, the wound grows from the inside out, with a high success rate, good protection of the anal function, and satisfactory appearance after healing. These are the advantages of traditional thread-hanging therapy. Traditional suture therapy often takes more than 1 or a half months to open all fistulas. At the same time, the drug line needs to be tightened several times after hanging. After hanging heavy weights on the drug line, the pain is greater and brings inconvenience to patients' lives and walking. These are the disadvantages of traditional thread-hanging therapy.

For this reason, since the 1960s, rubber bands have been gradually used instead of medical threads. Because the rubber band is low in cost, easy to obtain, and has its own contraction force, after hanging the string, by tightening the rubber band and using the contraction force of the rubber band itself, the fistula can be slowly opened without hanging an iron block on the line, and it is cut gradually. The effect is continuous, controllable, and rapid, which greatly shortens the time for the thread to cut off the fistula. It also simplifies the surgical procedures and post-operative care and facilitates patient activities after surgery. Such hanging lines are also called elastic hanging lines. However, the author believes that the use of rubber bands to replace medical threads is not perfect. The most obvious shortcoming is that the cutting effect of the rubber band thread-hanging therapy is not from the upward or downward, or from deep to shallow, but from the surroundings to the center. After the fistula and the sphincter are cut, the distance between the muscle ends is large, and the protection of the anal function is not as good as the traditional medicine thread-hanging treatment.

The use of ordinary surgical silk thread to replace drug thread hanging is another reform of the hanging line treatment method. However, at present, such thread hanging is hardly used for real thread hanging (tight thread hanging). It is mainly used for thread hanging and drainage. A total of 10–20 silk threads are used to hang the fistula and are knotted into a ring to prevent slippage. This kind of loose hanging thread has none of the traditional effects of the medical thread itself. Although Jiuyidan and other medicines can be attached to the wet silk thread when changing dressing, the adsorption effect of the silk thread is noticeably inferior to traditional medicine thread, and the thread is not as easy to loop as traditional threads or rubber bands.

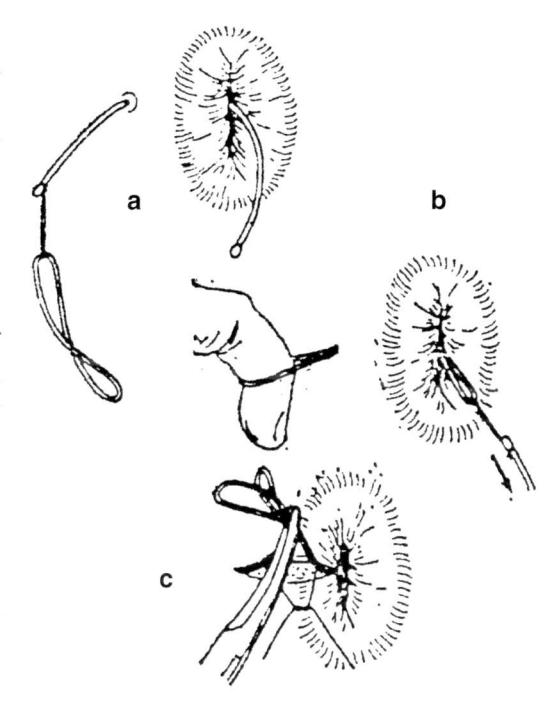

Fig. 8.9 Anal fistula low incision and high thread hanging therapy. (**a**) The probe enters the fistula, (**b**) pull out the rubber band, (**c**) cut the skin, tighten the ligation of the rubber band

The Transformation from Simple Thread-Drawing to Incision Thread-Drawing Therapy

Initially, when the thread-hanging method was used to treat anal fistula, the skin was not cut, but the whole fistula between the inner mouth and the outer mouth was hung with medicated thread and tightened, and heavy objects were suspended to enhance the cutting effect. In the process of slowly cutting the skin, muscles, etc., the patient suffered great and unbearable pain. At the same time, the threading process was long and so was the recovery time.

Since it was recognized that the incision of the skin and the fistula below the deep external sphincter muscle had little effect on anal function when the suture was hung, the original whole-layer suture was changed to incising the fistula below the skin and the external sphincter muscle, and only the fistula above the deep external sphincter was cut and hung (Fig. 8.9). This does not increase sphincter damage but can greatly reduce the suffering of patients and shorten the course of treatment. This treatment method of low incision and high thread hanging is still the main operative method of high anal fistula thread-hanging therapy today.

Change from Real Line to Virtual Hanging Line

Inspired by Parks's "Theory of Anal Crypt Gland Infection" and the surgical method of anal fistula with sphincter preservation, it was recognized that the complete elimination of the internal orifice, anal duct, anal gland abscess, and the maintenance of unobstructed drainage are the necessary conditions for the treatment of anal fistula, while the incisions of the sphincter were not absolutely necessary conditions for the treatment of anal fistula. The anal fistula can be cured without cutting the sphincter. Therefore, since the late 1990s, doctors began using the "false hanging line" (also known as floating hanging line, slack hanging line) method to treat anal fistula. Hollow suture is a method that does not tighten the rubber band or cut the fistula after

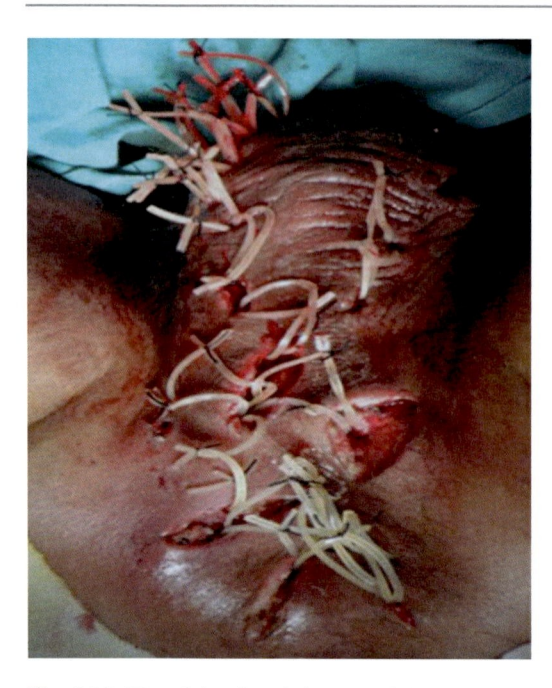

Fig. 8.10 Thread-drawing drainage and virtual thread-drawing therapy of anal fistula

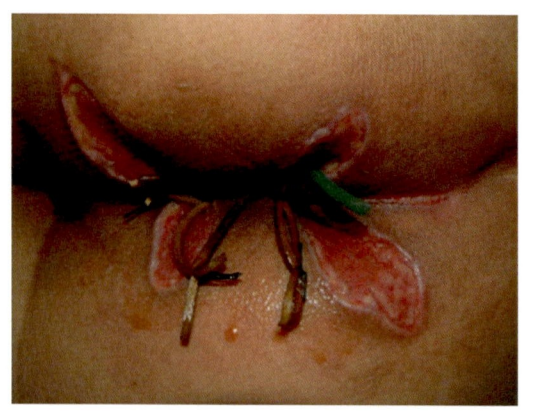

Fig. 8.11 Anal fistula catheterization therapy

hanging the thread in the fistula and only uses the drainage effect of the rubber band to treat anal fistula (Fig. 8.10). In general, secretion gradually decreases in the fistula cavity until there is no more purulent secretion left. When the purulent cavity shrinks, the elastic band that loosens the thread is gradually removed.

After adopting the method of virtual line, the anal sphincter and its function can be better protected, and the number of incisions and tissue damage can also be reduced. However, some patients still were not cured after the removal of the floating thread, and the recurrence rate of the virtual line was higher than that of the real line. That is, the main disadvantage of the virtual line therapy is that the cure rate is not as high as that of the real line therapy.

Change from Thread Hanging to Drainage Tube

In the process of using thread-hanging therapy, it was found that in some cases, the fistula was located high and even extended to a plane that was difficult to perform thread hanging (such as the prostate or an even higher plane), or the distance between the fistula and the rectum was too large and the tissue was thick, so the difficulty of thread hanging and the potential injury it could cause were both large. At this point, the biggest difficulty of the thread-hanging operation was that the line cannot be drawn from the rectal cavity after being hung in a high position. Even if the line can be drawn, there is still a concern that it will be extremely difficult to stop the bleeding if bleeding occurs at the artificial internal orifice. For such anal fistulas, doctors used drainage tubes or infusion straps in the high fistula (Fig. 8.11). When changing the dressing every day after defecation, first wash the wound cavity with normal saline or metronidazole solution. When the secretions in the lumen of the fistula lessen and become clear, withdraw the drainage tube by a small amount (0.3–0.5 cm) outward each day, until all the secretions are withdrawn. Therefore, this method is widely used in the treatment of similar fistulas, with a very high success rate, and has gradually become a routine practice in the treatment of anal fistula.

The author believes that the essence of the drainage tube method is the virtual hanging method, and its principle is to create the necessary conditions for the healing of the high fistula through drainage. When using this method to treat anal fistula, the anal sphincter is basically not damaged, and normal tissues are not cut open, which reduces the damage to anal function. However, there is also the disadvantage that the cure rate of this form of relaxed hanging therapy is lower than that of real hanging therapy. Suitable candidates should be selected, the hardened fistula wall should be removed as much as possible during the operation, and the blood supply and repairing ability of the tissue should be improved in order to improve the success rate of drainage tube therapy.

Change from the Drainage Tube Method to Virtual and Real Thread Hanging
The essence of the drainage tube method is the virtual thread hanging method. Although this reduces the damage to anal function, this also has the disadvantage that the cure rate is lower than that of actual thread-hanging therapy.

Director Zheng Lihua summarized a method for treating high anal fistula that combined virtual and real thread hanging based on years of clinical experience. This method is mainly aimed at high anal fistula with a fistula position higher than the anorectal ring, or high anal fistula with a high blind end position. The fistula above the inner opening and within the range of infection of the anorectal ring was firmly connected with the silk knot during the operation, and the high infection lesion above the anorectal ring was partially cut off by the strangulation force of the silk thread. About 7 days after the operation, some infected lesions in the upper part were cut off, and the ligation line became loose. The silk thread was used to continue drainage of necrotic infected tissues, and granulation took place. This innovation completely relieved the pain of postoperative thread tightening.

At the same time, the rubber band was replaced by silk threads. The multistrand silk wire has a more smooth drainage effect, stronger cutting force, and faster cutting speed than the rubber strip, and the patient's pain is significantly reduced. In view of the biggest difficulty in the operation of line hanging, that the hanging line cannot be drawn from the rectum cavity after high line hanging, director Zheng used the method of guiding through the intestinal cavity with the index finger and pulling out the silk line with the rubber band to accurately locate the hanging line position. During the operation, avoid bleeding at the artificial stoma after tightening the surgical knot. The clinical application of virtual combined with real thread hanging simplifies the operation process, and has achieved success in the treatment of high and complex anal fistula.

8.2.2.3 Therapeutic Principle of Thread Hanging
Currently, there are five main therapeutic principles of hanging line therapy (Fig. 8.12).

The Effect of Slowly Cutting
By means of the tight line contraction or elastic force, compression ischemic necrosis can be generated locally in the cut tissue, which will slowly disconnect and fall off, thus replacing the use of a knife with a line. In this process, sphincter separation and tissue fibrosis repair are carried out at the same time so that the broken end of the separated muscle has an attached fulcrum, and the broken end of the separated muscle is connected with the new scar tissue in the middle to form a ring structure again, which can still maintain functions such as anal constriction. Hu Bohu and Shi Zhaoqi conducted experimental studies on incising and hanging canine anal sphincters. The results show that the width of scar between the ends of incisions in the hanging group was significantly smaller than that of the cutting group, and the influence on the static pressure and systolic pressure of the anal canal was significantly reduced compared with that of the cutting group too. This shows that although thread-hanging therapy can also damage anal function in a degree, it is to a lesser extent, and on the whole, it can better protect the anal function.

Foreign Body Irritation
Medicine thread or rubber band, as a foreign body, can stimulate local tissues to produce an inflammatory response. Inflammatory stimulation can cause the sphincter to be severed and broken and to adhere to or fix onto surrounding tissues.

The Drainage Effect
When the hanging line is placed in the anal fistula wound cavity, it has a good drainage effect,

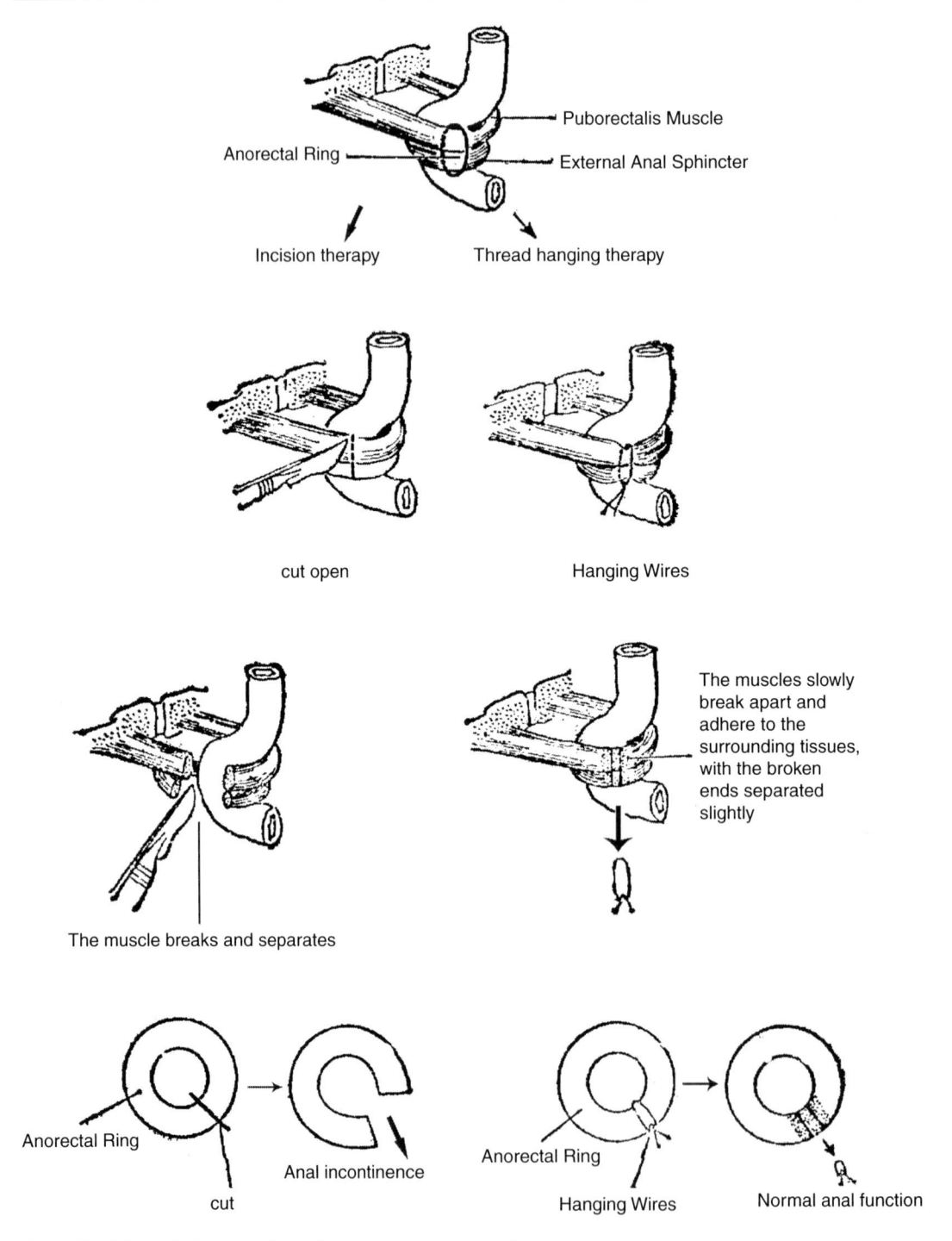

Fig. 8.12 Schematic diagram of thread-hanging therapy principle

which can make the secretions in the wound cavity flow out along the hanging line (rubber band) without accumulating, so that the wound surface is kept clean, thus creating ideal conditions for healing. For Crohn's disease patients and some others that are not suited to open surgery, the hanging line drainage can greatly reduce inflammation of the tissues around the anal fistula, thus creating the conditions necessary for future surgery.

Marking Function
It can indicate the relationship between the outer orifice and the inner orifice and indicate whether the fistula has been completely cut. Therefore, it has a marking function.

Medicinal Effects
The traditional Chinese medicine thread has certain medicinal effects because it is cooked with medicine that can reduce swelling, remove necrotic tissue, and promote muscle growth. This is the advantage of using traditional medicine thread over rubber band or silk thread. As there has been little clinical use of the medicine line therapy contemporarily, many methods of cooking the thread properly have been lost. Lu Jingen and others adopted modern silk thread as the thread-hanging material and added some drugs on the silk thread to play a similar role as traditional medicine threads, inheriting some characteristics of traditional thread-hanging therapy. However, the author believes that this still cannot fully encapsulate the advantages of traditional medicine lines.

8.2.2.4 The Main Surgical Methods Used in Thread-Hanging Therapy

Low-Position Incision and High-Position Thread-Hanging Technique
Referred to as incision-hanging technique, or external incision and thread-hanging technique. It is suitable for high simple and high complex anal fistula. It is also recommended for patients with weak sphincters or female anterior anal fistula.

Key points of operation: the treatment of fistulas below the deep part of the internal orifice and external sphincter is basically the same as that of anal fistula incision or internal orifice incision. After cutting the low-level pipeline, before using the high-level pipeline to hang the line, treat the inner opening first. Cut the skin of the anal canal, internal sphincter, and external sphincter below the inner opening, scratch and remove the infected anal glands and the hardened and proliferated tissues around them, trim the wound, and treat the mucous membranes on both sides of the inner opening and the adjacent anus. The sinuses are ligated with thick silk threads to enlarge the wound surface of the internal opening and facilitate drainage.

For the fistula above the deep part of the external sphincter, use a ball-head probe with a rubber band at one end to explore the deep fistula, gently insert it into the top of the tube along the lumen, and pull it out after the top of the tube penetrates the rectal wall (if the patient has a perforation, the probe can pass into the rectum through this perforation). Pull the probe, together with the rubber band, out of the anus and tighten the thread appropriately (Fig. 8.13). In anal fistula with a particularly high position, because of the deep tube, it is difficult to pull the probe deep into the high fistula through the rectal wall. Some people have proposed that with the aid of instruments, a probe or a vascular clamp can be inserted from the rectum and pulled out of the anus through the fistula.

For nonmain duct wounds of patients with complex anal fistulas, part of the wounds should be sutured if necessary to reduce the wound surface area and shorten healing time.

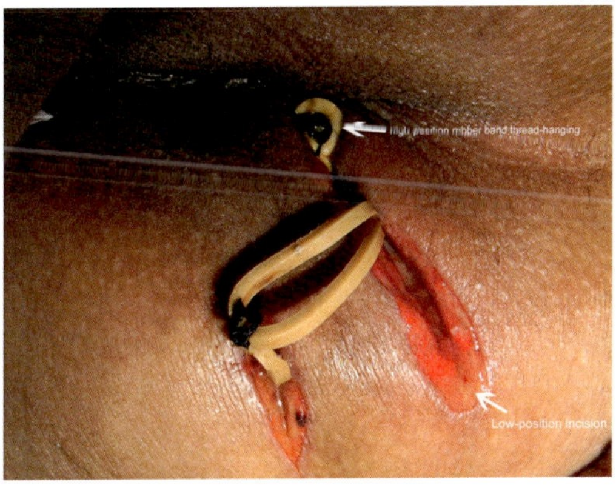

Fig. 8.13 Low-position incision and high-position rubber band thread-hanging therapy for anal fistula

Low-Position Incision and High-Position Virtual Thread Hanging

Also known as low-position incision and high-position loose thread-hanging technique, or called low-position incision and high-position floating thread-hanging technique, it is an advancement based on incision and thread-hanging therapy. Surgical style: it is suitable for the treatment of high anal fistulas and abscesses.

Key points of operation: it is basically the same as the low-position incision and high-position thread-hanging technique. The only difference is that the thread is not tightened after it is threaded. The two ends of the pulled-out rubber band are loosely ligated to form a rotatable ring. When changing the dressing each day, one must rotate the rubber band ring and flush the fistula cavity with a liquid such as metronidazole or normal saline.

It should be noted that the low incision and high loose thread-hanging technique has higher requirements for the right candidate than low-incision high-thread-drawing. If the fistula wall is thick, blood supply is not good, there are many scar tissues after multiple operations, or if tissue healing ability is poor, the former treatment will easily fail. Therefore, the loose thread-hanging technique is suitable for the cases of anal fistula with thin tube walls, good blood supply, tissue regeneration, and healing ability. For anal fistulas with thicker walls, sometimes it is necessary to use virtual thread therapy instead. In order to improve the success rate of the operation, the wall must be trimmed to remove the hardened wall and improve the healing conditions of the fistula lumen.

Combination of Virtual and Real Thread-Hanging Techniques

The combination of virtual and real thread-hanging methods is an innovative treatment that combines the advantages of the gradual strangulation effect of real thread hanging and the postoperative drainage characteristics of virtual thread hanging. It is suitable for high anal fistulas, including high simple anal fistulas and high complex anal fistulas, and it is also applicable to refractory anal fistula with repeated attacks.

Operation points: the specific method is that during operation, make a radial incision to the inner mouth from the dentinal line, about 3–4 cm in length, and the incision position is generally on the same side as the outer opening to fully drain the infection foci at the inner opening. Cut the inner opening, extending 0.5–1.0 cm upward, and extend downward to the outside of the anal margin. Use curved hemostatic forceps to probe the upper end of the high fistula from this incision until the top of the fistula is reached. Use your fingers to reach into the intestinal cavity for guidance, and the tip of the forceps to penetrate the stoma of the intestinal wall. Withdraw the finger, use 4–10 gauge silk threads, tie one end to the fingertip, and put it into the intestinal cavity. Open the hemostatic forceps to clamp the thread, draw the silk thread from the intestinal cavity through the fistula, gather the two ends, and fix it with a knot. Routine cleaning and dressing should be changed once a day after the operation. Vaseline gauze is drained, and the gauze is applied and fixed. About 7 days after the operation, the silk thread is loose, and the virtual thread is drained at this time. After the granulation tissue fills the fistula, it can be removed on the 20th day of the operation (Fig. 8.14).

It should be noted that the combination of virtual and real thread hanging is divided into two stages: intraoperative real thread hanging and postoperative virtual thread hanging. Intraoperative actual threading is the same as high thread hanging. Low-position incision and high thread hanging can be used. The difference is that in the postoperative virtual thread hanging, the ligation thread is loose, the thread is not tightened, and the thread is removed after 7 days after the operation so that the ligation thread plays the role of virtual hanging and drainage. At 20 days, the suture is removed according to the granulation filling of the fistula cavity.

Tunnel Thread-Hanging Surgery

In the 1980s, the Department of Traditional Chinese Medicine Surgery of Longhua Hospital applied thread-hanging therapy to the treatment of anal fistula for the first time in China. This sur-

8 Surgical Treatment of Anal Fistula

a Schematic diagram of high anal fistula

b Cut the inner opening, extend 0.5–1.0 cm upwards, extend downwards to the outside of the anal verge

c Use vascular forceps to penetrate the topn of the fistula into the intestinal cavity, and introduce

d The silk thread is drawn from the intestinal cavity through the fistula and then tied and fixed

e About 7 days after the operation, the silk thread was loose, and the virtual thread was continued to be drained at this time

f After the fistula granulation tissue is filled, remove the hanging thread on the 20th day

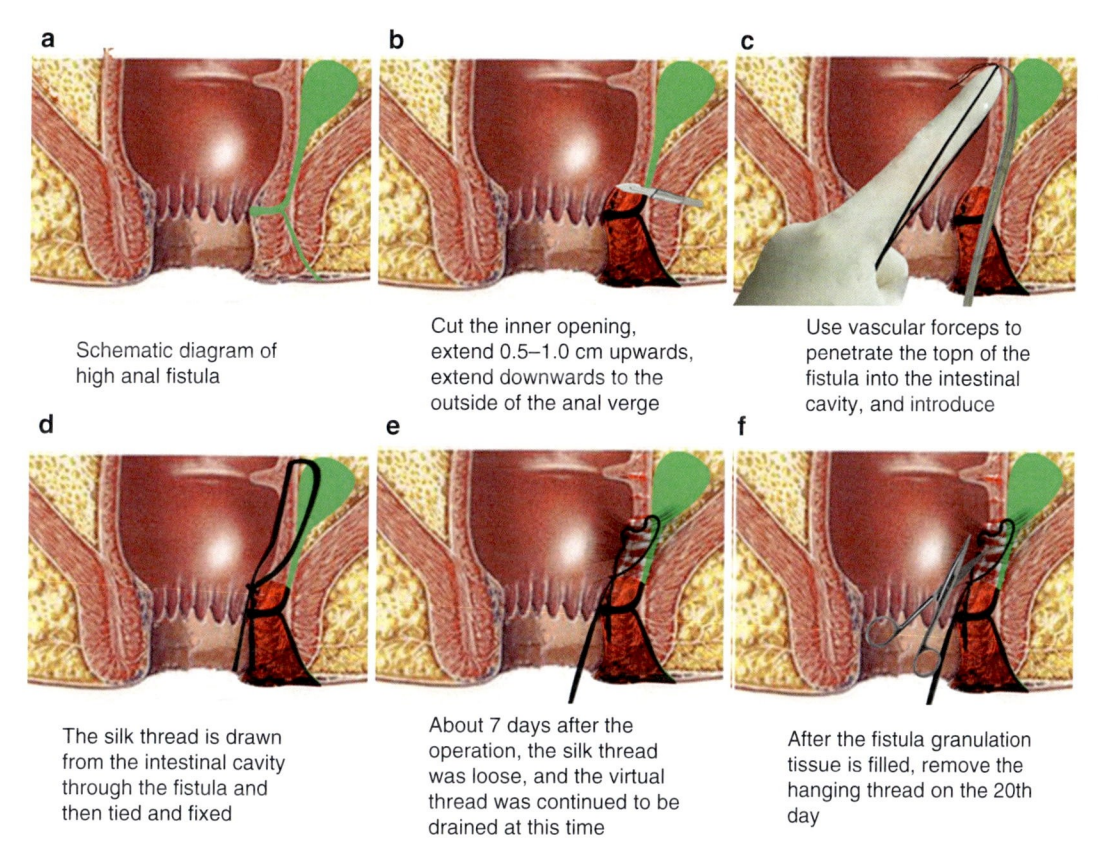

Fig. 8.14 Schematic diagram of anal fistula. (**a**) Schematic diagram of high anal fistula. (**b**) Cut the inner opening, extend 0.5–1.0 cm upwards, extend downwards to the outside of the anal verge. (**c**) Use vascular forceps to penetrate the top of the fistula into the intestinal cavity, and introduce 4 silk threads under the guidance of the fingers. (**d**) The silk thread is drawn from the intestinal cavity through the fistula and then tied and fixed. (**e**) About 7 days after the operation, the silk thread was loose, and the virtual thread was continued to be drained at this time. (**f**) After the fistula granulation tissue is filled, remove the hanging thread on the 20th day

gical method is mainly suitable for low simple anal fistula and low complex anal fistula.

Key points of operation: after probing and locating the fistula, an appropriate incision is made to the outer opening, and the necrotic tissue inside the fistula is scraped with a curette. Introduce ten silk thread strands into the pipe with a ball-head silver wire. The two ends of the silk thread are knotted in a circular ring shape. The length of the silk thread in the pipeline is preferably less than 5 cm. If the fistula is long and deep, the thread can be dragged in segments to keep the thread slack (Fig. 8.16). Fumigation, washing, and dressing change are started on the first day after surgery, once in the morning and once in the evening. There tends to be more pus and rotten tissues in the lumen in the early stage. After washing with normal saline, Ba er Dan mixed with the silk thread can be dragged into the lumen. About 10–14 days later, when there is no longer any obvious purulent secretion overflow in the lumen, the silk thread can be removed by batch stitching. After the silk thread is removed, you can choose whether to flush out the wound or not according to the cleanness of wound secretions and close the cavity by compressing with a cotton pad.

Towing line therapy achieves the purpose of treatment by removing the internal orifice and primary lesions and removing the ducts. It treats the inner and outer openings and the fistula under the premise of protecting the normal tissues of the anus as much as possible. This operation organically combines incision, drainage, removing decay, and cotton pad compression. It does not need to cut the skin directly and does not need to remove too much muscle tissue, thus avoiding damage to the tissues around the anal fistula.

Attention should be paid to the following points during the towing line operation:

1. Improve preoperative examination: through examinations including intracavity ultrasound, MRI, and colonoscopy, a comprehensive understanding of the primary internal orifice of the fistula and the path and potential cavities of all branches of the fistula can be made. The methods of anorectal pressure measurement and patient anal function score were used to objectively evaluate the patient's defecation function and anal sphincter function.
2. Correct handling of the internal opening: the internal opening of glandular anal fistulas is mostly located near the dentate line. After clearing the internal opening and surrounding inflammatory tissue, appropriately incise the tissue below the internal opening to the skin of the anal margin to facilitate drainage. For example, although the high sphincter anal fistula passes through the deep part of the external sphincter muscle, the inner opening is still near the dentate line. Therefore, for this type of fistula, it is not necessary to blindly protrude from the deepest part of the fistula and thus forming an iatrogenic false pathway. The internal opening can be appropriately incised to the corresponding groove between the anal marginal sphincter to ensure adequate drainage of the deep duct.
3. Reasonable design of incision and thread setting: the incision position is usually designed according to the length and shape of the fistula, and the incision should be larger than the cross section of the fistula, generally 1 cm × 1 cm, to ensure smooth drainage. The number of silk threads used depends on the size of the fistula lumen. If the diameter is less than 1 cm, ten wires can be used; if the diameter is greater than 1 cm, more than ten wires can be used. The length of the tow line (the silk thread placed in the cavity of the fistula) is generally controlled within 5 cm, and there should be no residual cavity. If the pipeline is too long, it can be treated by the segmented towing method.
4. Postoperative dressing change: when changing dressing after the operation, first flush the lumen with normal saline, and at the same time rotate the silk thread placed in the cavity to wipe off any pus attached, and then the anticorrosive drug Jiuyi Dan should be mixed with the silk thread and gently dragged into the lumen. When the secretion on the silk thread is significantly reduced, the anticorrosion medicine can be stopped. For those who have more necrotic tissue in the fistula wound or for patients who cannot relax during dressing change, the silk thread can be used for treatment in the early stage, and the silk thread can be replaced with a scalp needle tube with a small hole during the later period, and a syringe can be used to flush out the necrotic tissue. This method can not only completely change the dressing but also alleviate patient suffering.
5. When to remove the thread: the lumen of the fistula begins to shrink about 1 week after the operation, and part of the silk thread can be removed at this time. In general, when the local granulation tissue is bright red and the secretion is clear and viscous from about 9 to 11 days after surgery and combined with local ultrasound examination that shows the diameter of the lumen to be less than 0.5 cm, all the silk threads can be removed, and the sore cavity can be scraped with a curette until there is fresh bleeding.
6. Posttreatment care after the tow line is removed: after the tow line is removed, defecation can begin to be controlled, preferably to once a day, and at the same time, cotton pad compression should begin. A small piece of cotton or gauze pad is used to press on the affected area, and external adhesive plaster or bandage is moderately used. Pressurize vertically to shrink and bond the lumen, and finally achieve the purpose of healing. Generally, such compression should last for about 7 days, and the cumulative amount of time spent should be no less than 4 h/day.

The most important material in thread-hanging therapy is silk thread. As a medium, it can drain the necrotic tissue in the fistula lumen. At the same time, the thread can carry anticorrosive drugs into the lumen to accelerate the erosion of the tube wall. In addition, in the early postoperative period, according to the growth rate of granulation tissue and the shrinkage of the lumen, several strands can be properly removed, which can maintain thorough drainage and prevent false adhesion. However, if the drag line is removed too early, the necrotic tissue in the lumen has not been thoroughly removed, and the drag line is placed for too long and leads to fibrosis, recurrence of the fistula can occur. Therefore, finding the most appropriate time to remove the tow line is the main factor that affects the success of the tow line therapy. On the other hand, the pus and rot-removing medicine Jiuyi Dan is the medicinal pill with the least amount of mercury and has the effect of "corroding and decomposing, without sacrificing muscle." Mixing the Jiuyi Dan with silk thread and dragging and creating friction during dressing change can make contact with the wall of the tube in all directions and place the medicine in the lumen. The silk thread allows the poison to escape with the pus, which is not only conducive to the decomposing of the pus but also aids in the growth of new muscles. It has a synergistic effect. However, reports have found that improper use of Jiuyi Dan can cause liver and kidney damage. Despite this, the wounds treated with thread-hanging therapy are nonopen wounds, and long-term, high-dose use is avoided in clinical use, so Jiuyi Dan is only absorbed in small quantities and has no obvious effect on liver and kidney functions. For patients with abnormal renal function, it is not recommended to use Jiuyi Dan during the thread-hanging treatment, and the fibrotic fistula wall tissue should be removed as much as possible during the operation.

A retrospective analysis of the failed cases of thread-hanging therapy found that for anal fistulas or abscesses above the levator ani muscle and whose internal orifice is in the rectum, the effect of thread-hanging therapy alone is not sufficient. Thread-hanging therapy is suitable for fistulas and abscesses with a large range in the horizontal direction, while treatment of deep fistulas and abscesses in the vertical direction need to be combined with catheter drainage and negative pressure suction.

Traditional Medicine Thread Hanging

This is a traditional Chinese medicine treatment of anal fistula. It can be used for the treatment of all types of anal fistulas, and it is currently rarely used in clinical practice.

Key points of operation: use a ball-tip probe with a medicine thread at the other end to penetrate from the outer opening, go deep along the pipeline, and pull the thread out through the inner opening, and finally lead the medicine thread out of the anus. Then tighten the medicine thread, tie a slipknot, and hang heavy objects such as iron blocks onto the end and tighten the medicine thread once a day when changing the medicine.

The traditional thread-hanging technique is painful and takes a long time for the thread to cut the skin. At present, this original method is no longer used much in the clinic. Generally, the skin and subcutaneous tissue are incised, and the external sphincteric fistula is incised and then threaded so as to alleviate the painful shortcomings of using the thread alone to cut the skin and subcutaneous tissue and shorten the time to cut all the fistulas.

Drainage Tube Therapy

This surgical method is an anal fistula treatment method developed on the basis of anal fistula virtual thread drainage. Suitable candidates for the incising and threading of anal fistula mainly include those with particularly deep and complex anal fistulas and when the fistula lumen is far away from the rectal cavity and thread hanging is very difficult to carry out or even technically impossible.

Key operating points: the treatment of the internal opening, primary lesions, sphincter, etc. is basically the same as that of anal fistula incision and threading, except that the thread is not threaded through the rectal wall, but a suitable drainage tube (straight type hose, stamen type catheter, T-shaped hose, etc.) is placed in the high fistula wound cavity (Fig. 8.11), usually to the degree that it can be rotated appropriately, and rinse with hydrogen peroxide and then normal saline to ensure smooth drainage, then suture the hose to the peripheral skin of the anus to prevent it from falling off. After the operation, the drainage tube is used for flushing the fistula lumen every day until there is no longer much secretion in the fistula lumen left and there are no obvious floccules. The catheter should be withdrawn a little (about 0.3–0.5 cm) every day. In general, the catheter should be removed 2 weeks after the operation. After extubation, cotton pad compression therapy can be used to accelerate the closure of the wound cavity until the fistula cavity is fully healed.

Since the fistulas of patients using this technique are more complicated and the position is deeper, the residual fluid in the lumen should be drawn back as much as possible after flushing, and the patients should be told to stand upright and walk slowly.

The advantages of catheter drainage are little tissue damage and fast healing and can better avoid postoperative anal incontinence, stenosis, deformity, and other complications so as to better protect anal function.

Long-Term Drainage and Thread-Hanging Operation

This operation is mainly used for the treatment of Crohn's disease anal fistula and the hard-to-cure high complex anal fistula, not for the purpose of curing completely, but for the purpose of reducing symptoms, maintaining remission state, reducing inflammation of the fistula, or creating the conditions for possible future operations.

Key operation points: it is basically the same as the traditional technique of thread hanging, except that the material used is a special drain line.

The University of Minnesota Affiliated Hospital reported 55 cases of anal fistula secondary to Crohn's disease that were treated by thread drainage. Among them, 22 cases of high complex anal fistula and 19/22 cases of perianal lesions remained in the static stage after thread drainage. White (1990) believed that thread drainage was effective in treating Crohn's disease anal fistula. Williams (1991) reported on 23 cases of anal fistula with Crohn's disease that were treated by thread drainage and the recurrence rate was 39%.

Ren Donglin believes that long-term thread-hanging drainage can prevent the expansion of infectious lesions and control the formation of acute stage abscesses, thus improving the quality of life for extremely complicated cases of anal fistula that are "incurable" or too expensive to treat. "Stabilizing" fistulas are as important as healing fistulas in these cases. In addition to serving as a bridge for radical surgery, the drainage line is also the most effective and appropriate lifelong treatment for some special cases.

Although the treatment of complex anal fistula by thread drainage protects the integrity of the sphincter and does not cause anal incontinence, its success rate decreases with the extension of follow-up time and the efficacy is uncertain. Therefore, before choosing to go ahead with thread drainage, adequate communication with the patient should be done to make sure the patient is thoroughly aware of the procedure and outcomes, and the patient's choice and opinions should be respected.

8.2.2.5 Some of the Academic Controversies Surrounding Thread-Hanging Therapy

Although it has been widely used in the clinic, there are still some controversies surrounding the practice.

Under What Circumstances Should Thread-Hanging Therapy Be Used?

Ren Donglin believes that, in clinical practice, the vast majority of high complex anal fistulas do not require thread-hanging treatment because thread-hanging therapy itself may bring a longer treatment time, greater pain, and other problems. Therefore, the choice of whether or not to use thread-hanging therapy depends on finding the most suitable candidates with the correct indications. Because of the modern-day advances made on the anatomy of anal fistula resection, the treatment of pathological changes has become more thorough, muscle protection more precise, and internal search and processing more accurate, coupled with a better understanding of the function and role of the anorectal ring. Some cases that had to be treated with thread hanging in the past can now directly undergo open surgery, and only when the fistula is extremely complex and completely or mostly transverses the anorectal ring, thread hanging is now used.

In the author's opinion, it is safer to use thread-hanging therapy for most high complex anal fistula, even in cases of stiffened anorectal ring fistula. The use of line therapy can also play a role in stimulating the growth of granulation, drainage, and marking; advantages that the incision method does not have and at the same time reduces the pain brought to patients during the filling and drainage strip process when the deep wound cavity's dressing is changed. Because in this method drainage is good, it is conductive to healing. For female anal fistula in a front location, if the position is deep, even if it is below the external sphincter, it is best to use thread-hanging therapy.

Pang Wenbin, Li Ruiji, and others advocate that for pediatric anal fistula, no matter low or high, it is better to treat with incision and thread hanging. It is considered that the use of thread-hanging therapy has the following advantages: (1) drainage is unobstructed to prevent wound infection and adhesion. The rubber band used to hang the thread can not only open the fistula slowly but also has a good drainage effect; even though the wound is often contaminated with feces, infection will not occur. The thread incision forms an ulcer wound that is not easy to adhere to, and after the rubber band falls off, do not put in gauze strip drainage. (2) The pain is mild and completely tolerable for ill children. Anal sensory nerve receptors mainly distributed in the skin layer, subcutaneous tissue, and muscle layer are not very sensitive to pain. When hanging the thread, a small incision is made in the anal skin. The thread is hung on the incision to avoid ones that are sensitive to pain, so the pain was mild, and mostly painkillers are not needed. (3) Simple wound care. Due to drainage patency, the wound is not easily infected and does not easily stick together. Clean the anus every time after defecation with potassium permanganate solution. In addition, for older children, postoperative dressing change is needed, but most children can be nursed by parents alone and the healing process is smooth. (4) The wound on the thread line is relatively narrow, so the scar is small after healing and will not cause anal deformation.

Which Is Better, the Traditional Medicine Thread or the Rubber Band Cord?

The indications for traditional thread hanging and rubber band hanging are basically the same. However, traditional hanging line therapy uses a medicine line or silk line when hanging, and a heavy weight needs to be hung onto the end, so it has a stronger cutting ability; therefore, it is also called the gravity hanging line. On the basis of the traditional technique, the rubber band is used to hang the line. After changing to the rubber band, the contraction force of the rubber band is used to replace the pulling force of the weight. Therefore, the technique of thread hanging with a rubber band is also called the elastic string technique.

In the author's opinion, elastic cord hanging is more convenient than the traditional gravity cord hanging, as there is no need to tighten the cord every day. However, in the treatment mechanism and treatment effect, there are obvious differences between the two. The traditional gravity line is hung from bottom to top and from the inside to the outside to gradually cut the fistula. That is to say, the wound surface grows from deep to shallow and from the inside out after the thread is hung and can achieve the following: "the drug line drops daily, the intestinal muscles grow, gradually grows from a shaded location, water flows down the line, not through the sore opening, goose tube elimination." The wound heals gradually from deep to shallow and from top to bottom. However, although the elastic thread-hanging technique also has the drainage effect of "water flowing by line," because the cutting direction is to the center from all around, the wound surface grows slowly after the complete strangulation, so it cannot achieve the effect of "the drug line drops daily, the intestinal muscles grow, gradually grows from a shaded location." At the same time, the control of the gravity hanging method is better, and the cutting force can be adjusted at any time, so it can be temporarily removed at night for a break and let the patient can have a good rest. Therefore, the author thinks that with regard to the treatment effect, the gravity hanging method is still better than the rubber band technique. That said, using a rubber band is less painful and has a shorter course of treatment than traditional gravity thread hanging.

The current high anal fistula clinical operation done in conjunction with real and virtual thread hanging is an innovative combination that, according to its founder Zheng Lihua, its advantages are as follows:

1. It maximizes sphincter function and protects normal tissue. It not only guarantees the cutting of the inner mouth, rectum ring, and the infected site but also does not completely cut off the anal straight ring, with less tissue damage and less postoperative scarring. There is no postoperative scar deformity, anal deformity, displacement, and other sequelae.
2. Two-way isobaric drainage in the rectum is achieved. During operation, the doctor cuts 0.5–1 cm upward through the opening of the anal fistula, removes it from the hyperbaric area, and makes an artificial opening at the top of the fistula into the intestinal cavity so that the upper and lower ends of the fistula are in the same pressure area, forming a two-way isobaric drainage, which is conducive to adequate drainage of the secretions.
3. The use of silk threads instead of rubber bands. Compared with rubber bands, silk threads have thinner fibers, a firmer binding effect, and faster cutting force. However, their stimulation effect is less than that of rubber bands, which is not only beneficial to the drainage of secretion, but also to wound healing, and can also act as a marker for dressing change and oil gauze filling after surgery
4. Hanging the lines but not tightening them not only greatly reduces the suffering of patients but also reduces the cost of medical care.
5. The natural closure of the lumen is achieved through granulation filling. The cavity left behind after the removal of the virtual line drainage is narrow and thus is easier to heal.
6. The operation is more doable, clinical treatment effect is satisfactory, prognosis is good, and it is easy to be widely applied.

How Much Muscle Tissue Should Be Used When Hanging Up the Line?

Ren Donglin put forward hanging the thread on a small area of muscle and not a large muscle bundle. This requires that the lesion should be opened as far as possible during the operation, and only the muscle part should be treated with the hanging line so as to make the purpose of the hanging line more clear. For a large bundle of tissue, hanging in groups of pairs can be used. Hanging in groups can solve the issue of the incomplete cutting of large bundle muscle tissues and the need to re-tighten the line. When there are two areas that need to be cut and then have the line hung at the same time, the surgeon can first tighten one line, let the other line be floating, and when the first tightened line cuts open the area, tighten the floating line.

In author's opinion, the thread should be hung to the top of the fistula, without leaving a space, even if it is in a large bundle. In this way, all fistulas can be hung open to avoid poor drainage and the existence of dead cavity in the top. Avoid bleeding when the rectum mucosa is cut open directly. Because the upper mucous membrane is fast to open, even hanging to the top does not affect the rate of cutting tissue. For large bundles of tissue, it is possible to tighten the wires appropriately after hanging the lines on a large bundle. If the tight line is not cut during the operation, it can be tightened again after the operation.

Is the Real Thread Better or the Virtual Thread Better?

Until the 1990s, thread-drawing therapy was mainly applied to the treatment of high fistulas and abscesses above the external sphincter, using the tight thread method (solid or real line method). Since then, according to the principle that thread hanging can play a role in drainage, thread-hanging therapy is not only used for high anal fistulas and abscesses but also used widely in the treatment of low anal fistulas and abscesses.

More recently, it is not the tight line hanging method that is used most often but the "slack hanging," "virtual hanging," or "floating hanging" method. This is a major advance in the use of thread-hanging therapy.

At present, the fistula and abscess cavity below the external sphincter can be treated by virtual drainage. That is, according to the length or scope of the fistula or abscess, make one or more incisions, and use rubber band virtual drainage between adjacent incisions. For the fistula set deep and above the external sphincter or with many abscess cavities, the real line treatment is used more often, but virtual line treatment is also sometimes used. There is no uniform standard at home or abroad, and choosing which method mainly depends on the treatment concept and methods of the surgeon.

We believe that in the treatment of high anal fistula, the virtual hanging method is more suitable for anal fistula above the deep external sphincter muscle and for anal fistula patients with thin tube walls, small lumens, short pipelines, unobstructed drainage, less scarring from previous operations or on surrounding tissue, and no systemic basic diseases such as diabetes and tuberculosis. For those with thicker and longer canal walls, larger lumens, obstructed drainage, many previous operations or local anal scar tissues, or other systemic circumstances, the virtual hanging method should be avoided. If the tube wall is thick or there is a lot of scar tissue at the operation site, the hardened tissue of the tube wall must be removed as much as possible.

In terms of practical application, the real hanging method has higher cure rate and better thoroughness than the virtual hanging method, but the virtual hanging method has better protection of anal function, less postoperative complications, shorter course of treatment, and less pain.

We commonly use the method of suspension in the treatment of the external sphincter high above and deep below the fistula. Methods: the superficial part of the main pipe corresponding to the inner opening is radially cut, and the upper part of the main pipe is hung up. The abscess cavity of the branch tube is not extensively excised or incised, and several small radial incisions are made according to the drainage requirements, scrape out the necrotic tissue in the fistula cavity, and then rubber bands are hung into the fistulas between the corresponding incisions to form a loose ring. The drainage effect of the rubber bands is used to successfully discharge the secretions in the wound cavity (Fig. 8.15). There is no need to place drainage strips in the lumen after the operation. Only children's scalp needle tubes with the needles removed are needed to be placed in the lumen during dressing change, and the dirt in the lumen is washed with normal saline or metronidazole solution. When the lumen shrinks, the main duct is cut, and the wound surface is close to healing, remove the loose rubber bands and continue to flush the fistula cavity until it cannot be flushed through anymore. Usually, in 1–3 days of removing the line, the branch canal or purulent cavity can no longer be flushed through, and the wound begins to close and gradually heals.

This kind of relaxed hanging method using the rubber band has a continuous drainage effect, will not slip, and does not need to be replaced. It can also be placed in small tube cavities that cannot use drainage strips, and compared with other drainage materials, it has a better drainage effect, has lighter pain, and is easy to carry out. This type of relaxed hanging drainage method changed the traditional arc-shaped incision of the tube or purulent cavity method, which would produce a large wound surface and thus a larger injury, and thus correcting these faults.

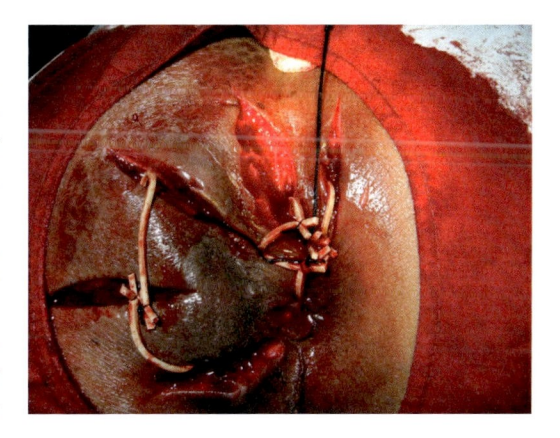

Fig. 8.15 Loose threaded in the branch tube for drainage in complicated anal fistula

How to Tighten the Thread? When Should the Line Be Tightened?

The mechanism of thread-hanging therapy in curing anal fistula mainly depends on the strangulation effect of the thread, which causes hung tissue to gradually die and fall off due to ischemia. In the process, the rubber band, as a foreign body, can stimulate the growth of granulation tissue at the broken end of the muscle, and the broken end will gradually be adhered and fixed by the hyperplastic scar tissue. This will not cause the decline of anal encircling function and even maintains the basic anal encircling function. Studies have shown that after cutting and hanging the line, the sphincter end will ultimately fix the surrounding tissue through focal fibrosis. The thread hanging method is superior in that the cutting method leaves a large scar between the two muscles and the distance between them is large, whereas the thread hanging method leaves only a small scar and the distance is small.

In order to allow a sufficient amount of time for the new tissue to grow, fill, and adhere to the broken end of the muscle cut through strangulation, the cutting speed must be controlled. This is mainly achieved by controlling the level of tension and the timing of hanging the thread so that the rubber band falls off after an appropriate amount of time and not too early. If the thread is too tight and falls off too fast, although the course of treatment is shortened, the muscle tissue is cut off too early, and the tissue between the broken ends of the cut muscle has not had enough time to grow, so the broken ends of the muscle do not have enough adhesion and fixation ability. In this case, retraction can easily occur. Results showed that on the one hand, anal sphincter contraction weakened, and on the other hand, because of muscle retraction and the increased space between the muscle ends, muscle contraction of the anal canal ring decreases, which in turn decreases anal constriction and makes it difficult to satisfactorily control stools and the emission of gases and liquids. Anal leakage of air and fluids can occur together with other complications sequela.

Ren Donglin points out that cutting and thread-hanging therapy is widely used in the treatment of high transsphincter type anal fistula or upper sphincter type anal fistula, and cure rates are relatively high. From the perspective of clinical experience, the first stage of cutting and thread-hanging therapy is often accompanied by obvious postoperative pain, the rapid and uncontrollable cutting of muscles, and insufficient drainage of deep gap abscesses. Compared with the simple fistula incision treatment, the primary incision and suture treatment also has a higher recurrence rate and decreased anal function rate. Not only that, but the indications for this type of thread-hanging therapy often overlap with the indications for multiple "sphincter retention techniques." Therefore, he does not advocate this type of cutting and thread-hanging therapy. It is suggested that the staged incision and thread-hanging therapy can play the role of both gradual myotract incision and long-term abscess drainage. It is more effective to cut the thread after the perianal incision has significantly reduced in size and the deep acute stage abscess is completely controlled. The treatment can be performed in the form of single-strand lashing, moderate tension maintenance, and regular tightening or changing of the threads. It can also be completed through the combination of multistrand thread hanging, first-stage high drainage thread hanging, and second-stage low cut thread hanging. According to relevant literature, the cure rate of this treatment method can reach more than 90%, and the risk of anal function decline is greatly reduced.

Regarding when the line should fall off, most experts think that it should be controlled to 10–14 days or above, and then use subdivided tensioning. Yu Baodian, Cao Lei, and others believe that the earliest time for it to fall off should not be less than 7 days; generally between 12 and 15 days is appropriate, and more than 2 weeks is too long. Zhu Bingyi et al. believe that, in the 14 days or so after hanging the line, foreign body stimulated fibrosis reaches a peak, and at this time tighten the line and let the line fall off. Premature falling off should be prevented; otherwise, there will be insufficient fibrosis at the ends of the broken sphincter muscle, so there will not be enough adhesion and will likely reopen and cause anal incontinence or anal canal defects. Xiong Lagen and Xiong Jinglan believe that the fistula could be completely opened, and the rubber band could come off by itself 10–12 days after the thread-hanging surgery. If the fistula has not opened 12–14 days after the operation and the rubber band cannot come off by itself, the rubber band can be removed by opening the fistula. It is believed that if the fistula is opened too late, the growth of wounds inside and outside the anus will be different, and a wound with insufficient drainage will be formed in the anal canal, which will prolong treatment time. A study conducted by Kou Yuming and Nie Weijian noted that the timing of when the elastic band falls off is the comprehensive result of thread tightening and its healing effect. There is an association between the time of elastic band shedding in the treatment of high anal fistula and postoperative anal function. When the timing of elastic band shedding ranges from 11 to 16 days, the Wexner score and the change rate of rectal and anal pressure measurement after recovery are significantly lower than when the timing of elastic band shedding is less than 10 days. Both the Wexner score and anorectal pressure measurement play a significant role in the assessment of anal function. The sensitivity of anorectal pressure measurement is better assessed by comparing the change rate of anorectal pressure measurement before and after surgery. After recovery, there was a linear correlation between the Wexner score and the rate of changes in rectal and anal pressure measurement, and this was consistent with the anal function assessment.

Ding Zemin argues that the high complicated anal fistula should not be tightened intraoperatively and that it should only be tightened or drawn when the wound granulation tissue grows close to the thread. In this way, the wound growth materials will be enriched, and the anal function will not be greatly affected even if the wound is tightened. At the same time, when the thread is tight, Ding believes that the principle of "a small amount and high frequency" should be followed, and try to cut the thread in one direction only so as to prevent adhesion or defects.

Li Chunyu et al. advocated that for anal fistula with a relatively high position, the time of tightening line should be delayed, and the slow cutting and continuous drainage effect of the hanging line should be used to reduce the scope of inflammation and reduce the size of the wound cavity through only tightening line a little at a time. The first tightening should occur 10–14 days after the operation when the rubber band is loose and has no cutting effect. However, do not tighten the thread too frequently or too tightly. It is best to let the rubber band fall when the branch duct is healed, and there are no more wound cavities. The most ideal timing for this is usually around 18–25 days. In the case group they treated, the earliest time the rubber band fell off was in 15 days, and the longest time was in 41 days. In 17 cases, the line fell off after tightening once; in 58 cases, it fell off after tightening twice; and in 43 cases, it fell off after tightening three times.

Li Jingxiang et al. proposed that retraction force should be used to tighten 1/4 width of the wrapped muscle bundle and proposed the use of subdivided tightening. The healing of the tissue at the blind end was observed when dressing was changed on the tenth day after the operation. If the surrounding tissue healed to the top level of the hanging rubber strip and the drainage is smooth, the rubber strip should be removed. If the drainage is poor, make the first tightening of the line (tighten the rubber strip) and tighten 1/4 width of the muscle bundle again. The wound drainage and healing were observed after 7 days of dressing change. The treatment method is the same as above. They believe that the use of subdivided tightening is favorable because of its weak cutting effect, the fact that the broken end muscle head is fixed firmly and not easy to retract so that the local scar tissue of the anus becomes narrower, and that the shape of the anal canal does not change much so that the effect on anal control function is minimal. When applying subdivided tightening, the elasticity of the rubber band should be correctly mastered. The elastic band should be relaxed and hung up first and then tightened according to how the wound is healing. The disadvantage of subdivided tightening is that the course of treatment is relatively long.

It is worth noting that the anal canal tissues in children are tender, the sphincter bundle is small, the fistula is easy to be cut, and the time it takes for the line to fall is shorter than that of adults. Therefore, for children with high anal fistula, the time it takes for the line to fall should not be too fast so as not to cause anal incontinence.

But there are also advocates for tightening the line only once and an early opening of the fistula. Li Bonian advocated that only the mucous membrane and a small amount of anal epithelium should be retained when dealing with the tissue in the rectal ring area within the hanging line area. For a hanging width less than 5 cm, generally tighten the line once, and it can fall off after 2–3 days. They believe that because there is little or no muscle tissue in the line, patients do not have too much pain when the line is tight. Because the mucous membrane and a small amount of anal epithelium are retained, the appearance of the anus after healing is better protected, and the anal defect is small, thus avoiding the occurrence of anal leakage, air leakage, thinning, and uncontrollable sequelae. However, the author does not agree with this and believes that hanging open the muscle in such a short period of time, in theory, does not constitute gradual strangulation. It becomes similar to one-time incision, so what effect does hanging the line have? Can good anal function be maintained after this type of thread hanging? This is all worth contemplating.

How to Use Multiple Thread Hanging?

For anal fistulas with multiple high fistulas, multiple suture methods are often used in clinical treatment.

Bai Liansong and some others believe that if there are two or more main pipes, tie one first, let the rest hang, and tighten slowly to prevent the rubber bands cutting off the anorectal ring at the same time and thus affecting the function of the anal sphincter muscle. When there are multiple hanging lines, the time it takes for the rubber bands to fall off is usually 4–5 days.

Li Bainian believed that for more than two internal orifices, if the internal orifices are not in the same vertical direction along the intestinal cavity, the lines can be hung at the same time, but after the operation, the lines can be tightened separately so that they do not fall off at the same time. This is to prevent multiple sphincter cuts at the same time and the destruction of the anal containment function that causes anal incontinence. If the internal orifices are in the same vertical direction along the intestinal cavity, the line can be hung between the two mouths or between the lower internal mouth and the anal margin. Make sure to time the tightening of the threads correctly, first tighten the line between the two internal mouths, wait for it to fall off, and then tighten that between the internal mouth and the anal margin. This can effectively move the location of the two internal mouths so that during healing, they become one. This therefore converts high complex anal fistula into high simple anal fistula and thus reduces the degree of anal defect.

When Should the Virtual Hanging Line Be Removed?

Li Chunyu and Jiao Fang suggested that the virtual hanging line should be removed 3 days after the operation. This may be related to a large number of drainage incisions and the length of these incisions. Their specific methods are to enlarge the external opening; the length of the incision should be less than that of the artificial incision of the main pipeline. Use hemostatic forceps to destroy the branch pipe, scrape with curettage, remove the necrotic tissue in the branch tube, and make the drainage between the main branch tube unobstructed. Then, the incision between the main tube and the branch tube should be loosely ligated with an adhesive film strip, and the drainage strip is to be removed 3 days later. If the branch tube is long and is a curved fistula, a radial incision could be made in the middle of the branch tube so that the distance between the two incisions is about 2.5 cm so as to facilitate washing and dressing change. It should be noted that radial incision is often used instead of arc incision.

The author advocates that the virtual hanging line should be removed in 7–14 days. Indications for removal: when there is less wound secretion and the color is clear, the wound pus should be removed, and fresh granulation, narrowing of the cavity, and greater resistance to rubber band rotation should take place (Fig. 8.16). If double-stranded rubber band virtual seton therapy is tied,

8 Surgical Treatment of Anal Fistula

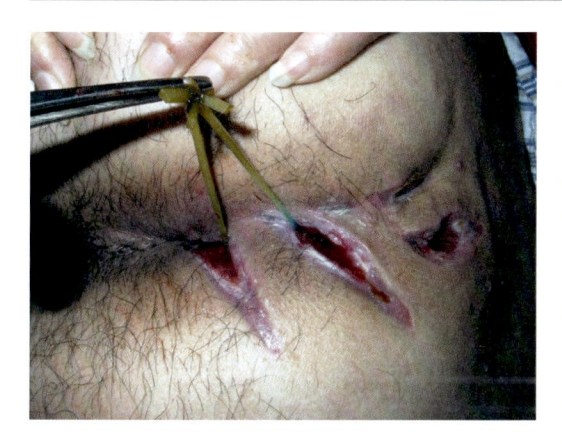

Fig. 8.16 Indications for removal of drainage line

the single strand should be dismantled first, and another rubber band should be dismantled after 3–5 days. The specific application should also be based on the individual wound growth conditions and so on. Before removing the virtual hanging rubber band, rinse and rotate when changing dressing. After the removal, the wound should be rinsed for 1–3 days according to the growth condition of the wound. Meanwhile, the cotton filling method should be used to compress the wound cavity after the removal of the virtual seton and accelerate its closure.

8.2.2.6 Evaluation of Thread-Drawing Therapy

In the treatment of high anal fistula, thread-drawing therapy can make the cut end of the anal sphincter adhere to form a ring, maintain the integrity of the anorectal ring, avoid the destruction of the circular structure of anal sphincter caused by one-time incision of the anal sphincter, and preserve certain anal function, thereby minimizing the damage to the anal function, and avoid or reduce the occurrence of anal incontinence. At the same time, through the drainage effect of thread hanging, it is also conducive to the drainage and repair of the anal fistula wound.

After all, thread-drawing therapy severs the anal sphincter, which will still cause a certain degree of damage to the anal sphincter. If the thread is too tight and the falling off time is too fast, there will still be a certain degree of anal incontinence, and there will be anal leakage, leakage of air or loose stool that cannot be controlled, and other symptoms. At the same time, cutting the muscle tissue with the rubber band will cause severe anal pain, which will last for at least 1–2 days. If thread drawing with a medicated thread, it often needs to be tightened several times, and there is also some pain.

8.2.3 Anal Fistula Sphincter Retention Surgery

The anal fistula retention sphincter surgery is a kind of surgical method that does not cut the anal sphincter as much as possible and still cures anal fistula. It has been developed for more than 60 years.

8.2.3.1 Origins and Development

In 1956, Eisenhammer found that most anal fistulas formed abscesses between the internal and external sphincters, so it was put forward that the intermuscular abscess was regarded as the root cause of the anal fistula. In 1961, Parks clearly pointed out that the root cause of the anal fistula is the result of the further development of the abscess between the internal and external sphincters formed after an anal gland infection. The anal gland is present in the internal sphincter and its lateral longitudinal muscle fibers and is not distributed in the external sphincter. Accordingly, Parks proposed the "anal fistula removal method" by (1) resection of the anal crypt that caused the infection (cryptectomy) and (2) removal of secondary abscess or fistula (fistulectomy) to radically treat the low intermuscular fistula.

Parks's "fistula removal method" was introduced in Japan in the late 1960s. The earliest to carry out this type of surgery were Takao Moriya, Yukio Sumikoshi, Masahiro Takano, etc. In the process of carrying out anal fistula retention sphincter surgery, Japanese scholars have made continuous improvements and reforms on this surgical procedure, forming a variety of surgical methods, such as fistula ligation resection, mucous flap or skin flap elapse coverage, intersphincter resection of intermuscular abscess, muscle flap filling, etc. At present, anal fistula retention sphincter surgery is still commonly used in Japan.

In the treatment of anal fistula in China, the application and research of surgical methods of sphincter retention surgery for anal fistula came relatively late due to the leading position of thread-hanging therapy or thread-hanging therapy by incision and corresponding academic viewpoints. In the mid-to-late 1980s, the Japanese anal fistula retention sphincter surgery was introduced in China and gradually become widely adopted. On the basis of this, combined with the improvement of thread-hanging therapy, medicine twist-off tube method, etc. was formed the anal fistula sphincter retention operation with Chinese characteristics. But on the whole, sphincter retention surgery for anal fistula in China is not as common and is not standardized. The common problem is that there are many names of the same operation. Parks's "fistula removal method" has many different names in the literature, such as tunnel-type anal fistula resection, fistula removal, anal fistula digging, etc. At the same time, there are problems with reports of efficacy and complications that are less objective. Almost all the reports said that the operation they carried out had no complications and the effect was very good, which was a prominent phenomenon. In the past two decades, there have been more and more exchanges between the Chinese anorectal discipline and foreign counterparts. Some foreign surgical methods for treating anal fistula are now being introduced and applied in China; for example, the use of mucous flap elapse surgery, intersphincter fistula ligation (LIFT surgery), and so on are now on the same page as foreign countries. This indicates that the treatment and research level of anal fistula in China is improving and progressing day by day.

8.2.3.2 The Main Method of Anal Fistula Retention Sphincter Surgery

Fistula Removal
Also known as fistula extraction, tunnel-type anal fistula resection, anal fistula digging. This kind of operation is basically based on the anal fistula digging operation of Parks.

Fistula Removal (Parks's Method)
Also known as fistula extraction and anal fistula digging, it is the procedure reported by Parks in 1961. It is suitable for the treatment of various anal fistulas and is most commonly used for the surgical treatment of low simple anal fistula.

Operation points: the inner mouth and its surrounding tissue are cut open and partially excised to completely excise the primary lesion between the anal gland and anal gland duct and the internal and external sphincters, and the wound surface is opened. Then, the external opening is excised from around the external opening, and the fistula in the external sphincter is tactically exfoliated from the outside to the inside of the fistula, and then dug out. When removing the fistula from the sphincter, be careful not to injure the external anal sphincter as much as possible. Drain the wound from the excavation opening (Fig. 8.17).

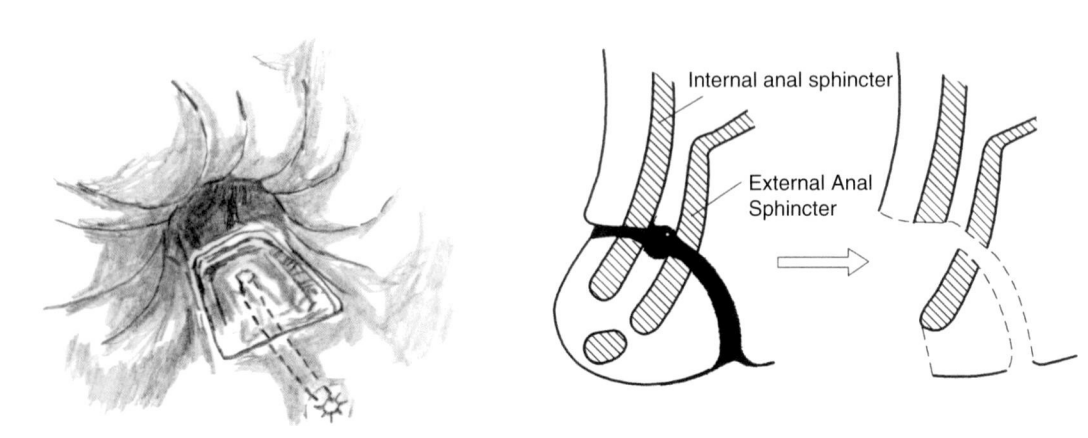

Fig. 8.17 Parks' anal fistula sphincter preservation surgery

The difference between fistula removal and fistulectomy is that fistulectomy is performed after cutting off the sphincter and then the fistula is removed. Fistula removal, however, does not cut the sphincter and removes the fistula from the sphincter.

Since Parks used this method to cure 38 cases of anal fistula, this procedure has become the basic procedure of modern sphincter preservation surgery and is widely used in clinical practice. However, Mann (1985) argued that Parks's method deviated from the principle of complete incision of the fistula from its base, and the recurrence rate of high anal fistula was high with this method. According to Domnule Iwatari's report, only two of the 54 patients who were treated with this method had a recurrence, but they had some shortcomings such as internal sphincter defects. Because defects in the internal sphincter may lead to underwear contaminated with feces and other symptoms, Domnule Iwatari believed that the anal fistula excavation of Parks is not a perfect operation.

Improved Fistula Removal

After anal fistula retention sphincter surgery was introduced in Japan, Japanese scholars generally believed that Parks's tunneling technique resulted in too much damage to the internal sphincter and was improved on by Yukio Sumikoshi and Junichi Iwatari (Fig. 8.18).

The improvement to Parks's trench-digging method is to remove the anal gland duct locally from the internal sphincter muscle, not to remove the anal internal sphincter muscle below the internal mouth, but only to remove the anal epithelium and subcutaneous tissue below the internal mouth, and then make an open wound with external drainage. In this way, the anal internal sphincter and its function can be preserved as much as possible to prevent complications such as dampness and leakage of the anus and sequelae.

Modified Fistula Removal and Internal Sphincter Invasive Suture

This is an improved procedure performed by Mr. Masahiro Takano and based on Parks's method. It is mainly for low anal fistula.

Operation points: first cut around the outer mouth of the anus, use Kocher to clamp the tissue at the outer mouth, and use scissors to peel the fistula from the surrounding adipose tissue until the outer edge of the external sphincter. Use a scalpel to cut along the inner mouth, clamp the inner mouth with a vascular clamp, and use a Kocher to clamp the outer mouth to pull both to confirm whether the two are connected together. Further peel off the fistula in the external sphincter until reaching the primary abscess, clamp the fistula and pull it outward, and observe again whether the inner mouth is concave. After confirming that the internal mouth and the primary

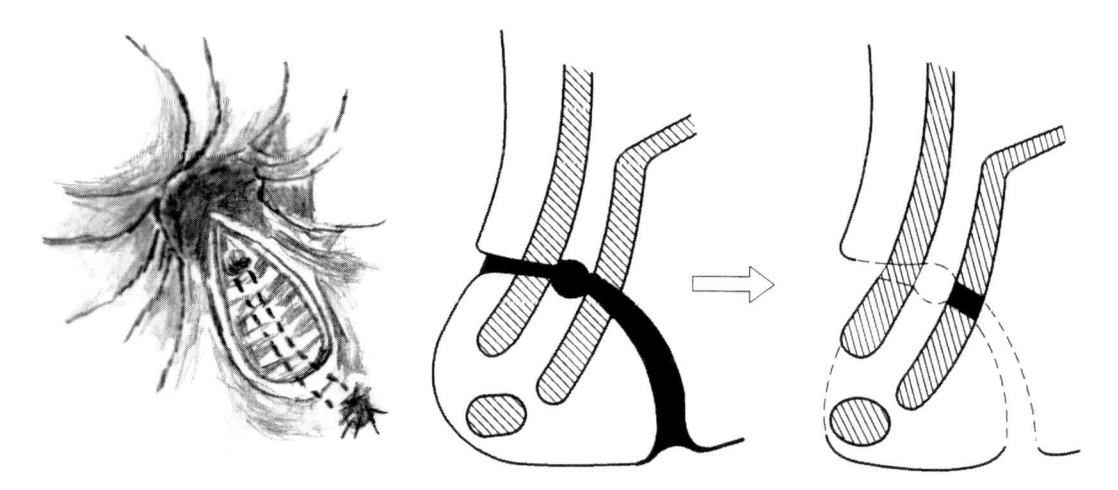

Fig. 8.18 Sumiko's and Iwataru's procedures for low intermuscular fistula

abscess are correct, the primary fistula is removed from the internal sphincter, and this continues until the primary abscess. Because the primary fistula is small, fracture must be prevented. The fistula is pulled from the outside and from the inside again to confirm that the fistula is stripped correctly. For the wound holes produced after the fistula in the internal sphincter is removed, the 2-0 Vicryl line is used to transverse suture every few millimeters, and generally about three to six stitches are sutured. Extend the wound of the inner aperture outward as a drainage window. The wound surface of the lateral excavation fistula is not sutured, and the drainage is opened (Fig. 8.19).

The characteristics of this operation are that (1) it does not injure the sphincter muscle, the anal sinus (inside the mouth). (2) Only the fistula is excised, and the sphincter and other normal tissues are retained. (3) The wounds generated after the excavation are extended outward and the drainage is opened. (4) The defect in the inner mouth is closed. (5) Adjacent lesions are removed. Therefore, this method can not only cure anal fistula but also protect the normal tissues and functions of the anus.

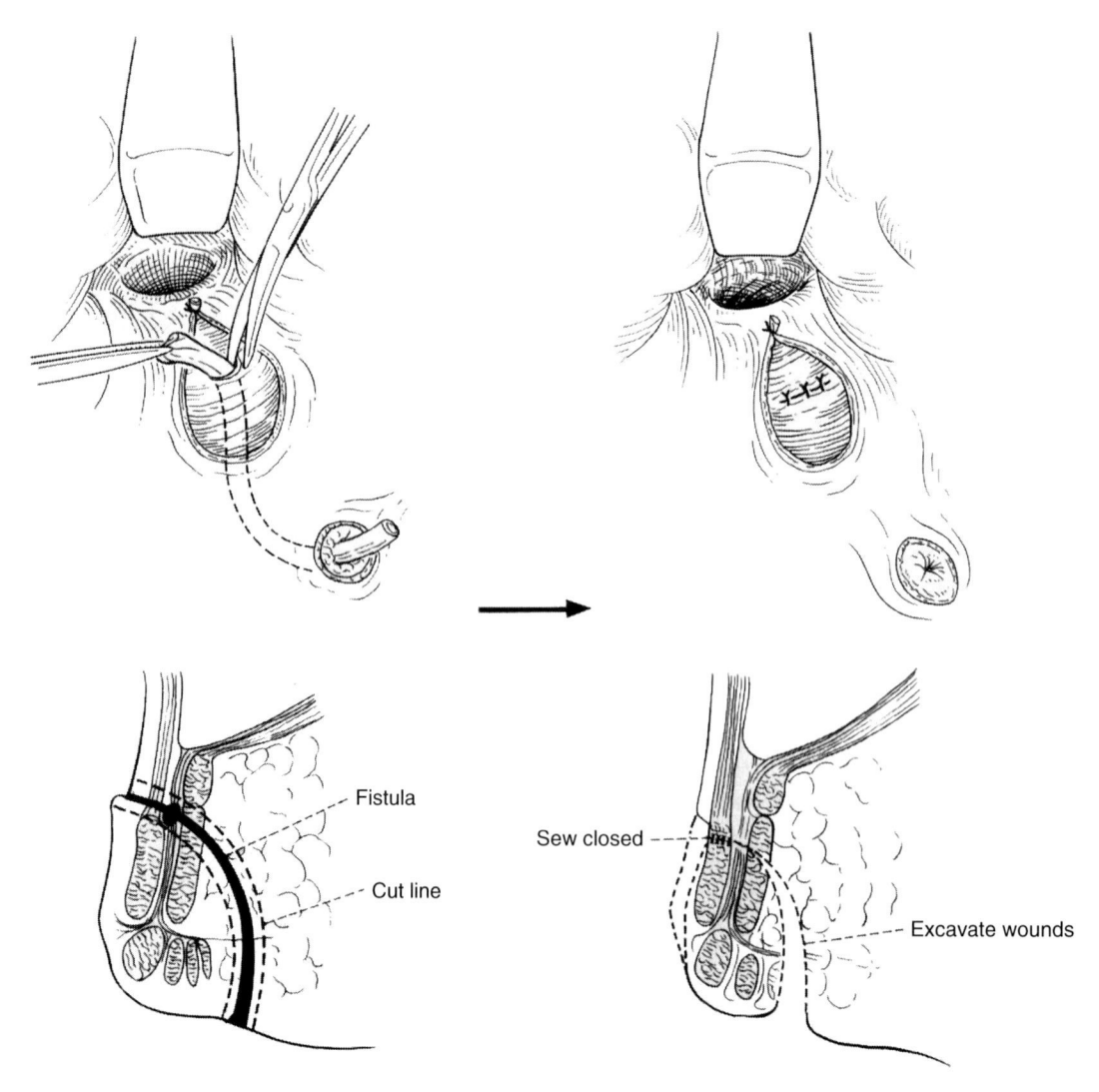

Fig. 8.19 Sphincter preservation operation for low intermuscular fistula. Excavate the fistula from the internal and external openings, until the entire fistula is excavated, and close the internal sphincter defect

For complex low intermuscular fistulas with multiple external orifices and fistulas, the fistulas between the primary abscesses between the external orifices and internal and external sphincters are respectively tactically exfoliated, and the remaining treatments are the same as the previous method.

Anatomical Radical Surgery (Takano)

Masahiro Takano introduced another low anal fistula retention sphincter operation method.

Operation points: first, the entire surface of the fistula is cut radially and shallowly; that is, the anal epithelium between the inner and outer mouths is cut, and use vascular forceps to hold the wound epithelium and pull it outward from the left and right to expand the opening surface. At this time, the subcutaneous mesh structure is exposed, do not damage it. After that, a circular incision is made around the outer mouth, and the outer mouth is held by a vascular clamp and then pulled outward to peel off the fistula from the outside to the inside, taking care not to injure the sphincter muscle. When the fistula is stripped to the primary abscess between the internal and external sphincters, the primary abscess should be firmly adhered to the surrounding tissue, and the fistula is peeled off from the surrounding normal tissue with capillary forceps and small scissors.

Turning to the anal procedure, we first use a capillary clamp to hold the inner mouth, cut the epithelium around the inner mouth, and then peel off the small fistula in the internal sphincter all the way to the primary abscess between the internal and external sphincter. Due to the small size of the fistula in this part, it is easy to fracture when peeling, so special attention should be paid to it.

Through the above operation, the entire fistula should have been peeled off from the sphincter, and the entire appearance of the fistula and its relationship with the surrounding tissue (especially with the sphincter) can be thoroughly observed, and the anal sphincter is preserved relatively intact.

After all the fistulas are removed, there are holes generated after the fistulas are removed, which can be sutured by using a Vicryl line with a needle in the internal sphincter muscle of the inner mouth, and the wounds generated after the lesions between internal and external sphincters are closed. After repairing the sphincter muscle, the anal epithelium is sutured to close the wounds in the anal canal, while the remaining wounds were drained (Fig. 8.20).

Coring-Out Method (Takao Moriya)

This method was founded by Moriya after learning in St. Mark's Hospital in the UK and returning to Japan. It is mainly used for the treatment of low intermuscular fistula.

Key points of operation: first, a few purse-string needles are buried around the inner mouth under the mucosa, and the knot is not tightened temporarily. From the outer opening, the fistula is peeled inward along its side, and the fistula in the external sphincter, the primary lesion between the sphincters, and the fistula in the internal sphincter are gradually peeled off. When peeling off to a thin layer of mucous membrane from the inner opening, the fistula is tightened outward, and the inner opening is concave outward. At the same time, the purse-string buried in the submucosal at the inner opening is tightened, knotted, and ligated. The previously dissected fistula is then removed from the submucosa. The wound cavity after dissection of the fistula is opened and drained through the external wound (Fig. 8.21).

Excision of Primary Anal Fistula Lesion with Preserved Mucosa (Yamamoto Method)

In 1980, Yasuo Yamamoto created this method, and it is mainly used for the treatment of low intermuscular fistula.

Key points of operation: starting from the external orifice, gradually remove the external opening, fistula, and the primary lesion between the muscles until the submucosa at the inner opening. Be careful not to damage the mucosa at the inner opening, and then use a gelatin sponge to plug and stop the bleeding and start gauze drainage in the wound cavity through the outer mouth (Fig. 8.21).

Yamamoto believed that the anal crypt does not have any significance other than as the initial a Low intermuscular fistula shape

b Cut the skin to expose the subcutaneous connective tissue

c Peel the fistula from the anus to the external sphincter

d Dissection and excision of the primary abscess between the internal and external sphincter

e Peel the internal opening from the internal sphincter

f Fistula removal

g Suture the wound on the inner side and open drainage on the outer side

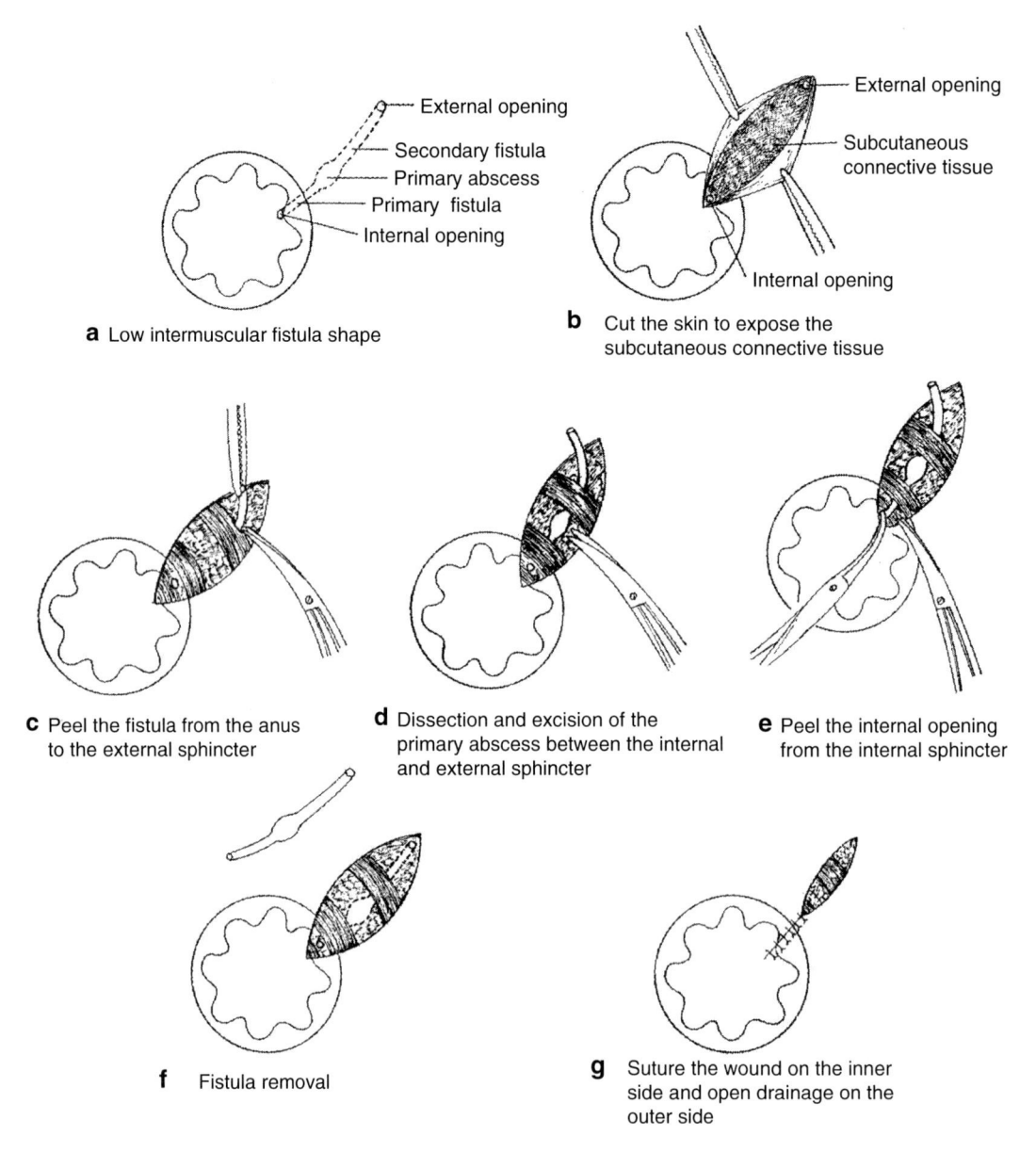

Fig. 8.20 Anatomical radical resection of low intermuscular fistula. (**a**) Low intermuscular fistula shape. (**b**) Cut the skin to expose the subcutaneous connective tissue. (**c**) Peel the fistula from the anus to the external sphincter. (**d**) Dissection and excision of the primary abscess between the internal and external sphincter. (**e**) Peel the internal opening from the internal sphincter. (**f**) Fistula removal. (**g**) Suture the wound on the inner side and open drainage on the outer side

route of infection. Once the inflammation goes deep to form an anal gland abscess, at this time, the anal gland is occluded due to inflammation, and the anal gland abscess constitutes the main body of the primary lesion. Only by excising the primary lesion can all inflammation subside and recovery be achieved. The fundamental shortcoming of anal fistula surgery in the past was that open wounds can easily cause a secondary infection. Resection of the anal crypt can cause a large internal opening in the anal canal, resulting in the failure to prevent secondary infection from occur-

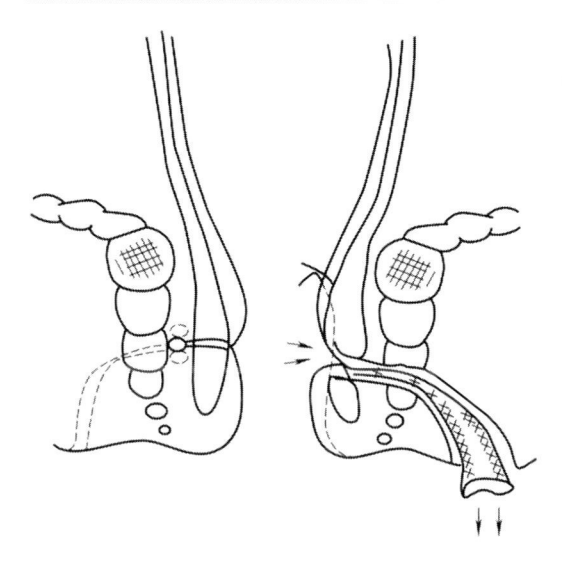

Fig. 8.21 Moriya Takao's coring-out method

ring in the anal canal. He believes that the idea of preserving the mucosa to cover and cut the fistula wound is theoretically and surgically feasible. Although the preserved mucosa is thin and almost transparent, it has many advantages. Even if part of the sphincter is cut, the anus function is completely normal, and the fine exhaust function is not abnormal. This shows that the function of the mucosal reflex sensor is also fully protected after the mucosa is preserved. In addition, wound healing is promoted by preventing separation and contamination of the wound.

According to Yamamoto's introduction, the operation only takes three to ten minutes to complete, and hemostasis is convenient and sufficient. The patient has no pain after surgery, can move freely, and can resume defecation quickly. The pain is light, and the wound will not be polluted by feces when defecating. The postoperative treatment is simple, and the patient can recover from the hospital and resume work quickly. After healing, scarring and anal deformation are mild, and there are no sequelae and complications. However, he did not talk about the recurrence rate.

Utui treated 37 cases of low intermuscular fistula and 2 cases of high intermuscular fistula with this method in 1982, and 33 cases were cured within 2 months and 6 cases were cured after 2 months. Among the 37 cases of low intermuscular fistula, 6 cases had recurrence (15.3%), and 2 cases had no recurrence after having high intermuscular fistula. Utui believed that mucosal preservation is the most advanced operation with minimal surgical damage, but there are many cases of surgical failure, and the indications should be strictly limited to low simple intermuscular fistula. In addition, this procedure is still worth discussing in terms of surgical techniques. Junichi Iwatari et al. reported a 37% recurrence rate in a group of patients treated with the procedure. Therefore, Iwadare believes that mucosal preservation is the worst method in terms of efficacy. He believes that the high recurrence rate of this operation is due to the unresected internal mouth, which in turn proves the importance and necessity of treating the internal mouth in anal fistula surgery.

Subcutaneous Primary Lesion Resection (Sumie Method)

This was reported by Shoji Sumie in 1979 mainly for low intermuscular fistula.

Key points of operation: first, make a small arc-shaped incision in the anal skin, and sneak through the anal canal to remove the lower end of the internal sphincter containing the fistula and the fistula between the internal and external sphincters. Then, the external mouth is excised, and the fistula is removed from the outer mouth to reach the internal and external sphincters. The primary lesions are treated and all the fistulas are removed. Then, the arcus incision of the anal margin is closed, and the wound is opened and drained at the outer mouth (Fig. 8.22).

Sumie's subcutaneous primary lesion resection is similar to mucosal preservation, except that Sumie advocates making an arc incision at the anal edge to remove the primary lesion from the anal canal subcutaneous. No recurrence was reported in 26 cases of anal fistula after the operation.

Preservation of High Intermuscular Fistula Sphincter Operation

This is suitable for the treatment of high intermuscular fistula. The high intermuscular fistula extends upward between the internal and external

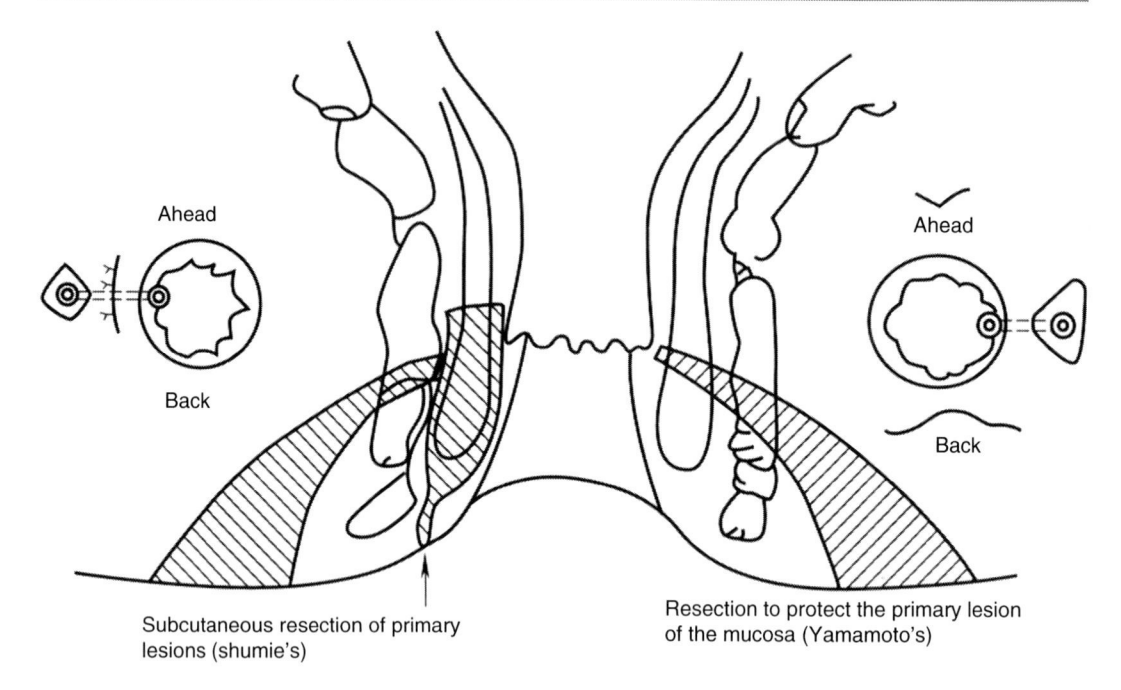

Fig. 8.22 Resection of primary mucosal lesions and subcutaneous primary lesion resection. Subcutaneous resection of primary lesions (Zhujiang's). Resection to protect the primary lesion of the mucosa (Yamamoto's)

sphincter and spirals upward, sometimes leading to rectal stenosis. This type of anal fistula has a high risk of anal incontinence if all fistulas are removed or opened. Takano believed that as long as the internal orifice, intermuscular primary lesion, and part of the low fistula are removed for this type of anal fistula, it is alright to make a wound that is drained outward.

Key points of operation: open the inner mouth, deal with the primary lesion, cut off the upward fistula appropriately, and drain the wound outward and downward. If the fistula rises in a spiral with rectal stenosis, use electrotome to cut several places in the middle of the fistula. As this operation may damage the superior rectal artery and vein, once the injury causes bleeding, hemostasis may be difficult due to the poor visual field, so it is necessary to pay attention to this. If the middle and upper rectum still has serious stricture, surgeons should not make a direct incision and should use the hanging line therapy (Fig. 8.23).

According to Masahiro Takano, for intermuscular fistulas that are very deep or high in position, there are sometimes residual terminal fistulas, and in most cases, these fistulas will naturally atrophy and then become occluded. If they do not heal in the long term, surgeons must undertake the second phase of the hanging line therapy.

Incision and Suture of Fistula Outside the Sphincter

This is suitable for high complex anal fistula. It was reported by Masahiro Takano with the purpose of opening all fistulas for necessary examination and treatment.

Key points of operation: the inner opening and the fistula between the primary abscess are stripped and removed from the anus to create a wound that is drained outward. For the fistula in the depth of the ischiorectal fossa or in the pelvirectal fossa, it is treated by incisions outside the sphincter and then curettage or excision. Most wounds outside the anus are sutured, or drainage strips are placed for open drainage (Fig. 8.24).

Ischiorectal Fossa Fistula Retention Sphincter Surgery

This is suitable for the treatment of total horseshoe-shaped anal fistula formed in the inner

8 Surgical Treatment of Anal Fistula   145

Fig. 8.23 Sphincter preservation operation for high intermuscular fistula. The fistula develops from the inner opening up to the intermuscular. For example, it is dangerous to cut the entire fistula during the operation. As long as the inner opening is removed, the wound surface with proper drainage is enough

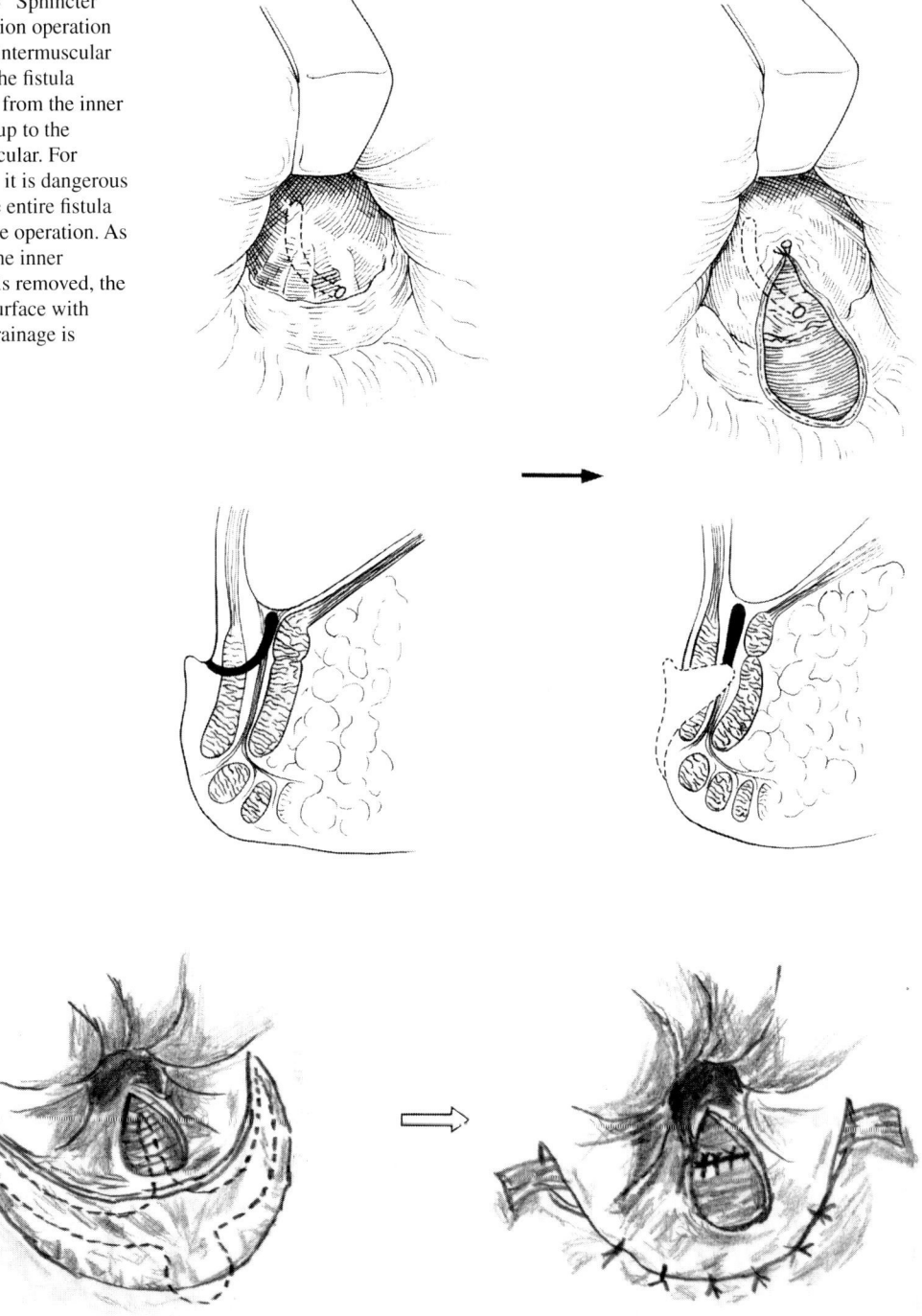

Fig. 8.24 Sphincter incision and suture for high anal fistula. Sneak peeling from the anus to remove the fistula between the inner opening and the original abscess and make a wound that drains smoothly outward. For fistulas in the deep ischiorectal fossa or in the pelvic rectal fossa, an incision is made outside the sphincter, and then scraped or excised. The wounds outside the anus are usually sutured or drained before being drained

mouth in the posterior middle of anus and is a fistula that spreads to both sides of the ischiorectal fossa.

Operating instructions: from the external opening to the direction of the primary abscess, peel off the fistula and resect it. If the fistulas extend to both sides, potential dissection of the fistulas is performed from both sides to the primary abscess. If there is no external orifice, bluntly separate the superficial part of the external sphincter right behind the anus to the postanal space, and peel off the primary abscess and resect it. Then the inner opening is excised, and the fistula between the inner opening and the primary abscess is removed from the surrounding internal and external sphincters. The incision of the internal sphincter is sutured horizontally with "0" Vicryl line to form an appropriate drainage wound. Open drainage of the wound should take place after resecting the primary abscess. For the wound cavity after a unilateral or bilateral fistula is removed, drainage strips are applied from the external orifice to allow open drainage (Fig. 8.25).

Pelvirectal Fossa Fistula Retention Sphincter Surgery

This is suitable for pelvirectal fossa fistula. The inner orifice and primary abscess of this type of anal fistula are mostly behind the anus, and it is mostly bilateral horseshoe-shaped anal fistula.

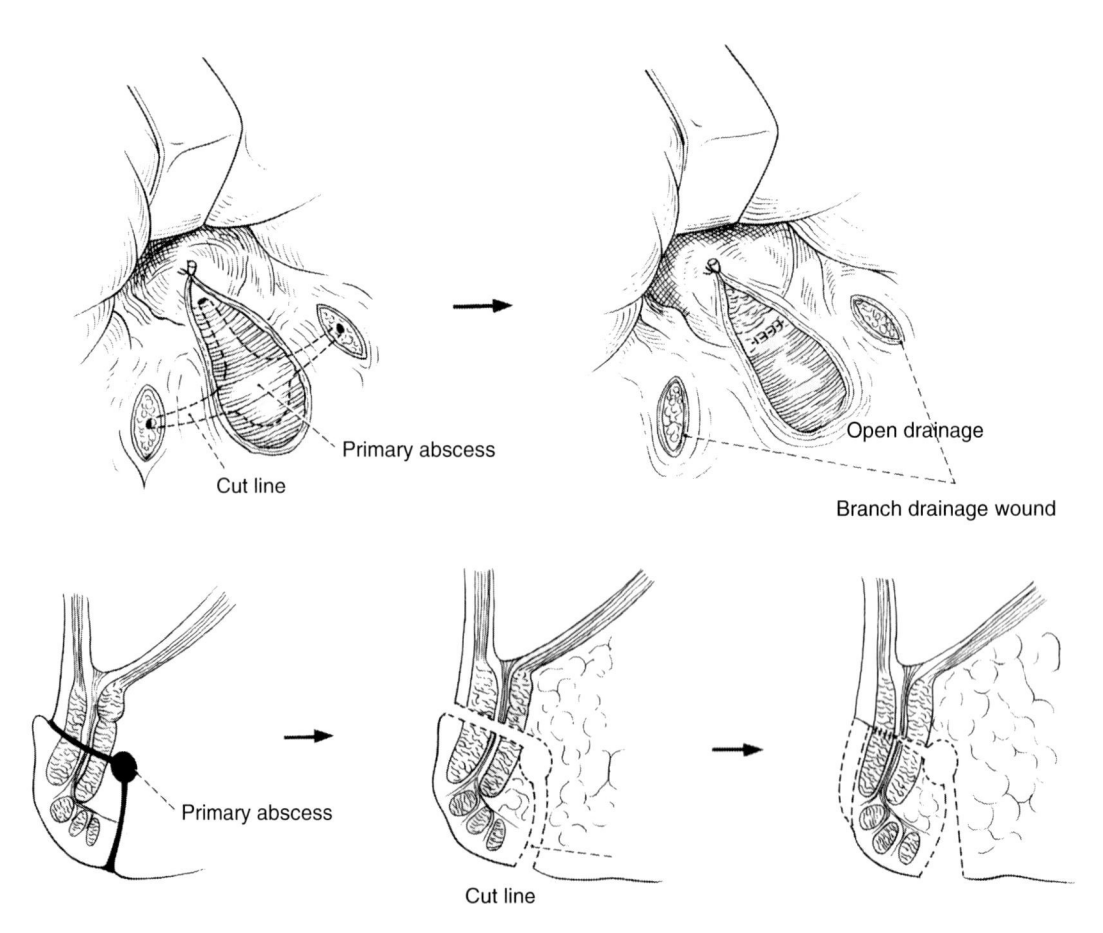

Fig. 8.25 Sphincter preservation operation for anal fistula of ischiorectal fossa fistula. Excise the internal opening in the anus, separate the internal and external sphincter from the posterior anus and enter the posterior space of the anus, and scrape with a curette. Suture the wound from the anus to occlude the wound after resection of the internal mouth. Under the premise of not damaging the sphincter, the fistula extended to the left and right ischiorectal fossa was cut and scraped or removed with a curette

8 Surgical Treatment of Anal Fistula

Operating instructions: peel off the fistula from the external opening all the way to the primary abscess between the muscles. When there is no secondary fistula, the skin between the anus and coccyx is incised longitudinally in the posterior midline and dissociated to its deepest parts. Since the deep lesions are located above the levator ani, below the sacrum, and in front of the coccyx, in order to thoroughly clean the primary lesions, the coccyx should be removed after separation if necessary and reach the lesions behind the rectum from above the sphincter. The lesions in the pelvirectal fossa are gradually stripped from top to bottom, excised, and opened for drainage.

Then, the primary fistula is stripped and excised from the inner opening. The inner opening is separated from the surrounding internal sphincter, and after clamping with a Cochle forceps, the fistula in the internal sphincter is dissected until the primary abscess is stripped and removed. Then, suture the wound in the internal sphincter of the inner mouth, and make the drainage wound of external drainage from the anus. Open drainage is performed on the wounds after fistulectomy of the external orifice and intermuscular abscess or after resection of the coccyx of the sacral anterior rectum posterior (Fig. 8.26).

Sometimes the fistula leads to the left and right sides of the anococcygeal ligament, and

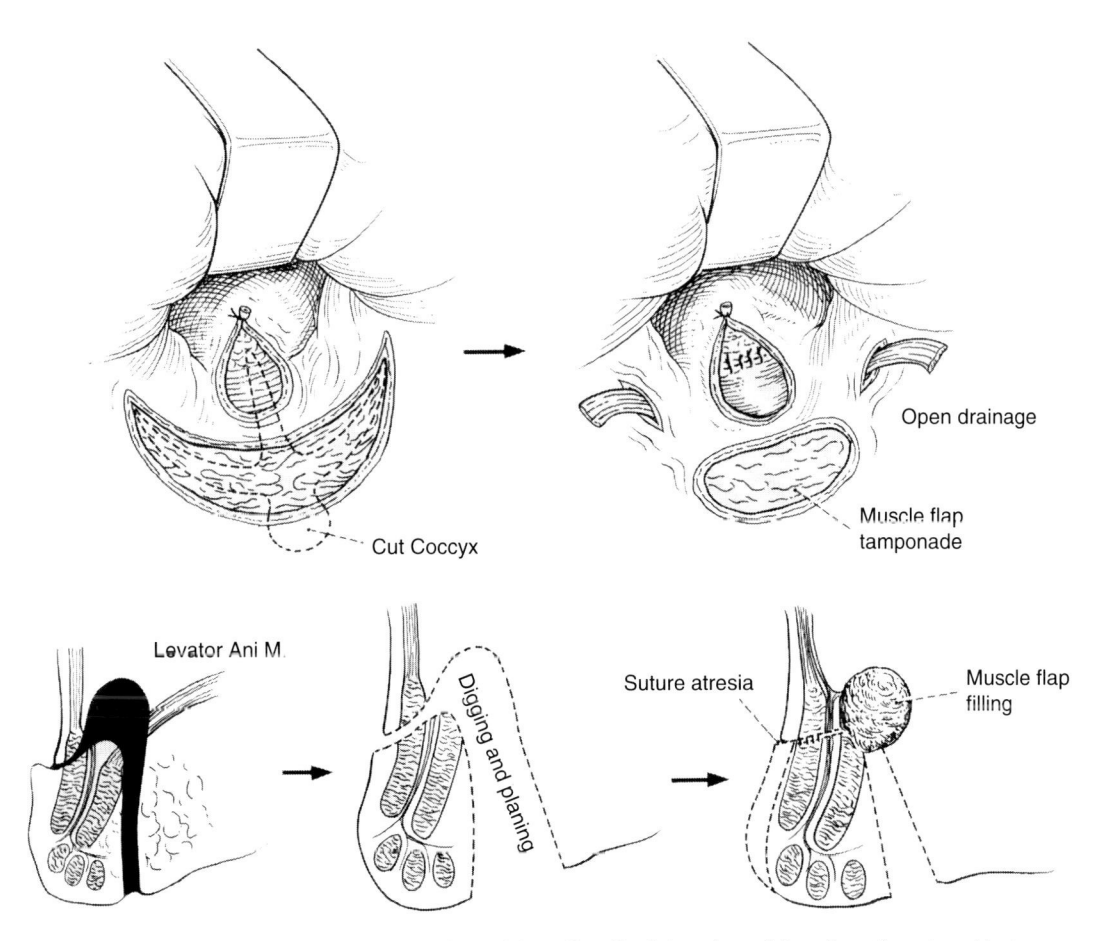

Fig. 8.26 Sphincter preservation operation for pelvic rectal fossa fistula. Excavate the fistula between the internal opening and the primary abscess from the anus, and use the method to suture the internal and external active muscles and the levator ani muscles to close the wounds. Cut all pelvic and rectal fossa from the outer sphincter arc, and scrape or excise. If there is a large wound after treating the fistula in the pelvic rectal fossa, the gluteus maximus flap can sometimes be used

sometimes it extends to the front of the sacrum. When handling such a fistula, it is necessary to prevent missing branches. If the wound after excision of the primary abscess is too large, it will prolong the healing time. The gluteus maximus can be used as a pedicled muscle flap to fill the wound. Because these deep anal fistulas are likely to be associated with canceration and Crohn's disease, it is necessary to send the fistula removed for pathological examination.

Anal Fistula Muscle Flap Filling Surgery

This is mainly aimed at the treatment of high anal fistula (especially open surgery) when there are large tissue defects and prolonged healing time, anal local blood circulation is poor, anal deformation is obvious, cavity cannot be completely closed, or there are other noticeable issues. The purpose of filling the tissue defect produced by the operation with the muscle flap is as follows: (1) filling the dead space; (2) using the blood supply rich in the muscle flap, absorbing the secretion of the abscess and the necrotic tissue, and exerting the internal drainage effect, so that the dead space gradually disappears; and (3) using the muscle flap to block the traffic between the internal and external wounds so that the muscle flap acts as a barrier between the intestinal cavity and the lesion, preventing feces from contaminating the wound and thus promoting healing. It is suitable for complex anal fistula, high intermuscular fistula, ischiorectal fossa fistula, and so on. The muscle flap filling method is recommended in Japan by Iwatari, Kono, and Takano.

Main operating points:

1. **Muscle flap filling surgery of Kazuo Kono**

    Under general anesthesia and after disinfection, a small amount of skin is cut through the lateral skin of the external orifice, the incision is extended upward to the anorectal, and the diseased anal sinus and mucosa in the inner mouth are removed. The diseased tissues around the inner opening, including the anal recess adjacent to the inner opening, are also fully removed. The low wide upper narrow drainage wound exposes the internal and external sphincter muscle. Then, different muscle flap filling methods are adopted according to the position of the fistula and the amount of excision of the diseased tissue.

    (a) Type I (single muscle flap method)

    The primary lesion is found by separating the muscle space, the abscess cavity is curetted sufficiently, the granulation tissue and necrotic tissue are removed, and the scar and hard wall of the cavity are excised or trimmed to soften the local area (Fig. 8.27). Care must be taken during the operation to protect the anal sphincter and mucous membrane as much as possible. When the fistula surrounds the rectum and causes rectal stenosis, as long as the longitudinal fistula is cut off, the rectal stenosis can be eliminated, and no fistula needs to be completely removed. For the cavity formed between internal and external sphincter muscles during surgery, a segment of the subcutaneous of the external sphincter near the cavity can be separated to form a single pedicled muscle flap, and then the muscle flap can be inverted 180° from the outside to the inside to fill the cavity and fixed to the internal sphincter with catgut suture (Fig. 8.28).

    (b) Type II (double muscle flap method)

    In the same way as in the usual anal fistulectomy, the external sphincter is cut and the lesion is cleaned. For the defect caused by the treatment of the lesion, the two ends of the subcutaneous of the external sphincter are cut, and each is made

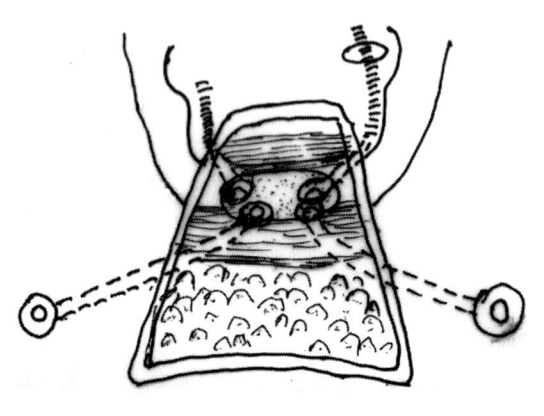

Fig. 8.27 An indication of the treatment of primary lesions with muscle flap filling

8 Surgical Treatment of Anal Fistula

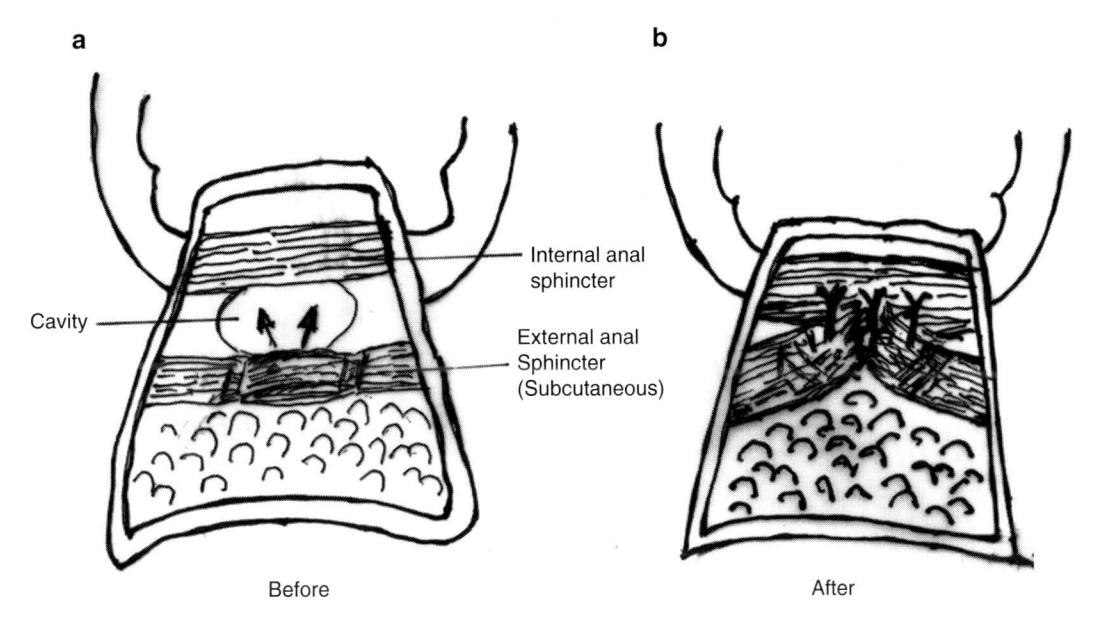

Fig. 8.28 Muscle flap filling operation type I. (**a**) Before. (**b**) After

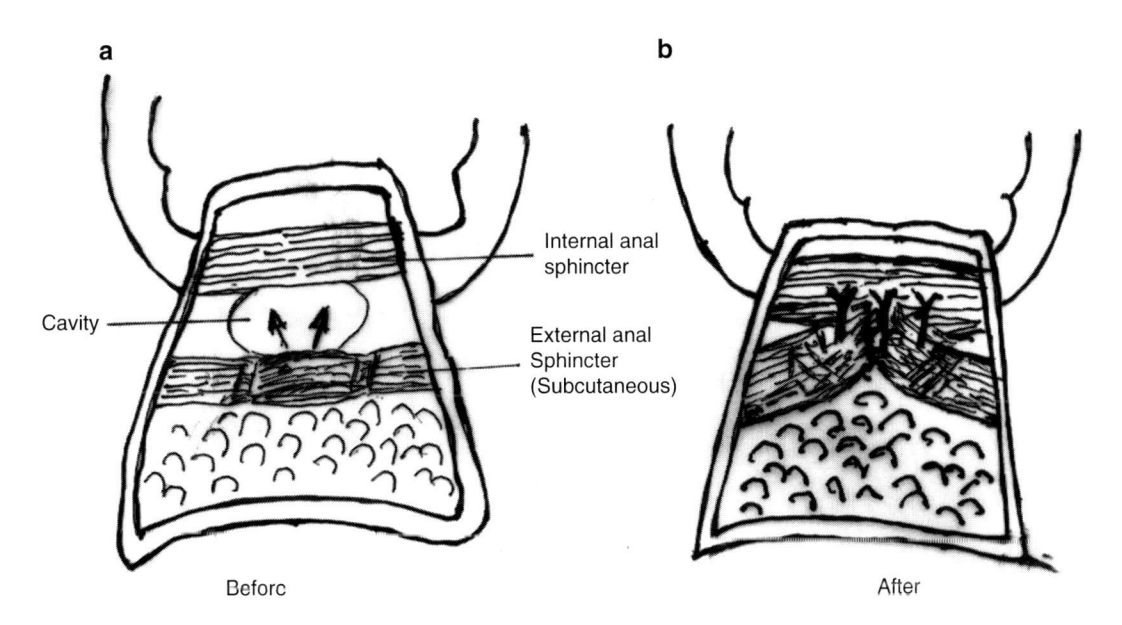

Fig. 8.29 Muscle flap filling operation type II. (**a**) Before. (**b**) After

into a pedicled muscle flap, and then the muscle flap is pulled to the center to be filled in the defect, sutured, and fixed on the internal sphincter (Fig. 8.29).

(c) Type III

When the outer orifice is far from the anus and adjacent to the lateral side of the external sphincter, it can scratch and peel off the fistula from the outer opening and remove the primary lesion until reaching the outer sphincter muscle. After the primary abscess is cleaned, a part of the tissue of the subcutaneous of the adjacent external sphincter is separated to form a pedicled muscle flap, which is inserted into the cavity 180° outward (rear), sutured and fixed on the subcutaneous tissue (Fig. 8.30).

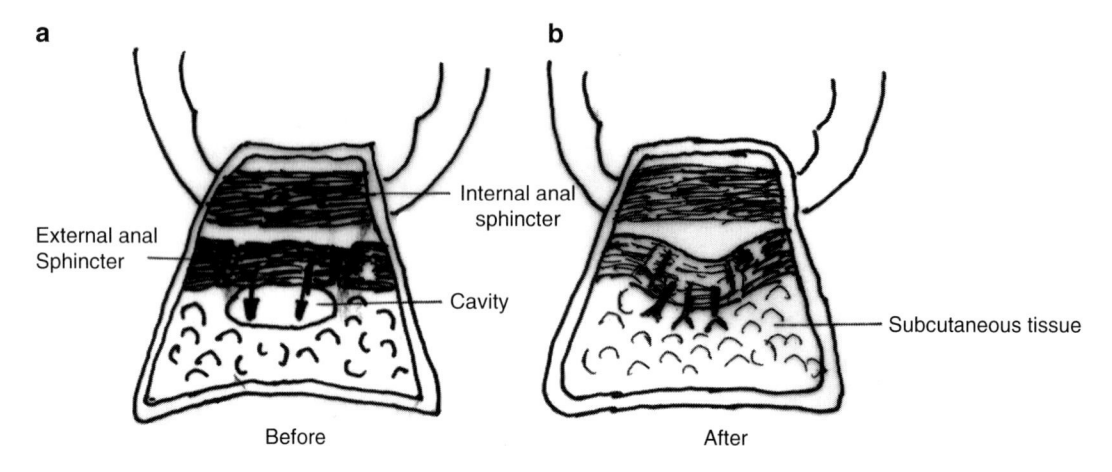

Fig. 8.30 Muscle flap filling operation type III. (**a**) Before. (**b**) After

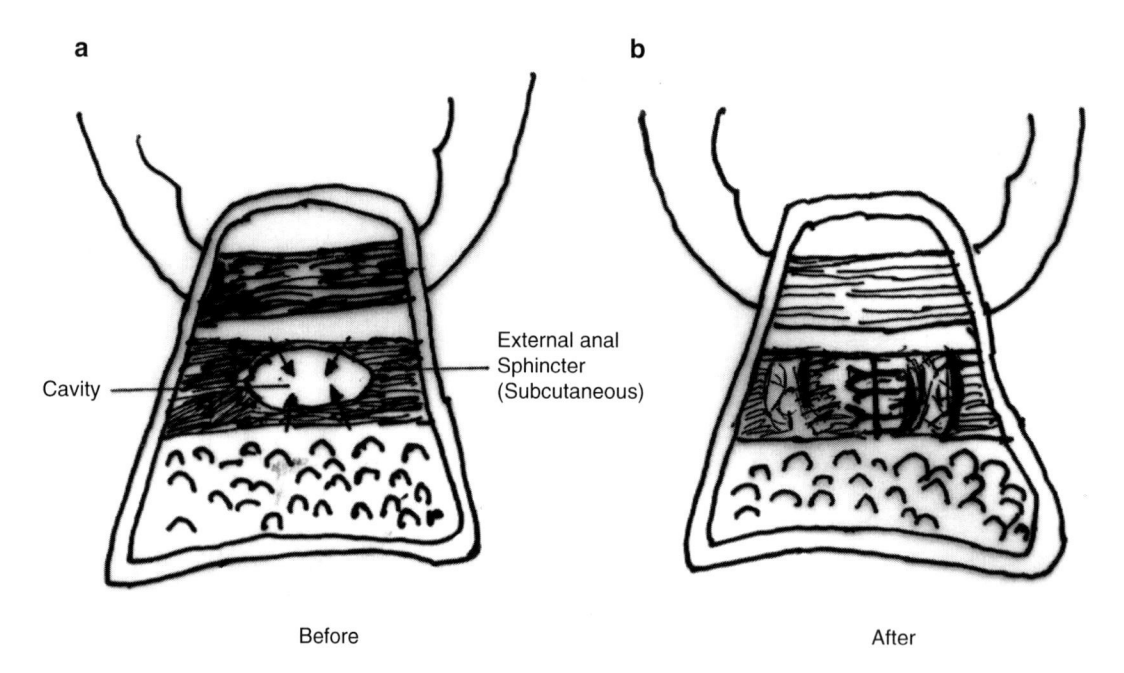

Fig. 8.31 Muscle flap filling operation type IV. (**a**) Before. (**b**) After

(d) Type IV (wrapping method)

For cases where the fistula is located in the middle of the external sphincter, after treating the primary lesion of the fistula, the dead cavity appears in the middle of the external sphincter. The method is to cut the subcutaneous of the external sphincter around the cavity to form a muscle flap, take the cavity as the center, fill the muscle flap as if wrapping a parcel, and fix it in the dead cavity (Fig. 8.31).

(e) Type V (using the gluteus maximus)

In cases where the lesion is too large, the cavity left after the treatment of the lesion is also large; or there is external sphincter atrophy; or after many operations in the anus, the scar is severe, especially in the subcutaneous of the external sphincter, there is a serious scar, and it is difficult to use the external sphincter subcutaneous to obtain a muscle flap. Therefore, a gluteus maximus muscle flap can be used.

Cut the scar first and find the lesion and then remove it. Then extend the anal margin incision, expose and separate a portion of the gluteus maximal muscle bundle on the left side, and make a pedicled muscle flap of sufficient length. Between the incision scars, the muscle flap is pulled and filled in the dead space that appears after the lesion is removed, sutured, and fixed on the internal sphincter (Fig. 8.32). In the preparation of the gluteus maximus muscle flap, it is necessary to pay attention to the deep and upper part of the gluteus maximus muscle, which is rich in blood vessels and nerves. However, what is needed to make the muscle flap is the part of the muscle of the gluteus maximus near the anus with a diameter of 2–3 cm. So there is no need to worry about damaging blood vessels and nerves.

After the pedicled muscle flap is fixed in the cavity with the above methods, the wound becomes flat. Next, the margin of the mucosal incision is fixed to the internal sphincter by continuous overlocking suture with catgut and cover most of the suture line of the muscle flap. Continuous suture of the easily bleeding submucosa is also a measure to prevent hemostasis. In order to prevent blood and fluid accumulation in the residual cavity, drainage strips can be placed in the mouth outside the anal fistula or the newly opened small incision for drainage (Fig. 8.33).

Two to four days before the muscle flap filling operation, diet control and bowel preparation should be done. Antibiotics should be taken orally to prevent infection within 1–2 days before sur-

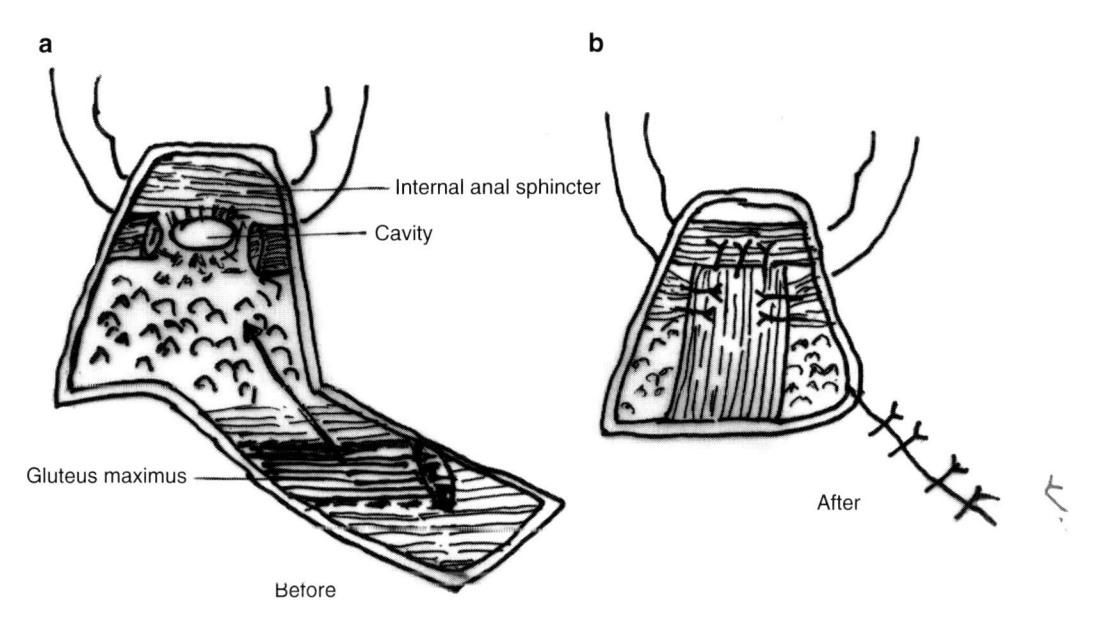

Fig. 8.32 Muscle flap filling operation type V. (**a**) Before. (**b**) After

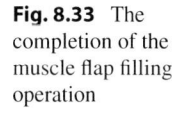

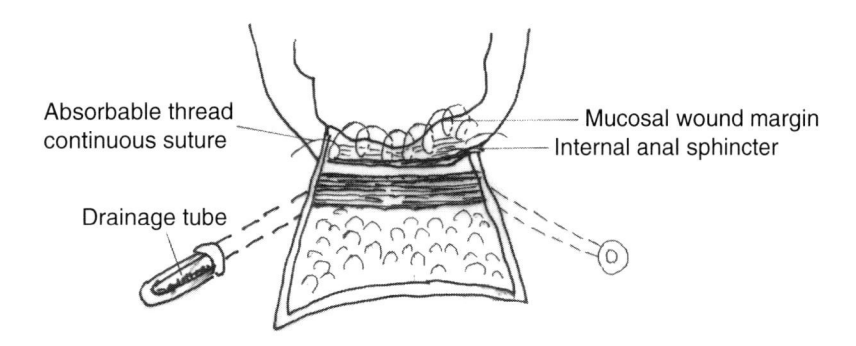

Fig. 8.33 The completion of the muscle flap filling operation

gery. Antibiotics should be continued for 2 weeks after surgery to prevent infection and contribute to the survival of the transplanted muscle flaps. A slag-free diet is given 2–3 days after the operation, and opioid tincture or codeine phosphate is given orally for 1–2 days to control defecation. A bath or sitz bath can be taken 2–3 days after the operation to clean the wound surface.

The wound is usually healed about 2 months after the operation, the induration basically disappears, the scarring and deformation of the anus are very light, and the softness is maintained. Among the 168 patients with muscle flap filling performed by Kono, 11 patients had the following problems: there were four cases of recurrence (2.4%), of which three cases were cured by the second operation and one case was planned for a second operation. Residual abscess occurred in three cases (1.8%), all of which were cured by simple incision and drainage. One case (0.6%) had residual induration swelling and was cured by local injection of antibiotics. One patient (accounting for 0.6%) had partial necrosis of the muscle flap and was cured by removing the necrotic part of the muscle flap. Two cases (1.2%) had residual blood and were cured by cutting and clearing the blood. The survival rate of the muscle flap is very high, and there are no cases of complete failure due to incomplete filling and suture of the muscle flap, or the muscle flap came completely out of the dead space and must be removed. The prevention measures for the above problems are as follows: the pedicle of the pedicle muscle flap should be broad enough to maintain adequate blood supply; a drainage strip should be placed between the muscle flap and the dead space for drainage 2–3 days after surgery.

2. **Muscle flap filling surgery of Masahiro Takano**

This is suitable for the treatment of whole horseshoe-shaped anal fistula with the inner mouth at the back.

Main operative points:
(a) Filling method I

The diseased tissue between the posterior inner port and the primary abscess is removed, and the drainage wound is made in the same way as the Hanley procedure. The muscle flap is used to fill the fistula hole leading to the bilateral branches (Fig. 8.34).

(b) Filling method II

Without cutting the sphincter, the diseased tissue between the internal opening and the primary abscess is removed from the anus and the defect is filled with a muscle flap (Fig. 8.35). The subcutaneous portion of the external sphincter can be used for filling, but the subcutaneous portion of the external sphincter is thin and superficial, so it is not enough to use as a filling material, so it is better to use the superficial portion of the external sphincter as the filling material.

Internal Sphincterotomy (Eisenhammer Method)

Eisenhammer put forward the theory of "intermuscular fistula abscess" in 1958. Based on this theory, for the treatment of intermuscular abscess

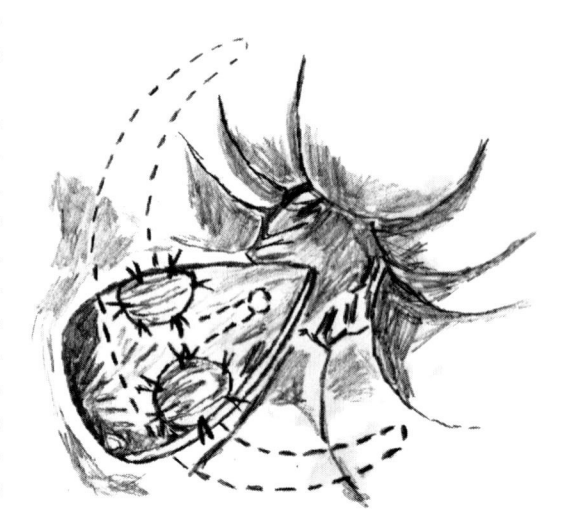

Fig. 8.34 Muscle flap filling of ischiorectal fossa fistula
1. The internal mouth and the primary abscess were incised to make a drainage wound and open drainage. Fill the wound with a nearby muscle flap to prevent dirt from invading, and insert a drainage strip at the end of the fistula to drain

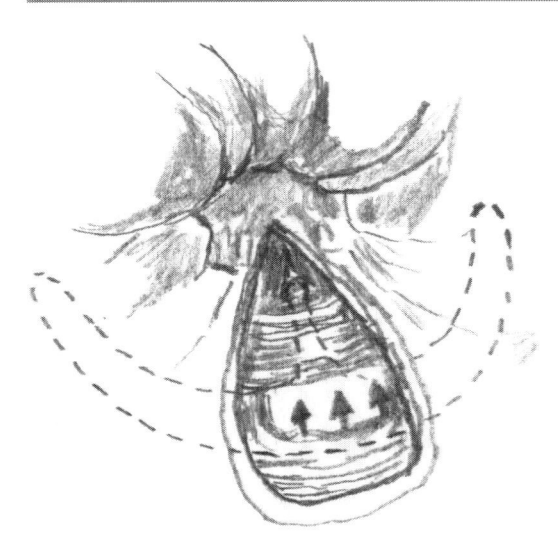

Fig. 8.35 Muscle flap filling of ischiorectal fossa fistula 2. The part between the internal mouth and the original abscess was stripped sneakily from the anus, and the muscle flap taken from the surrounding was transferred to the dead space to be sutured and closed

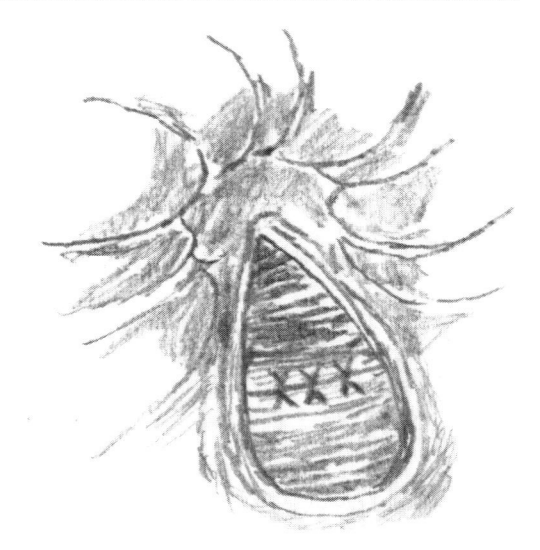

and anal fistula, he advocated the incision of anal crypt and intermuscular abscess from the anus and performed anal drainage without cutting the external sphincter but only cutting off part of the internal sphincter.

Operation points: open the anus with a two-lobe anoscope, expose the inner orifice area, gently hook the inner opening position with the crypt hook, and cut the inner opening and the inner end of the fistula under the guidance of a crypt hook. The length of the incision is 1.5–2 cm, scratch the tissue, and trim the wound. When the posterior hoof-shaped fistula is long, the incision is cut in the posterior middle inner mouth area, and then the incision is cut at a distance of 1 cm in each of the two sides of the pipe. The subcutaneous tissue is separated and the fistula is punctured, and a curette is inserted into the fistula to scrape the anal incision and the distal end of the fistula. The wound is open, and no drainage strips are placed.

Detachment Therapy (Insert Medicine Therapy)

This is one of the traditional Chinese medicine treatments. It is a corrosive drug wrapped with fine cotton paper, such as Hydrargyrum oxydatum crudum, Hydrargyrum chloratum compositum, or Kuzhisan, and rubbed into a medicine twist. Or the above drugs plus appropriate excipients are used to make medicine sticks or medicine nails. The medicinal twist or medicine nail and the medicine stick are inserted into the fistula tube to make the tube wall corrode and fall off, and the purpose of curing the anal fistula is achieved.

The treatment of anal fistula by the method of detachment therapy was first recorded in the book "The Peaceful Holy Benevolence Formulae" in the Song Dynasty. It describes the method of treating the anal fistula by dissolving arsenic in yellow wax and rubbing it into a sliver and putting it into the hemorrhoids' tube. By the Ming and Qing dynasties, detachment therapy was widely used to treat anal fistula. For example, in "Puji Fang" the paper twist of Danfan San (Chalcanthite, keel, huangdan, snake exuviate, musk) was put into wounds, and this was the earliest record of the medicine twist without arsenic. "Wai Ke Qi Xuan" detailed the preparation method of the medicinal twist: first probe the size and depth of the pipeline with a probe, and then apply the medicinal twist according to the condition of the pipeline, and the principle of later dressing change is adopted. The treatment of anal fistula by "San pin yi tiao qiang" medicinal strip created by "Orthodox Manual of External Diseases" had a great impact on later generations. The Qing Dynasty's "Wai Ke Da Cheng" specially introduced the technical requirements and prognosis of inserting a medicine nail and the result of the misuse of ointments. According to the book, "do not insert the medicine into the bottom of the tube, such as a hole depth of one inch, the insertion depth is preferably 0.7–0.8 inches for the degree, insert it twice in the morning and evening, …. When it is observed that there is no carrion in the wound and its surroundings, switch to Shengji powder. When the pus is thick, use pearl to promote healing. Do not stick the ointment for fear that it will drain and the wound will recover slowly."

Commonly used drugs for the detachment therapy include Hong Sheng Dan and Bai Jiang Dan that are sold in pharmacies. No. 1 detachment nail, No. 2 detachment nail, and shengji nail are self-made, and these are all from the book "Treatment of Anorectal Surgical Diseases with Integrated Traditional Chinese and Western Medicine."

The No. 1 detachment nail consists of Baijiangdan 6 g, red powder 9 g, cinnabar 4.5 g, coptis 9 g, raw gypsum 18 g, toad venom 1.5 g, and daemonorops draco 9 g. The medicine is mixed and ground into a fine powder and is added into 80% japonica rice and 20% rubber powder to make an adhesive agent. The ratio of the powder to the adhesive is 5:1. Mix it evenly to make a nail with a length of 1.5–5 cm and as thick as a matchstick and make spares. It has the effect of eliminating necrotic tissues and promoting granulation and is anti-inflammatory and analgesic when used in anal fistula treatment.

The No. 2 detachment nail consists of 3 g of red powder, 3 g of frankincense (roasted), 9 g of myrrh (roasted), 3 g of realgar, 6 g of Cortex Phellodendri Chinensis, and 6 g of Procaine. The production method is the same as that of the No. 1 detachment nail. After the detachment therapy, the tube wall falls off, and it can be used if there is dirt and necrotic tissue in the wound.

The Shengji nail consists of musk; ampelopsis japonica 3 g each; pangolin 6 g; catechu, Bletilla striata, and Angelica dahurica each 3 g; cinnabar; and mercurous chloride and ivory 1.5 g each. The production method is the same as that of the No. 1 detachment nail. It has anti-inflammatory and analgesic effects and is used for promoting tissue regeneration for astringency. It is used in patients with anal fistula wall already falling off, and the wound surface is clean without necrotic tissue after detachment therapy.

Detachment Nail Detachment Therapy

This is suitable for the treatment of low simple anal fistula (straight fistula) and complex anal fistula.

Operating points: use a syringe with a thin plastic tube and fill it with hydrogen peroxide and saline and thoroughly flush the fistula. Then, the detachable nail is inserted into the fistula to make the whole fistula filled with medicine nails. When inserting the nails, attention should be paid to making the detachable nails not exceed the inner opening so as to prevent drugs from corroding the surrounding of the inner opening and enlarging it. Cut off the excess medicine nails at the outer orifice to make them flush outside. After covering the sterile gauze, fix them with adhesive tape to prevent the nails from coming out. The medicine nails should be replaced once a day, and the fistula should be thoroughly flushed when the nails are changed so that the medicine can fully touch the tube wall. This operation is carried out until the fiber granulation tissue of the fistula wall is corroded and peeled off by the detachment nail (generally in 4–5 days). The signs of complete detachment of the fistula wall are that (a) no more purulent secretions are flowing out of the fistula; (b) pain is obvious when inserting the nails; and (c) bleeding easily when touching the lumen.

Detachment Therapy with Detachment Nail and Hardening Injection to Seal the Internal Orifice (291 Hospital)

This is suitable for high anal fistula and posterior horseshoe anal fistula.

Operating method: this method is based on the detachment therapy and involves injecting hardener around the inner opening to promote the adhesion and closure of the inner opening and improve the curative effect of detachment therapy. First, the fistula is detached with a detachment nail. After the fibrous granulation tissue is removed from the fistula wall, the internal orifice is closed. Closing method: when injecting Xiaozhiling liquid with a syringe, choose a fine needle, and inject two to three points around the inner mouth, inject 0.5 ml of medicine at each point, and then put on Vaseline yarn. If one closure is unsuccessful, the second closure can be made. After closure of the internal orifice, the fistula is not completely healed. Shengji nails should be inserted at the internal orifice to promote the growth of fresh granulation, which takes about 4–5 days.

Notes: (a) For complicated anal fistula or horseshoe fistula, the proximal canal can be incised by retaining the anorectal ring (the incision site is within the anal skin line). (b) The external opening should be enlarged to facilitate the insertion of nails. (c) Avoid inserting nails too deep to avoid corroding the inner mouth and causing inner mouth enlargement, thus affecting the sealing effect.

Detachment Therapy with Medicinal Twist and Then Suturing the Inner Mouth (Affiliated Hospital of Chengdu College of Traditional Chinese Medicine)

This is an improved anal fistula detachment therapy based on the traditional detachment method. After removing the primary lesion, the internal orifice is sutured directly to prevent contamination and infection of the wound by feces. Purulent scavenging drugs are used to remove the fistula wall and necrotic tissue, reducing the possibility of recurrence, thus improving the cure rate and better protecting the anal function.

Operating points: carefully ascertain the position of the inner and outer ports, running pipeline, etc. The anal canal is pulled open with an anal retractor to fully expose the inner orifice. With the inner orifice as the center, an oval incision is made in the size of 1 × 1.5 cm. The mucosa, submucosa, internal sphincter, and internal and external sphincters are incised gradually. Open the primary lesion located in the intermuscular tissue from the inside of the anal canal. The necrotic tissues in the primary lesions are scraped with a small curette. The infected anal sinuses, anal glands, anal ducts, and proliferated and thickened intermuscular tissues are removed and rinsed repeatedly with normal saline. Fissures in the internal sphincter are sutured intermittently with 0/3 intestinal suture to close the medial end of the fistula. Then the upper mucosa of the medial wound is freed properly to form a pedicled mucosal flap. The mucosa flap is sutured with the anal skin below by 0/3 intestinal thread or No. 1 silk thread to seal and cover the inner orifice wound. For the remaining fistulas, a small curette is inserted into the fistula to scrape the necrotic tissue in the fistula lumen, with emphasis on the main canal, large branches, and dead lumen. If there are several external holes, they shall be dealt with separately in the same way. If the proximal part of the superior sphincter fistula (posterior horseshoe anal fistula) is curved and difficult to scratch, it can be cut at the bend of the canal behind the anus and scratched in segments. Then, depending on the size and depth of the pipeline, select the appropriate Ke Long Ben Jiang Dan medicinal twist to insert into the pipeline through the outer opening, leaving 0.5-cm-long drug twist at the outer end for easy removal when replacing, and pay attention to protecting the normal tissues around the outer opening to prevent them from being corroded by the Danyao. If the outer opening has been closed, it can be cut into a small hole and then have the medicine nail put into it with a ball-head probe, taking care not to cause a false path. If there is connective tissue hyperplasia around the outer orifice, it can be cut by appropriate trimming or a small circular incision along the outer edge. Finally, Vaseline yarns are placed in the anus to cover the wound surface of the inner mouth, and external tower-shaped yarns are applied and fixed as pressure bandaging. A fluid diet is administered for 2 days after the operation, stool control should last for 2–3 days, and antibiotics should be used appropriately. The dressing is changed once a day, and arnebia oil yarn is used for drainage in the anal canal. Change the Ke Long Ben Jiang Dan medicinal twist on the outside of the pipeline until the pus is removed and then stop using the twists. It usually takes 4–6 days for the twist to be used. Then change the Shengji powder or let it heal naturally.

Internal Orifice Incision and Pipeline Drainage with Medicated Thread (Li Yunong)

This is suitable for complex anal fistula with multiple external orifices and curvature of the fistula canal, accompanied by many branches, and the external mouth distance from the anal margin is above 5 cm.

Operational essentials: under the local anesthesia of the anal margin, the infiltration anesthesia is performed with procaine or lidocaine containing a small amount of adrenaline around the fistula. Dye the fistula with methylene blue mixed with hydrogen peroxide. If the inner opening is in the posterior position, open the inner mouth, anal recess, and part of the anal internal anal sphincter, and open the deep postanal space. If the inner opening is elsewhere, only the inner mouth, anal recess, and part of the anal sphincter are incised. Use a soft probe with a round head to slowly penetrate from the outside orifice, through the stained inner orifice, and scratch fistula with a curette. Scrape all the stained tube wall granulation, extract the probe, and lead the medicated line into the fistula, loosely ligate both ends of the drug line, dry the gauze locally, then wrap it with an absorbent cotton pad, and fix it with adhesive tape. Hot saline sitz bath is used after defecation after the operation. Change the medicated line one time on the second day after the operation, and withdraw the medicated line on the second day after indwelling. The incision is dressed daily with Jiuhua ointment gauze until the wound healed.

Ligation of the Intersphincteric Fistula Tract (LIFT)

In 2007, Thai doctor Rojanasakul and others introduced a new type of sphincter preservation surgery, namely ligation of the intersphincteric fistula tract (LIFT), in the *Thai Medical Association Journal*. After the publication of the paper, it attracted the attention of the Center for Colorectal Surgery and Pelvic Floor Diseases at the University of Minnesota Hospital, and it conducted a multicenter study of LIFT surgery in the United States to promote this new technology. LIFT surgery has a high application value for mature low sphincter anal fistula and mature and unbranched high sphincter anal fistula. LIFT surgery is seen as a first-line treatment and as important as fistula incision and thread drawing.

Operation points: use spinal anesthesia or general anesthesia, take the prone folding knife position or lithotomy position. First, hydrogen peroxide is injected from the external opening of the anal fistula to identify the internal opening, and then a probe is used to probe in from the external opening and pierce out from the internal opening, and this is used as a sign for the fistula. An arc-shaped incision about 2–3 cm long is made along the outer edge of the internal and external sphincter groove. The combination of sharpness and bluntness separates the internal and external sphincter groove. Fully expose and free the fibrotic fistula, and the fistulas are clamped and ligated as close as possible to the inner orifice (internal sphincter) of the intermuscular fistulas. Cut off the intermuscular fistula and remove any excess remaining parts of the fistula. Then, clamp, ligate, or suture the external opening of the intermuscular fistula, and use the absorbable suture to close the defect of the external sphincter at the external opening of the intermuscular fistula. The external orifice of the anal fistula and the fistula outside the sphincter are excavated down the tunnel, and the wounds are opened for drainage (Figs. 8.36 and 8.37).

A systematic analysis of the study of LIFT surgery for anal fistula by Yassin et al. showed that the success rate after summarizing the data was 71%. A total of 183 patients were evaluated for anal function, and 11 (6%) had mild anal incontinence. A randomized controlled trial with the repair of shift muscle flap showed no statistical significance in the difference of success rate between the two. After stratified analysis, the cure rate of LIFT surgery in high complex sphinc-

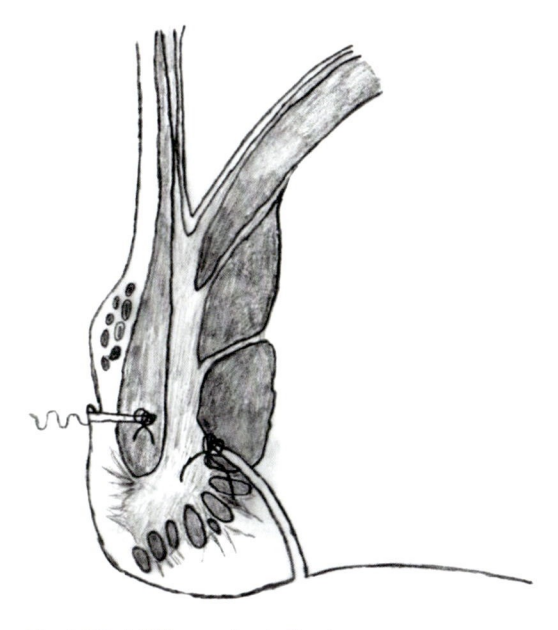

Fig. 8.36 LIFT operation indication

ter anal fistula and recurrent anal fistula was only 50 and 33%, and most of the failed cases occurred within 6 months after surgery. In another meta-analysis of LIFT surgery, the cure rate was 76.5% with a median follow-up period of 10 months, the decline rate of anal function was 0, and the incidence of postoperative complications was 5.5%. It was also reported that LIFT surgery combined with biological patch or anal plug technology (bio-lift or LIFT plug) could not improve the success rate of anal fistula surgery. There were also reports of using LIFT surgery combined with repair of shift muscle flap or intraoperative thread drawing for anal fistula, which did not improve the success rate of treatment. Comparing the effect of preoperative thread-drawing drain and preoperative, nonthread-drawing drain, there was no statistical significance in the difference of success rate between the two.

a. Incision between the internal and external sphincter
b. Pick out the fistula after separating the muscle
c. Tie the medial end of the intermuscular fistula
d. Removal of part of myocardial duct
e. Suture the lateral end of the intermuscular fistula
f. Suture the wound between the sphincter muscles

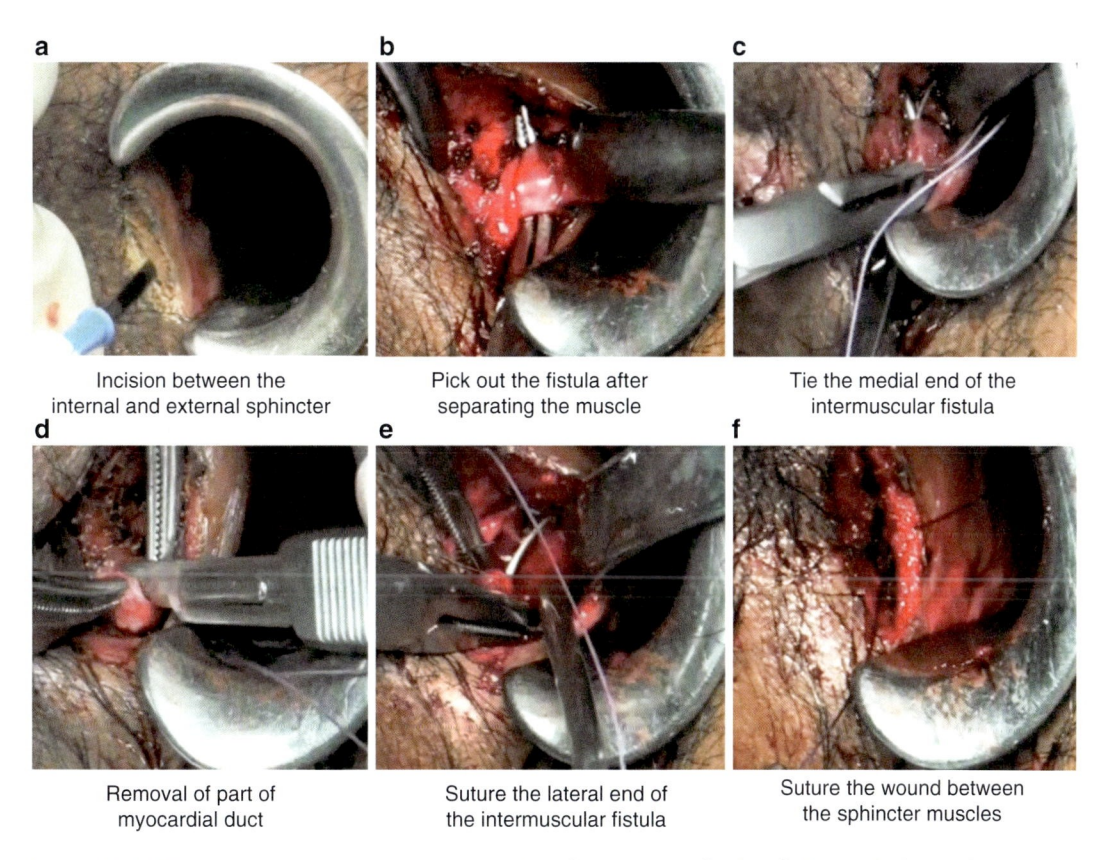

Fig. 8.37 LIFT procedure. (**a**) Incision between the internal and external sphincter. (**b**) Pick out the fistula after separating the muscle. (**c**) Tie the medial end of the intermuscular fistula. (**d**) Removal of part of myocardial duct. (**e**) Suture the lateral end of the intermuscular fistula. (**f**) Suture the wound between the sphincter muscles

Shao Wanjin believed that the types of anal fistula failure treated by LIFT surgery are diverse, and the causes leading to the continuous existence or recurrence of anal fistula may be the untreated internal mouth, residual fistula between sphincters, and secondary infection between the sphincters. The history of perianal abscess incision and drainage or the history of anal fistula surgery and the number of fistulas and external orifices had no significant effect on the outcome of LIFT surgery for high sphincter anal fistula. It is suggested to ligate or suture the internal sphincter as close as possible to the inner mouth. Resecting the residual sphincter fistula as much as possible can reduce recurrence. Flap drainage between the sphincters can reduce the chance of secondary infection; full-thickness suture of sphincter intermuscular wounds can reduce the occurrence of incision dehiscence.

Ren Donglin et al. believed that complex anal fistula in a high position behind the anal canal is often associated with the involvement of the posterior deep sphincter gap and the superior puborectalis gap. Most of the recurrence cases after LIFT surgery are due to residual secondary infection in this deep space. The causes of residual infection in the posterior deep sphincter space and superior puborectalis space may include the following two reasons: (a) the position of the first-stage drainage of the hanging line is low so that the acute stage abscess of the two deep muscle gaps is not well drained and relieved. (b) In the second LIFT surgery, the longitudinal free layer of the sphincter gap was insufficient, and the chronic fistula located in the deep slant to these two deep muscle gaps was not completely eradicated.

How to improve the LIFT operation method and improve its cure rate so that it can be more effectively applied to the treatment of high complex anal fistula, etc., still needs further exploration.

Fibrin Glue Sealing

Medical bio-protein glue is a biodegradable, absorbable biological preparation. The prepared biological protein glue is injected into the fistula to fill the defect tissue and seal it. A biological structure is established in the fistula, and the new granulation tissue accelerates growth along the structure. The bio-protein glue gradually degrades, and the fistula is eventually filled with fresh granulation tissue.

Main operative points: preoperative bowel preparation is performed according to routine colorectal surgery. Spinal anesthesia or epidural anesthesia is used to completely relax the pelvic floor muscles and sphincters. Routine skin and anorectal cavity disinfection is carried out and fully dilates the anus. Preoperative ultrasonography, contrast imaging, and magnetic resonance examination are performed to determine the direction of the fistula, its position, and the orientation of internal and external orifice. First, the expansion of the external opening of the main and branch canal and the external opening of the blind cavity is performed. In some cases, a paracanal stoma is also required. The inner wall of the fistula is scraped to the internal opening with a curet to scrape away the rotting flesh and unhealthy granulation tissue of the fistula wall. The anus hook is used to expose the inner orifice, and use a probe to reach out from the inner opening. With the inner opening as the center, the inner opening and surrounding mucous membrane tissues are resected, and the infected anal sinus, anal gland, and glandular duct are completely removed until healthy tissue is exposed. Repair and separate the mucosa, submucosa, and some muscular-layer tissues in the inner opening, and make them into the upper and lower labellum. The fistula and orifice are repeatedly rinsed with hydrogen peroxide, metronidazole injection, and gentamicin injection, and wiped dry with a sterile gauze. Stitch the muscle layer with a 3/0 absorbable thread "8." The fibrin glue is injected from the inner opening or the united main external orifice tube under direct vision until the inner and outer orifices overflow. After observing for a moment, the upper and lower label-like mucosal muscle flaps are sutured with absorbable line in the shape of a discontinuous number "8" and knotted to close the inner mouth. Fibrin glue is injected into each branch in the same way, the wound and external orifice are covered with saline gauze, and the wound is fixed with an external gauze pad.

Rehydration only after surgery, and fasting is for 3 days. Keep the anus and wounds clean, and disinfect the wounds daily. Mucosal protection suppositories are inserted into the rectum, and antibiotics are administered intravenously for 6–7 days. Prevent dry stools and prohibit strenuous activities within 1 week of surgery.

According to domestic reports, the cure rate of anal fistula treated with fibrin glue is more than 90%. However, according to reports in previous literature, the healing rate of anal fistula treated with fibrin glue ranges from 14 to 90%, and its recurrence rate ranges from 15 to 86%. The overall efficacy is not satisfactory. A retrospective analysis of all cases of fibrin glue-treated composite anal fistula by the Department of Anorectal Surgery at the University of Washington School of Medicine was undertaken. Patient statistics, treatment history, surgical information, and early postoperative follow-up were obtained from the patient's medical records, and telephone interviews were used to identify the cure and recurrence of anal fistula and even further treatment. Fishery's accurate detection was used for data analysis. Results: a total of 42 patients received this treatment between 1999 and 2002, including 19 males, aged 20–76 years. The causes of anal fistula were 22 cases of anal cryptitis, 13 cases of Crohn's disease, and 4 cases of ileal storage anal anastomosis. Types of anal fistula were divided into 33 cases of intersphincter fistula, 3 cases of transsphincter anal fistula, 2 cases of upper sphincter anal fistula, and 3 cases of rectovaginal fistula. Initially, most patients had anal fistula healing, but the recurrence rate was high. The cure rates according to the cause were anal cryptitis 23%, Crohn's disease 31%, and ileal storage anal anastomosis 75%. According to tissue classification, the cure rates are intersphincter fistula 33%, transsphincter anal fistula 0, sphincter superior anal fistula 0, rectovaginal fistula 33%. The cure rate for patients who had not received treatment before was 38%, compared with 22% for those who had previously received treatment. Eight patients were treated with fibrin glue again, but only one was cured. The average follow-up period of anal fistula healing was 26 months. Therefore, fibrin glue is considered to have a low success rate in the treatment of complex anal fistula, and most cases relapse within 3 months after surgery. However, due to its relative simplicity, fibrin glue closure is still recommended as a first-line solution for the treatment of complex anal fistula. The main points that should be mastered in this operation are that (1) incision is made in the lower fistula and drainage should be unobstructed; (2) scratch the open fistula and cavity until the microvessels of the tube wall ooze blood. After the removal of necrotic tissue and debris, rinse with hydrogen peroxide and normal saline, and dry the residual liquid in the fistula and cavity. (3) The configured fibrin glue is injected from the deep part of the open pipe to fill the pipeline and the cavity without leaving a residual cavity.

Fibrin glue is composed of two reagents, A and B. Reagent A mainly contains high concentrations of fibrin and blood coagulation factor X III, while reagent B mainly includes prothrombin and calcium chloride. After the A and B reagents are in contact, the prothrombin activation is converted to thrombin, which hydrolyzes fibrinogen and converts it into fibrin. At the same time, in the presence of calcium ions, thrombin can activate blood coagulation factor XIII and finally form a stable insoluble fibrin multi-body, which can bind tissues and block defects and can also stimulate the growth of capillary endothelial cells and fibroblasts. The fibrin network is used as a scaffold to form fresh granulation tissue, which promotes wound healing and accelerates fistula closure. Fibrin glue has good histocompatibility, rarely produces severe allergic reactions, has no invasiveness, and does not affect the normal function of the sphincter.

The use of fibrin glue alone has a weaker blocking force on the inner mouth. The method of fibrin glue sealing and inner mouth suture fixation can enhance the blocking force and block the communication between the fistula and the intestines so as to create the necessary conditions for healing the fistula.

Biological Patch Filling

A biological patch refers to a patch of tissue taken from the same or different species. After decellularization treatment, the various cells contained in the tissue are removed and the three-dimensional framework structure of the extracellular matrix is completely preserved. It is a biological material that can be used to repair human soft tissues. The main component of a biological patch is protein, and its repair mechanism is "endogenous tissue regeneration," which induces stem cells to enter the biological patch and secrete extracellular matrix, gradually replacing the degraded implants. Biological patch filling is essentially a new material application. It is based on the thorough removal of the internal mouth and the fistula. The biological patch is used to fill the fistula after the closure of the internal mouth in order to cure anal fistula. At present, it is mainly used for the treatment of simple anal fistula and rectovaginal fistula. The current report shows that it is mostly used in the treatment of low anal fistula in the nonacute inflammatory phase and complicated anal fistula with a single fistula. There have also been successful reports on the treatment of complex anal fistula with multiple external orifices by biological patch filling of the branch canal.

Main operative points: make a circular incision at the inner and outer mouths, and then use a curette to dig deep into the canal cavity to fully remove the fibrous tissue and carrion in the tunnel, and cut off some of the wall if necessary. Then, rinse the wound cavity with metronidazole solution, etc. and dry it with gauze. The bio-patch is then trimmed to the appropriate size, and the bio-patch is rolled up with a silk thread and pulled into the anus from the outer mouth. For patients with complex anal fistula with two external orifices and sinus channels, the patch materials are cut into two forks and two sinus channels are filled, respectively. It is sutured with 2-0 absorbable suture and fixed on the submucosa at the inner mouth to seal the inner mouth. Cut off the excess patch from the outer mouth of the anus, and open the wound at the outer mouth without suturing. Control defecation within 24 h after surgery, and have a semifluid diet on the second day after surgery. Postoperative routine use of antibiotics should last for 3–5 days usually in the form of intravenous drip of second-generation cephalosporin antibiotics. Warm bath and dressing change two times a day should be carried out for a few days after the operation.

Note:

1. It is important to choose the indications and timing of treatment carefully. It is recommended to perform the surgery after inflammation of the tissue around the fistula has completely subsided for 3–6 months, as this is expected to improve the success rate. In the treatment of rectovaginal fistula, a fistula diameter of ≤1.5 cm is appropriate.
2. The bio-patch should be soaked in 0.9% physiological saline for one to two minutes before being placed in the fistula. According to the diameter and length of the fistula, the biological patch should be trimmed to an appropriate size, and the biological patch is closely fitted to the wall of the fistula without tension. Excessive biological patch will form foreign body stimulation, which is not conducive to the degradation of the biological patch and tissue growth, and too little biological patch can easily fall off.
3. Effective fitting of the biological patch to the tissue is the key to the survival of the biological patch and the success of the operation. After the patch is placed, it can be rotated 90° clockwise or counterclockwise to ensure that the patch fits better with the tissue. The patch should be properly sutured and fixed with the rectal muscle layer. Several stitches are used to fix the submucosa at the inner mouth with 2-0 absorbable suture. Under the induction of the reticular scaffold, the local granulation tissue secretes the extracellular matrix as quickly as possible, gradually replacing the degraded implant. The composition of the bio-patch is a copolymer of polylactic acid and polyglycolic acid, which can be gradually hydrolyzed and absorbed in about 14 days in the body, and no stitching is required.
4. When used for the treatment of rectovaginal fistula, the rectal side fistula is mostly the primary site, so the intraoperative suture closes the high-pressure fistula on the rectum side. The vaginal fistula is opened without suture

to facilitate drainage and reduce the chance of infection.

According to Wang Zhenjun's report, a small amount of pale yellow secretion exuded from the outer mouth of the fistula within 1–3 days after the fistula was filled with the acellular dermal matrix material. The healing time of fistulas was 7–14 days, with an average of 12.1 days. Postoperative follow-up was conducted for 3–6 months (all cases lasted for more than 3 months and 70% cases lasted for more than 6 months), 40 patients were cured in the first stage, 3 had delayed healing, and 7 saw recurrence. The anal fistula cure rate was 80% (40/50), and the recurrence rate was 14% (7/50), no anal malformation occurred, and anal sphincter function stayed normal. At present, it has been used to treat more than 1000 cases in China. Some hospitals have been following up patients for more than half a year, and the success rate is about 70%. It is believed that this minimally invasive, restorative treatment that does not impair the function and appearance of the anus, even if it fails, can be treated again with the same treatment after drainage, and there is still a similar success rate. Currently, doctors are trying to find ways to increase the success rate of treatment and reduce the recurrence rate. At the same time, the current bio-patch material is expensive, and ways of improving the cost-effectiveness of this treatment are worth looking into.

Endorectal Advancement Flap

Endorectal advancement flap (ERAF) is a method of treating anal fistula by using the mucous flap or mucous muscle flap above the wound of the inner mouth and moving it downward to cover the wound of the inner mouth after suturing and fixing it. This technique was first used by Noble in the treatment of rectovaginal fistula. In 1912, Eltmg applied the method to the treatment of anal fistula. In 1948, Laird improved it, and it is currently used to treat anal fistula, rectovaginal fistula, and rectal rectourethral fistula caused by various factors. In addition, it is also used for the treatment of anal canal stenosis, rectal cancer, anal canal defect, and anal fissure.

Main operative points: after successful anesthesia, the surgical field is fully exposed. Determine the position of the internal mouth and completely remove the inner mouth and surrounding diseased tissues. A "U"-shaped mucosal flap is made above the inner mouth, and the exfoliated mucosal flap includes the mucosa, the submucosa, and a portion of the internal sphincter, which together forms a mucosal flap with a bottom wider than the top (the bottom is about two times wider than the top). After suturing the sphincter gap at the inner mouth, the mucosal flap is pulled down to cover the sutured wound. The mucosal flap is properly freed to relieve tension, and the flap is then sutured with the surrounding tissue with absorbable sutures (Fig. 8.41). The fistula can be removed by tunneling, and the fistula can also be closed by suture after resection.

Pay attention to the following three aspects during surgery:

1. Exposure of the surgical field: because most of the ERAF operation is done in a narrow anorectal cavity, good exposure of the surgical field is very important. According to the position of the inner mouth, choose the position that is advantageous for the operator. If the inner mouth is on the back side of the anus, the lithotomy position is used; if the inner mouth is on the front side of the anus, select the prone position. Both the Parks *retractor* and the Lone Star *retractor* can help to expose the surgery field. However, the continuous pulling of the anorectal sphincter by the Parks retractor may cause the anal function to weaken, while the Lone Star retractor does not.

2. Freedom and thickness of the advancement flap: a good blood supply and tension-free suture are the necessary conditions for the ideal healing of the flap. Therefore, the mucous flap should be free to move upward at least 4 cm, and ensure that the base (head side) width of the flap is twice the length of the top (tail side).

   Some doctors like to use partial-thickness flap with a small amount of internal sphincter muscle. A full-thickness flap containing the mucosa, submucosa, the full-thickness internal sphincter, and part of the rectum annulus muscle or a mucosal flap without the muscularis are selected for coverage. Some studies have found that compared with full-thickness flap, a mucous flap is more prone to necrosis in the early postoperative period (within 3 months), leading to surgical failure, and this may be related to poor blood supply and the inability to form a strong anti-infection barrier. The full-thickness flap has higher requirements for the surgeon, and a certain degree of surgical risk in the freeing of the full-thickness flap, while the partial-thickness flap operation is relatively simple and safe. Considering that the muscle structure of the female perineal body is relatively weak, it is better to choose the mucous flap without a muscular layer for female anterior fistula.

3. Treatment of the fistula and the external orifice: the fistula treatment methods described in the literature include coring out or core fistulectomy and curetting. To avoid iatrogenic damage to the sphincter during the treatment of the fistula, the fistula between the outer mouth and the external sphincter can be treated by coring out, and the fistula through the external sphincter can only be curetted. After excision of the glandular crypt and epithelial tissue around the internal orifice, the defect produced here can be sutured intermittently with a 2-0 or 3-0 absorbable suture. This will support and protect the rectal flap that covers it. Injecting physiological saline from the outer mouth can verify whether the suture is secure. Postoperative wound drainage at the external mouth should always be kept unobstructed to prevent local infection from accumulating at the suture, resulting in surgical failure. Most doctors use open drainage, but Uribe et al. used a vacuum suction-assisted approach for closed drainage, and this also achieves a higher cure rate.

Jarrar et al. summarized the treatment principles of mucosal advancement flap surgery as follows: the precise anatomic morphology and position of anal fistula are defined before the operation. The fistula inflammation should subside by adequate drainage. Close the inner orifice firmly by layered suturing. Avoid the occurrence of dead space, tension, and ischemia. The treatment of the fistula should also be just right to prevent abscess formation. In addition, careful hemostasis should be paid attention to during the operation. The rectal mucosa or skin flap used for repair must have a wide base, a wide pedicle, and a good blood supply. Stitching should completely eliminate tension.

In order to improve the success rate of mucosal advancement flap surgery, it is very important to choose the appropriate indication. This requires a healthy rectal tissue to cover and repair as the advancement flap. Therefore, patients with Crohn's disease with active inflammation or active proctitis are not suited to the advancement flap treatment. Jarrar et al. believed that local infection not under control was the main reason for the failure of the mucosal advancement flap operation. He advocated routine preoperative thread-drawing drainage for 6 weeks to fully achieve fistula fibrosis. Van der Hagen et al. believed that for refractory anal fistula, the initial hang-line drainage can reduce the inflammatory response before the final surgery, regardless of whether or not the fecal bypass is performed, thereby achieving a better therapeutic effect. Many studies have shown that the recurrence rate of mucosal advancement flap surgery treatment for Crohn's disease anal fistula is higher than that for glandular anal fistula. Sonoda et al. believed that even if there is no evidence of inflammatory activity in the rectum, patients with anal fistula who need to take large doses of hormones should not receive ERAF treatment.

The advantage of mucosal advancement flap surgery is that the free rectal mucosal flap or mucosal muscle flap is used to cover the wound at the inner mouth to close the high pressure end of the fistula so that the enteric contents or bacteria cannot enter the fistula, thus making the lateral fistula gradually shrink until it closes. The advantages of this technology are that the integrity of the anal sphincter is maximally protected, thereby protecting its function. The healing time is short, postoperative pain is light, and the diversion stoma can be avoided. Even if the operation fails, it will not affect further reoperation.

The cure rate of treating anal fistula with the mucosal advancement flap to cover and close the internal mouth is 67.0–80.8%. Through literature research, Jacob et al. conducted a retrospective analysis of anal fistula cases operated on from 1950 to 2009 according to surgical methods and concluded that the rate of anal incontinence after treatment of anal fistula with fibrin glue and rectal advancement flap is lower than that of other surgical methods. Uribe et al. observed 90 cases of patients with complex anal fistula treated with fistula resection and rectal advancement flap to close the internal orifice, and the maximum resting pressure and maximum systolic pressure of the anal canal after the operation were significantly reduced, and the recurrence rate was low. Abbas et al. treated 36 patients with complex anal fistula with rectal advancement flap and observed the long-term efficacy. Results: two patients were unhealed, and all the others were cured. Mitalas et al. found that the success rate after the first ERAF failure was the same as that after the second ERAF failure (67% vs. 69%), and the overall success rate of the two repairs was 90%. Jarrar et al. treated 21 patients with failed initial treatment of ERAF with more than one repair advancement flap treatment, and the cumulative success rate reached 76%. Stremitzer et al. performed ERAF on nine patients who had previously failed treatment with a success rate of 78%. Mizrahi et al. also obtained similar results using the same strategy. The patient should be evaluated for etiology, imaging, and anal function before reoperation. If there are concerns about tissue blood supply and tension, a full-thickness flap can be used as the covering tissue to improve the treatment success rate. Some authors believe that after the failure of the mucosal advancement flap treatment, a wide scar is formed in the surgical area. To ensure a good blood supply, it is recommended to adopt a full-thickness flap tissue when repairing again. In order to avoid mucosal ectropion, some authors chose the advancement flap during the second repair, which also achieved a high cure rate.

In China, Li Shengming retrospectively analyzed 23 patients with high anal fistula treated with transanal rectal mucosal advancement flap internal mouth repair. All the patients were cured. Hooker et al. treated 15 patients with high anal fistula with the flap of the distal end of the inner mouth advancement inward and closed the internal mouth. Compared with the traditional low cut high thread surgery, the former had shorter course of treatment, less pain, and no obvious complications. Gong Aimin reported that 20 cases of high anal fistula were treated with gluteus maximus muscle advancement flap, and the cure rate was 100%. In addition, it has been reported that the application of rectal mucosal advancement flap for the treatment of anal fistula in children has also achieved good results.

Wang Zhenjun believes that ERAF has the longest history in the clinical application of "retaining sphincter" technology in treating anal fistula. According to reports from different pieces of literature, the median cure rate of this surgical approach is about 70%. But technically, this surgical approach does not fall into the category of the "completely preserved sphincter technique." The process of dissociating the rectal flap requires the injury of part of the internal sphincter. Therefore, this surgical method also has a certain degree of influence on postoperative anal function. In some pieces of literature, the rate of decline in anal function can reach about 35%. In addition, ERAF surgery is also a skill-dependent procedure. Postoperative complications such as hematoma formation under rectal flap, rectal valve rupture, or necrosis are often closely related to the surgeon's experience and surgical skills. Although ERAF surgery and various modified procedures are relatively "minimally invasive" procedures that have long been clinically validated and proven effective, ERAF surgery has no significant advantage in the treatment of most cases of adeno-derived complex types of anal fistula compared with cutting in stages and the hanging line therapy. Therefore, Ren Donglin believes that ERAF should not be advocated as a first-line surgical method for the treatment of complex anal fistula. But for experienced surgeons, it is reasonable to select suitable patients for ERAF surgery.

Perianal Skin Advancement Flap Repair
This is a method for treating anal fistula by using the anal canal skin flap under the inner mouth wound surface and moving upward, covering the inner mouth wound surface, and suturing and fixing it, and the indications are the same as that of the mucosal advancement flap surgery. In the 1980s, the technique of the advancement flap was widely used in the treatment of anal fistula in Japan.

Operation points: make a trapezoidal incision in the perianal skin, the base should include the internal opening, and the side wall should include the external opening. Free the flap in the subcutaneous fat layer to ensure no tension, completely remove the fistula, move the flap to the proximal end, and suture and fix it with the mucosa above the anal canal inner mouth. The lower wound of the flap is opened and drained (Fig. 8.38).

Compared with the mucosal advancement flap, the skin advancement flap has a lower requirement for anal canal exposure, but the blood supply is relatively poor, and patients with skin inflammation and fragile skin are not suitable for treatment with skin advancement flap. In addition, after the skin advancement flap is used, feces can easily enter the wound surface below the suture between the flap and the rectal mucosa, leading to infection and thus failure of the operation.

In China, Song Yinggang reported that the short-term cure rate and long-term cure rate of 50 cases of complex anal fistula were 96% and 78%, respectively.

The author believes that both the rectal mucosal advancement flap and the perianal skin advancement flap to repair the internal orifice of the anal fistula are only the technical means of treating the internal mouth wound in the treatment of anal fistula, rather than an anal fistula treatment technique with an essential breakthrough in treatment principle. The key to the cure of anal fistula is the complete removal of the internal orifice and the primary lesion, and the treatment of the fistula and the external orifice in the sphincter. If these key steps are not handled correctly and are not in place, the anal fistula will not be cured even if the internal mouth wounds are repaired well. Therefore, we should avoid emphasizing the decisive effect of one treatment technique in the treatment of the efficacy, although one part of the procedure in the surgery will affect the overall efficacy.

Minimally Invasive Video-Assisted Anal Fistula Treatment
Video-assisted anal fistula treatment (VAAFT) is a technique that combines the concept of endoscopic surgery and the concept of minimally invasive treatment with the treatment of anal fistula endoscopic.

Operation points: anal fistula mirror and supporting equipment should be used to complete the operation. The set of instruments includes the anal fistula mirror, sealing rod, unipolar electrocoagulation, endoscopic grasping forceps, endoscopic brush, and three-leaf anoscope. The anal fistula lens is an 8° bevel mirror with an optical channel, operation channel, and perfusion channel. The two interfaces with valves are

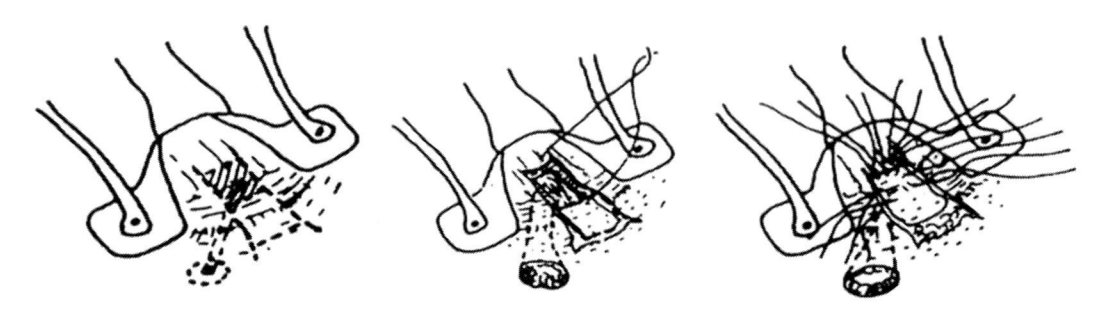

Fig. 8.38 Anal fistula moving flap repair operation

8 Surgical Treatment of Anal Fistula

connected to a 1.5% glycine solution and a vacuum suction.

The operation is performed under intraspinal anesthesia. According to the position of the external mouth, the patients are placed in the lithotomy position or the folding knife position. The surgical procedure can be divided into two parts: the diagnosis stage and the treatment stage.

1. Diagnosis stage: the goal is to accurately locate the internal orifice and explore the possible fistula branches and abscess cavity. Under the continuous perfusion of glycine solution, the anal fistula lens is introduced from the external mouth. Sometimes it is necessary to remove scar tissue around the external mouth to facilitate the insertion of the anal fistula mirror. Keep the sealing rod at the bottom of the display as a guide, and the fistula situation can be clearly presented on the display (Fig. 8.39). Introduce the mirror slowly until the position of the fistula end inner opening is found. At this time, the three-lobed anoscope is inserted, and the light source of the anal fistula mirror can be seen under the rectal mucosa, which is the position of the inner mouth (Fig. 8.40). Sew two to three stitches around the inner mouth to isolate the inner mouth. Be careful not to close the inner mouth at this time.

2. Treatment stage: the purpose of this is to destroy the fistula tissue from the inside, clean the fistula, and then finally close the inner mouth. The sealing rod is removed, and the electrocoagulation electrode is introduced. The fistula is removed from the inside to the outside under direct vision (Fig. 8.41), and the necrotic tissue adhering to the wall of the fistula is electrocauterized. Endoscopic brush or endoscopic grasping forceps are

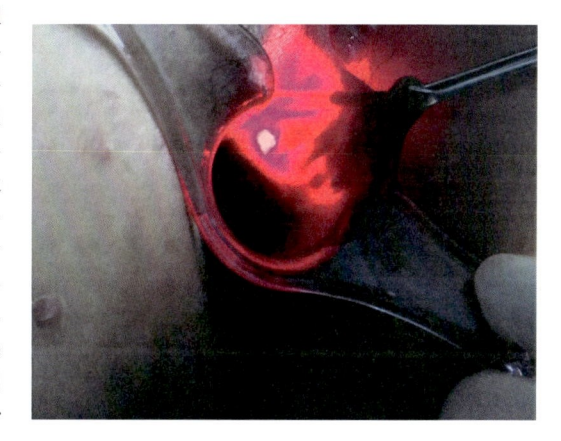

Fig. 8.40 Internal opening by video-assisted anal fistula treatment (VAAFT)

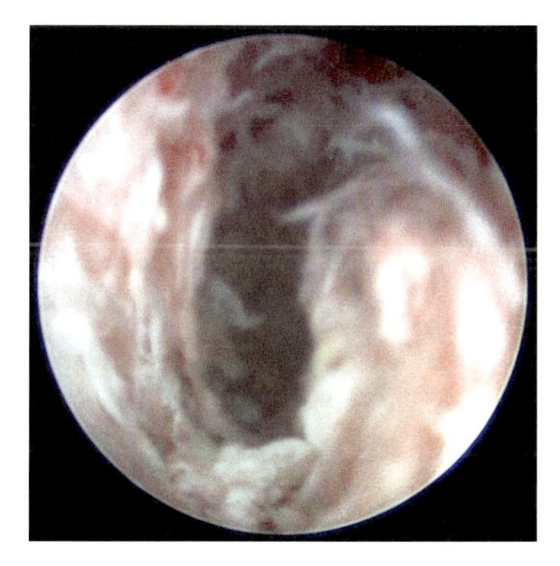

Fig. 8.39 Fistula seen by video-assisted anal fistula treatment (VAAFT)

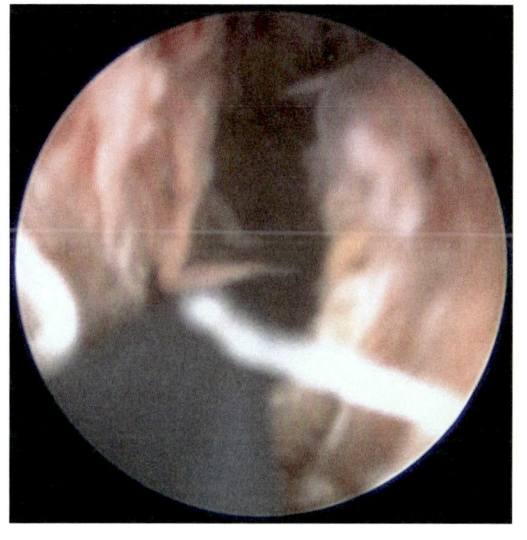

Fig. 8.41 Treatment of fistula under video-assisted anal fistula treatment (VAAFT)

used to remove necrotic materials. The exfoliated necrotic material can also be flushed into the rectal cavity through the inner mouth and discharged. Carefully explore to avoid missing possible branch fistulas and abscess cavities. After the fistula is cleaned, lift the inner opening and close it with a stapler or suture it with an absorbable suture. The biological protein glue is injected into the fistula from the outside mouth. The outer mouth is opened for drainage.
3. Postoperative treatment: a fluid diet is started six hours after surgery, and oral paraffin oil is administered at the same time. On the first day after surgery, the perineal dressing is removed, and a semi-liquid diet is given after defecation. Antibiotics are not routinely used after surgery. Different from traditional surgery, VAAFT surgery treats the fistula by endoscope without incision or resection of the fistula, so there is no obvious damage to sphincter function. VAAFT surgery can accurately locate the anatomical position of the internal orifice and fistula under the direct vision of the anal fistula mirror, and it is easy to find potential fistula branches and abscess cavities. The fistula wall is damaged by electrocautery, and the necrotic tissue is removed under the direct vision. The inner port is usually closed by a stapler or hand-stitched, and the inner port is further sealed by glue. Foreign literature has reported that VAAFT surgery has a high cure rate for complex anal fistula and can protect the function of the anal sphincter well.

In order to ensure the smooth operation of the VAAFT surgery and reduce postoperative complications, the following key points should be noted during the operation.

1. Exploration of the fistula: all possible fistula branches and abscess cavities are carefully explored to distinguish true fistulas and pseudofistulas. Granulation tissue with red edema can be seen in the true fistula, and the pseudofistula is white and has no edema.
2. Treatment of fistula: the wall of the fistula should be fully cauterized from the inside to the outside. Since the operation hole is located below the anal sinus mirror, the lower wall treatment is convenient, while the lateral wall or upper wall may need to be rotated completely to facilitate the treatment.
3. Processing of the inner mouth: use the three-leaf anoscope to expose and locate the internal orifice under the instruction of the anal fistula mirror. There is currently no clear evidence that Endo-GIA closes the inner mouth better than hand stitching, but Meinero et al. believe that the former may work better. Other researchers used rectal mucosal advancement flap or perianal advancement flap to close the internal orifice.
4. Prevention and treatment of postoperative complications of VAAFT: electrocoagulation can cause thermal damage to the normal tissue next to fistula granulation tissue, so the power of high-frequency electrotome should be about 40 W, and the monopolar coagulation mode should be used. The submucosal tissue around the inner mouth is relatively loose, and care should be taken to avoid the formation of false passages here. In addition, hypotonic glycine irrigating fluid often leads to edema in the surrounding tissue of the fistula and may also bring necrotic material in the fistula into the surrounding normal tissue resulting in delayed healing or recurrence of the fistula. Therefore, reducing perfusion pressure, shortening operation time, and avoiding the formation of false passages are helpful to reduce edema of the fistula's surrounding tissues and thus reduce the risk of postoperative infection.

According to Liu Hailong, of the 11 patients that successfully completed VAAFT surgery, 10 were treated with the suture method and 1 patient with Endo-GIA. The operation time was 42.0 ± 12.4 minutes, and hospital stay was 4.1 ± 1.5 days. One patient had anal hemorrhage after defecation on the third day after the operation. The rectal mucosal tear was seen at the internal suture after reoperation; the patient was discharged after the wound electrocoagulation occurred. During the follow-up period of 1.0–3.2

8 Surgical Treatment of Anal Fistula

months, eight patients were healed in the first stage, and the cure rate was 72.7% (8/11). There was no postoperative fecal incontinence. Among the other three patients, one patient who had received a total of five anal fistula operations developed perianal infection and received drainage treatment; two cases were unhealed and continued to be followed up. Liu believes that VAAFT surgery is a safe and effective minimally invasive procedure for the treatment of complex anal fistula.

Fistula Peeling

A visual rotary peeling knife is required for this surgery. The visual rotary planing knife is an anal fistula minimally invasive instrument that integrates LED light source, camera and image enlargement, planing, rinsing, and suction.

Surgical points:

1. Cut around the outer mouth, about 1.5 cm in diameter, and introduce a rotatable planing knife to the cutting area. Under the guidance of the LED light source, identify the tube wall and internal orifice tissues. The necrotic and fibrous epithelial tissue of the fistula wall are peeled to the intermuscular of the internal and external sphincters, the normal sphincter tissue is separated, the internal and external sphincter muscles are not damaged, and the fistula is removed to the internal mouth under the rectal mucosa. The normal sphincter tissue is isolated, the internal and external sphincters are not damaged, and the fistula is removed to the inner mouth of the rectal mucosa. The degree of gouging is determined by the fresh ruddy color and soft texture of the wound surface of the tube wall (Fig. 8.42). In the process of cutting the fistula, the visible rotary peeling can flush and suction at the same time to ensure the wound is cleaned.
2. Use a 3-0 absorbable suture around the inner mouth to make a purse of about 1 cm in diameter, with a little muscle layer, and the purse line is then tightened. The purse line is pulled into the cutter, cut, and closed after tightening.

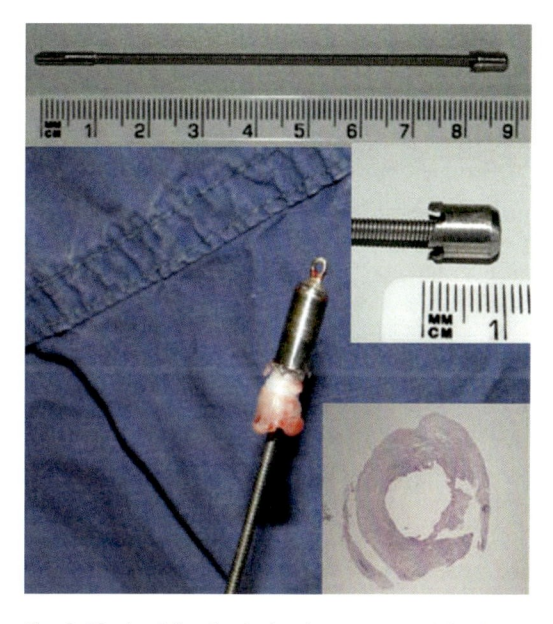

Fig. 8.42 Anal fistula planing instrument and fistula tissue under planing in VAAFT

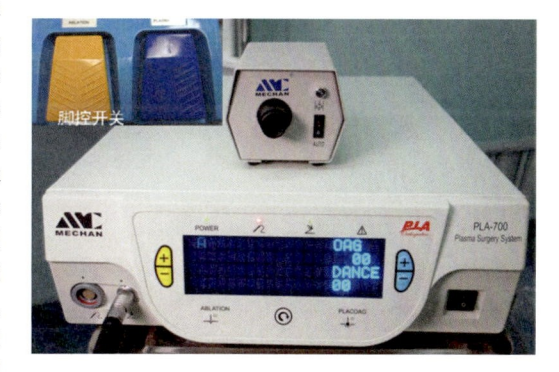

Fig. 8.43 Low-temperature plasma technology

Low-Temperature Plasma Knife Fistula Ablation

This is a treatment method of anal fistula by ablation of the whole fistula and the inner mouth with the help of a low-temperature plasma surgical system (Fig. 8.43). Low-temperature plasma radiofrequency is a 100-kHz segment of radiofrequency that excites the electrolyte into plasma. A thin layer of plasma with a thickness of 50–100 μm is formed in front of the electrode. The strong electric field enables the free-charged particles in the thin layer of plasma to gain enough kinetic energy to break the molecular bonds so that the target tissue cells can disintegrate as a unit of molecules and form molecular level cutting at low temperature. Plasma RF has the same "knife" cutting effect. Therefore, in the clinic it is also called the "plasma knife." The low-temperature plasma knife can precisely control the temperature at 40–70 °C, which ensures that the helical structure of the collagen molecule shrinks and maintains the vitality of the cells.

Operation points: To explore the fistula tract and identify the inner opening after routine disinfection and draping. Low-Temperature plasma knife is inserted into the fistula from the external opening, and the whole fistula is ablated gradually to the inner opening (Fig. 8.44). After the inner mouth is ablated, a radial incision is made from the inner mouth to the anal margin for drainage. Then, suture between internal and external sphincter with one to several stitches to close the channel between the internal mouth and fistula. After routine operation, control defecation for 2 days, use antibiotics as appropriate to prevent infection, undergo routine dressing change, and take out stitches after 7–12 days.

Compared with electrosurgery, laser, microwave, and other treatment methods, low-temperature plasma technology has the following advantages: the current does not flow directly through the human body, there is little tissue heat, a low treatment temperature, no direct destruction of tissues, and minimal damage to surrounding tissues. According to the introduction of Huang Dequan, after the treatment of anal fistula with low-temperature plasma technology, the patient has mild pain and mild postoperative inflammatory reaction. During the operation, the cutting of hemostasis can be completed at the same time. He treated 62 cases of high simple anal fistula from September to November 2015, respectively, using plasma ablation and the dissection and seton therapy. Results showed that the cure rate of both groups was 100% after treatment, while the former's postoperative pain score was significantly lower than that of the latter, and the wound healing time was significantly less than that of the control group.

Laser Fistula Ablation

Laser can be used in the treatment of a variety of diseases, including anal fistula. Previous lasers used for treatment have relied on radioactive energy. The use of new radiation-circumferential energy laser ablation for the treatment of anal fistula is currently only being attempted. At present, there are only a few related research articles, so this treatment method is not yet mature.

Operation points: a 15-watt probe is used to emit a 1470-nm wavelength laser, generating an energy of 100–120 J/cm^2 to treat anal fistula under general anesthesia.

A total of 50 patients, including 37 males and 13 females, were reported in the literature, with a median age of 41 (23–83) years. There were 10 cases of internal anal fistula of the sphincter, 34 cases of low sphincter anal fistula, and 6 cases of high sphincter anal fistula. The short-term outcome measures evaluated included the success rate of surgery, complications, pain scores, and length of time before resuming daily activities. The patient not having any complaints was the criterion for treatment success. The results showed that the success rate of this group of patients was 82%; all patients did not need to add peripheral analgesics. The median time to resume daily activities was 7 (5–17) days. The median follow-up time was 12 (2–18) months, and nine cases failed laser treatment and thus underwent further conventional surgery. This procedure is considered to be a safe

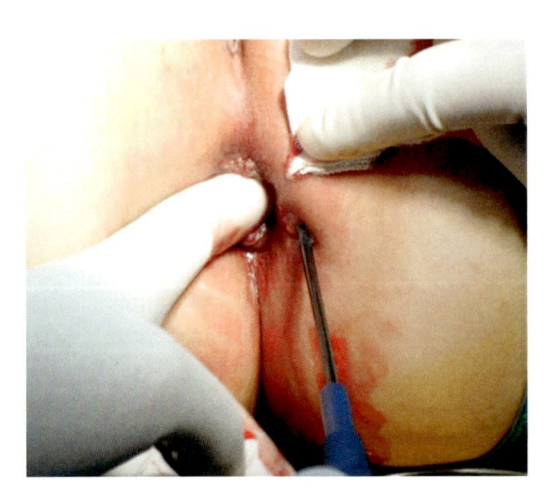

Fig. 8.44 Low-temperature plasma technology for anal fistula. The plasma knife is inserted into the fistula from the outer opening to dissolve the entire fistula and the inner opening

and effective method for the treatment of anal fistula that retains the sphincter.

8.2.3.3 Discussion on Some Problems in Anal Fistula Surgery

Clinical Significance of Sphincter Retention Surgery
Surgery in itself is a destructive treatment for any disease, which itself will cause damage to the body, so even anal fistula retained sphincter surgery will still cause some damage to the anal sphincter. Especially in high and complex anal fistula operations, in order to ensure the complete treatment and unblocked drainage, it is inevitable to cut or remove a part of the sphincter muscle, resulting in a certain degree of sphincter injury. The significance of anal fistula retained sphincter surgery is that on the basis of maintaining a high cure rate, it can significantly reduce the damage of the operation itself to anal function, and even after recurrence, there is a good functional basis for reoperation.

The Importance of Retaining the Internal Sphincter
In the earliest anal fistula retained sphincter surgery, when treating the internal mouth and intermuscular abscesses, it was advocated to remove the lower end of the internal sphincter of the internal mouth and then remove the primary lesion. However, this damage to the internal sphincter is large, and the postoperative defect is almost the same as that of anal fistula open surgery. Because the internal sphincter is a smooth muscle, it is weak but has a sustained contraction effect, is not controlled by consciousness, and can continue to close the anus becoming loose. When the internal sphincter has a defect, although the other muscles of the anus also have the effect of closing the anus, the external sphincter and other striated muscles are prone to fatigue, easy to loosen, and cannot continuously close the anus. At this time, there will be leakage of air and other substances, so it is easy for underwear to become dirty. Therefore, the fistula is removed from the internal sphincter to reduce damage to the internal sphincter.

However, according to the literature, the postoperative recurrence rate of the fistula removal from the internal sphincter is higher than that of the Parks procedure. The reason is that the Parks procedure for the intersphincter abscess and the resection of the fistula in the internal sphincter is performed under direct vision after excision of part of the internal sphincter, which can clear the primary lesion more thoroughly. However, the improved surgical procedure is performed under stealth by means of the sensation of the hand and the operator's experience, which may have residual effects and lead to recurrence. Therefore, for the fistula in the internal sphincter, many procedures for the treatment of high complex anal fistula are still treated by the Parks method, and the method of removing the fistula in the internal sphincter is used to treat mostly low intermuscular fistula.

Points of Attention When Dealing with Primary Intermuscular Lesions
In the excavation of the intersphincter abscess, it is done from the inner mouth, from the outer mouth, and also from the internal and external routes together. Masahiro Takano pointed out that the primary lesion between the sphincters is usually larger than the rest of the fistula (Fig. 8.45). If this feature is not known during fistula extraction, there may be residue due to the treatment not cleaning out the area thoroughly when the primary intermuscular lesions are treated, resulting in the recurrence of anal fistula. Therefore, more surgical methods use the method of cutting the internal and external sphincters to remove the primary intermuscular lesions through the incision, which can improve the thoroughness of the removal of the primary intermuscular lesions.

Wound Stitching Method
The Parks surgical method advocates open drainage of the wound in the anus, and most early preservation methods adopt the Parks method. Later, some people proposed the method of simply suturing the wound in the anus or covering it with an anal skin advancement flap upward so as to avoid the stimulation and pollution of feces on

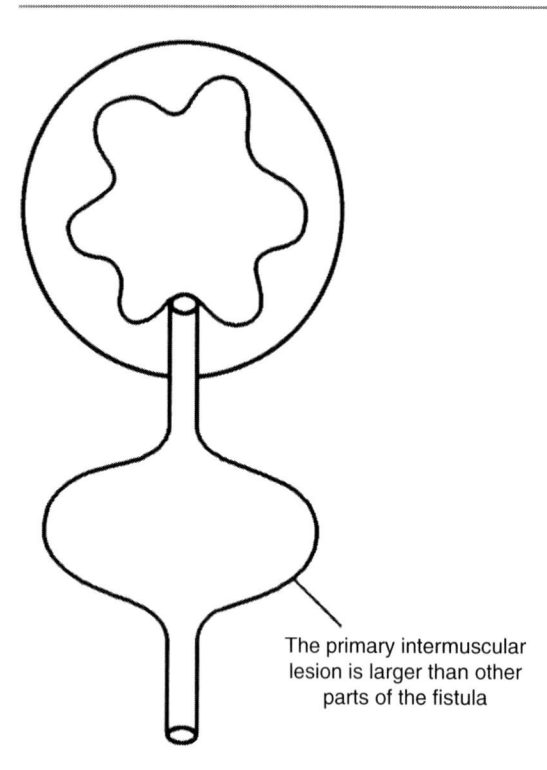

Fig. 8.45 Characteristics of primary lesions. The primary intermuscular lesion is larger than other parts of the fistula

the wound and promote the healing of the wound, but this failed to achieve the desired effect. On the contrary, due to incomplete coverage of the wound surface by the skin flap, there was a defect between the skin flap and the mucosa, and feces entered and formed infection lesions, which lead to the recurrence of the anal fistula. A further improvement is the combination of a mucosal-free flap for layered suture. That is, the fissure wound in the internal sphincter is sutured, and the mucosal epithelium is separated to eliminate the tension, and then the mucosal epithelium is sutured. At the same time, note that when suturing the mucosal flap, pay attention to adequately free it up (but pay attention to retain sufficient blood supply) to eliminate the tension during the suture.

Fistula Resection or Retention

In general, the fistula in the external sphincter will be scraped and preserved, and the small branch can be left untreated. When the fistula extends upward along the underside of the mucosa and causes rectal stenosis, it is generally believed that as long as the clearance of the inner mouth and the primary lesion is thorough, only longitudinal fistula cutting is enough to eliminate the rectal stenosis, and the anal fistula can also be cured. The residual fistula will gradually become fibrotic due to an infection-free environment, and finally it will be occluded, so there is no need to worry about them. Some people even think that keeping the fistula will improve the curative effect. But Takano believes that not all the fistulas can be left untreated. When the fistula is thick and deep, the contents of the cavity are dirty, and the surrounding inflammation is heavy, there are often cases of anal fistula recurrence or partial recurrence due to incomplete fistula treatment. At the same time, in deep complex anal fistula, the nature of the fistula is complicated, and there are cases of anal fistula caused by tuberculosis and Crohn's disease, as well as canceration. According to his report, in 19 cases of deep complex anal fistula surgery, one case of tuberculosis and two cases of cancer were found. Therefore, he advocates that for some high-complex anal fistulas, the fistula should be completely opened, which is convenient for a thorough examination and surgical treatment, as well as for collecting tube wall tissue for pathological examination. It can also be further treated according to the intraoperative pathological examination.

Suggested Reading

1. Takano Masahiro edited. Shi Renjie compiled. Essentials of diagnosis and treatment of anorectal disease. Beijing: Biomedical Branch of Chemical Industry Press, 2009, 132–166.
2. Huang Naijian. Chinese anoenterology. Jinan: Shandong Science and Technology Press, 1996, 745–766.
3. Cao Jixun. A new edition of Chinese hemorrhoidology. Chengdu: Sichuan Science and Technology Press, 2015, 166–170.
4. Ren Donglin, Zhang Heng. Some critical issues in the diagnosis and treatment of complex anal fistula [J]. Chinese Journal of Gastrointestinal Surgery, 2015, 18(12): 1186–1192.
5. Wang Yehuang, Wang Kewei. Analysis of Ding Zemin's clinical experience of incision suture therapy

for high complex anal fistula [J]. Jiangsu Traditional Chinese Medicine, 2015, (2): 1–4.
6. Li Chunyu, Li Yubo. Selection and techniques of anal fistula surgery [J]. Chinese Journal of Clinicians, 2015, (4): 20–21, 22
7. Zhang Hong. Surgical methods and efficacy analysis of low anal fistula [J]. Contemporary Medicine, 2012, 18(14):108–109.
8. YU Ting, CAO Yong-qing. Clinical common anal fistula surgery [J]. Medical Information, 2015, 28(7):338
9. Wang Chen, Yao Yibo, Dong Qingjun et al. Application and development of suture-dragging therapy for anal fistula [J]. Chinese Journal of Gastrointestinal Surgery, 2015, 18(12):1203–1206.
10. Chao Min, Peng Degong, Zhang Jingfeng et al. Treatment of low anal fistula with internal fistula incision (report of 40 cases) [J]. Shandong Medical Journal, 2009, 49(46):91–92.
11. He Xiaosheng, Cai Zerong, Lin Xutao et al. Comparison of the efficacies of seton drainage combined with different drugs in the treatment of Crohn's disease complicated with anal fistula [J]. Chinese Journal of Digestive Surgery, 2014, 13(8):604–606.
12. Wu Zuozhou. The History of Seton Therapy [J]. Jiangsu Journal of Traditional Chinese Medicine, 2006, 27(8):3–4.
13. Yang Bolin, Ding Yijiang. Suture therapy for anal fistula [J]. Journal of Coloproctological Surgery, 2005, 11(1): 79–81.
14. Shao Wanjin. Anal fistula seton therapy. Journal of Colorectal & Anal Surgery. 2006, 12(5) 326–327.
15. Nie Weijian. Clinical evaluation of the effect of traditional Chinese medicine hanging line therapy on the anal function of high anal fistula [D]. China Academy of Chinese Medical Sciences, 2011.
16. Shao Wanjin. The past, presence and future treatment of ligation of intersphincteric fistulous tract for the treatment of fistula in ano [J]. Chinese Journal of Gastrointestinal Surgery, 2015, 18 (12): 1200–1202.
17. Yu Hongshun, Wang Min, Duan Hongyan et al. Medical bio-protein glue for the treatment of high complex anal fistula [J]. Chinese Journal of Gastrointestinal Surgery, 2009, 12(5): 539.
18. Wang Xiaoyan's translation. Yu Dehong's proofreading. Treatment of composite anal fistula with fibrin glue has a low success rate [J]. Chinese Journal of Practical Surgery, 2004, 24(6):372.
19. Wang Zhenjun, Song Weiliang, Zheng Yi, et al. Clinical observation of anal fistula treatment with acellular extracellular matrix [J]. Chinese Journal of Practical Surgery, 2008, 28 (5): 370–372.
20. Wang Mingxiang, Dai Guangyao, Wang Hai et al. Observation of curative effect on the treatment of middle and low rectovaginal fistula with biological patch [J]. Hebei Medical Journal, 2011, 33(16):2473–2474.
21. Hou Chaofeng. Clinical study on the treatment of anal fistula with biological tissue patch filling [J]. Henan Journal of Surgery, 2010, 16(5):1–3.
22. Wang Zhenjun. Review and reflection on treatment of anal fistula [J]. Chinese Journal of Gastrointestinal Surgery, 2010, 13(12):881–884.
23. SONG Weiliang, WANG Zhenjun, ZHENG Yi et al. Clinical observation of allogenic acellular dermal matrix in the treatment of anal fistula [J]. Journal of Colorectal & Anal Surgery, 2009, 15(1):21–23.
24. Zhang Di, Zheng Xueping, Yu Suping et al. Clinical status of advancement flap patch repair in the treatment of high complex anal fistula [J]. Journal of Colorectal & Anal Surgery, 2011, 17(5):339–340.
25. Zhu Ping, Gu Yunfei. Application of endorectal advancement flap in the treatment of anal fistula [J]. Chinese Journal of Gastrointestinal Surgery, 2013, 16(7):696–697.
26. Song Yinggang, Gao Kun. Study on the effect of advancement flap and incision seton therapy on postoperative anal function of patients with complex anal fistula [J]. Guide of China Medicine, 2016, 14(6):70–70, 71.
27. Gu Yunfei, Pei Ping, Yang Bolin et al. A report of 17 cases of anal fistula treated with advancement flap with medicinal fuse half tube drainage [J]. International Journal of Surgery, 2010, 37(11):784–785.
28. Liu Hailong, Xiao Yihua, Zhang Yong et al. Primary efficacy of video-assisted anal fistula treatment complex anal fistula [J]. Chinese Journal of Gastrointestinal Surgery, 2015, 18(12): 1207–1210.
29. Zhao Risheng (translated), Wang Ting (revision). Laser fistula ablation: an anal fistula treatment method for retaining anal sphincter [J]. Chinese Journal of Gastrointestinal Surgery, 2014, (12): 1186–1186.
30. White RA, Eisenstat TE, Rubin RJ, et al. Seton management of complex anorectal fi stulas in patients with Crohn's disease. Dis Colon Rectum.1990;33(7):587–589.
31. Williams JG, Rothenberger DA, Nemer FD, et al. Fistula-in-ano in Crohn's disease. Results of aggressive surgical treatment. Dis Colon Rectum. 1991;34(5):378–384.
32. Mann CV, Clifton MA. Re-routing of the track for the treatment of high anal and anorectal fi stulae. Br J Surg. 1985;72(2):134–137.

Nonoperative Treatment of Anal Fistula

Renjie Shi and YiXin Zhang

Abstract

The nonsurgical treatment of anal fistula is suitable when the fistula cannot be cured, the patient is in poor health and temporarily inoperable, and it is also used for perioperative treatment. The nonsurgical treatment of anal fistula is mainly divided into internal treatment and external treatment. Traditional Chinese medicine has rich experience and characteristics in these two aspects. Internal treatment is to take medicine orally to eliminate the internal factors of the occurrence and development of anal fistula. Ancient Chinese medicine believes that some anal fistulas can be cured by internal medication. External treatment methods include dressing method, drainage method, fumigation and sitz bath method, washing method, cotton blocking method, dressing change method, etc. There are many targeted medicines in the treatment of postoperative wound in China, all made of Chinese herbal medicine as raw materials. These medicines have a significant influence on the prevention and treatment of wound infection and the promotion of wound healing.

Keywords

Anal fistula · Conservative treatment
Internal treatment · External treatment
Dressing method · Cotton blocking method
Dressing change

In principle, anal fistulas can only be cured by surgery, but not all anal fistulas are suitable for surgical treatment, and not all patients with this disease are willing to undergo surgical treatment. There are often patients who are unable to operate in time because of their physical condition, time schedule, economic reasons, lack of hospital beds, and so on. In such cases, in order to control or temporarily relieve the patient's pain, it is often necessary to use a nonsurgical treatment. These methods and drugs are also often used before and after operation to prevent and treat complications, accelerate wound healing, and improve curative effects.

9.1 Indications

1. Indications include patients with serious heart, lung, brain, liver, kidney, and other important organ diseases or other surgical contraindications. Whether they have absolute surgical contraindications or relative surgical contraindications, these patients are temporarily unable to have operation.
2. Patients with poor general condition, such as old and weak, advanced tumor, cerebral hemorrhage, and so on, cannot tolerate radical operation.
3. Patients with mental illnesses or patients who cannot cooperate with the treatment.
4. The intestinal lesions of Crohn's disease and ulcerative colitis complicated with anal fistula are not relieved, the tuberculous anal fistula has not received effective anti-tuberculosis treatment, or the normative treatment has not been completed.
5. Patients who have no time for an operation or are unwilling to operate for the time being.
6. Treatments for before and after anal fistula surgery.

9.2 Methods

The methods are mainly divided into two aspects: internal treatment and external treatment.

9.2.1 Internal Treatment

Traditional Chinese medicine believes that the occurrence and development of anal fistula have its inherent reasons and have always attached importance to internal therapy. For example, "Chuang Yang Jing Yan Quan Shu" said: "it is necessary to use warm tonifying agents to make up for its internal, and muscle-generating medicine to make up for its outside." "Dan Xi Xin Fa" said: "sores, first should take tonics to generate Qi and Xue, mainly with Shen, Zhu, Qi, Xiong, Gui, large dosage." "Xue Shi Yi An Wai Ke Shu Yao" said: "Nourishing vital energy and tonifying Yin essence is the main method of treating fistula." "Wai Ke Yi An Hui Bian" said: "therefore, the method of treating fistula, like the collapse of an embankment, or a leak in a house, if we do not make up for it, how can it be avoided?" The treatment of fistula requires enrichment Qi and blood first. Once Qi and blood become full, then vigor can be stored to stop leaking. The body can be harmless, body fluid is increasing day by day, and deficiency can be recovered. In the future, if the Qi Mai is empty for a long time, it will be filled with essence and marrow; if the stomach is weak for a long time, it will be fixed with sweet and warm drugs; Yin deficiency and yang hyperactivity will be accompanied by bitterness and firmness in Yin nourishing medicine; if the earth does not produce metal, use sweet and warm drugs to strengthen the middle energizer, accompanied by sour drugs. Among all the decoctions, lotus seed, *Euryale ferox*, *Terminalia*, and Zhongbai are all the drugs astring the kidney essence. These are all the methods to cure fistulas.

Even many Chinese medicine books believe that the use of drugs alone can cure anal fistula. "Yi zong Jin jian wai ke xin fa yao jue" said: "if hemorrhoids have passed through the intestines, dirt from the leak, take Hu Lianzhuidu pills with wine ... If the leak has a fistula, you miss a tube, take Huanglian closed tube pills, which can replace the operation." The "Surgical diagnosis and treatment of the book" said: "only to clear away the pathogens of dampness and heat, then the fistula can be cured completely." Although there are few cases of anal fistulas treated with drugs alone, with there being no official reports of this, the previous treatment experience in this area is still worth learning and requires us to carry out in-depth research.

There are also many different principles and methods of internal treatment in the previous dynasties' literature. "Ru men shi qin" said: "hemorrhoids leakage pain .... Treat it with the same method of treating dampness." "Introduction to medicine" said: "at first fistula with pus blood is damp-hot, as time goes, it becomes wet-cold. At the first stage we should cool the blood, clear heat and eliminate dampness. At the next stage we should dry tubes, take insecticide and warm-benefiting drugs." Generally speaking, the internal treatment of anal fistula in traditional Chinese medicine is mainly based on syndrome differentiation, sometimes combined with disease differentiation. At present, there are the following internal treatment methods commonly used in clinical practice.

9.2.1.1 Clearing Heat and Eliminating Dampness

Suitable for the syndrome of damp invasion of lower energizers. Symptoms: perianal ulcer, often overflow thick pus, white or yellow, local red, swelling, heat, pain obvious, and a fistula to the anus if you press. Can be accompanied by anorexia, stool discomfort, short red urine, heavy body, and other symptoms. Red tongue, yellow and greasy tongue coating, and slippery pulse.

Prescription: Bi Xie Sheng Shi Tang ("Yang Ke Xin De Ji") addition and subtraction. Commonly used drugs: Huangbai, Cangzhu, Jinyinhua, Pugongying, Zihuading, Bixie, Fuling, Zhizi, Cheqianzi, Baizhu, Yinchen, etc.

9.2.1.2 Heat-Clearing and Detoxification Method

Suitable for toxic heat flourishing syndrome. Symptoms: external fistula closed, local redness, swelling, and burning pain. Can be accompanied by fever, thirst to drink, dizziness, constipation, and short red urine. Tongue red with yellow coating, string, and rapid pulse.

Prescription: Xian Fang Huo Ming Yin.

Commonly used drugs: Jinyinhua, Fangfeng, Baizhi, Danggui, Chenpi, Zaojiaoci, Shenggancao, Chishao, and Zihuadingding.

9.2.1.3 Fuzheng Tuodu Method

Suitable for the syndrome of lingering pathogen due to deficiency vital Qi. Symptoms: perianal fistula with thin pus, dull pain, external anus skin dim, sometimes collapse and sometimes recovery, press harder, and always with tubes leading to the anus. Can be accompanied by fatigue, unglamorous complexion, shortness of breath, and so on. Light tongue with thin coating and soft pulse.

Prescription: Tuo Li Xiao Du Yin ("Jiao Zhu Fu Ren Liang Fang") addition and subtraction.

Commonly used drugs: Huangqi, Danggui, Chuangshanjia, Zaojiaoci, Chuanxiong, Baizhu, Fuling, Baishao, Shudi, Gancao, etc.

9.2.1.4 Nourishing Yin and Supporting Toxin Method

Suitable for yin fluid deficiency syndrome. Symptoms: perianal fistula depression, the surrounding skin color dark, pus clear, and always with tubes there leading to the anus. Can be accompanied by night sweats, restlessness, thirst, loss of appetite, and other symptoms. Red tongue with less or no coating and weak pulse.

Prescription: Qing Hao Bie Jia Tang ("Wen Bing Tiao Bian") addition and subtraction.

Commonly used drugs: Qinggao, Biejia, Zhimu, Dihuang, Mudanpi, Huangbai, etc. Artemisia annua, Biejia, Anemarrhena, Rehmannia glutinosa, Cortex moutan, Cortex Phellodendri, etc.

9.2.1.5 Tonifying Qi and Blood Method

Suitable for qi and blood deficiency syndrome. Symptoms: anal fistula for a long time, repeated attacks, ulceration is not fresh, and pus is not much. Often accompanied by emaciation, lusterless complexion, shortness of breath and laziness, pale lip and nail, loss of appetite, and so on. Pale tongue with white coating and weak pulse.

Prescription: Shi Quan Da Bu Tang addition and subtraction.

Commonly used drugs: Huangqi, Dangshen, Baishao, Baizhu, Fuling, Gancao, Shudi, Danggui, Chuanxiong, Chenpi, Shanzha, etc.

In addition, in order to control the development of inflammation, relieve pain, or prevent and treat postoperative infection before and after operation, appropriate antibiotics can be selected at the stage of acute inflammation of anal fistula. Commonly used antibiotics are penicillins, aminoglycosides, tetracyclines, and so on (generally when inflammation subsides or infection can be controlled). If sensitive antibiotics can be selected according to the results of pathogen culture and drug sensitivity test of fistula pus, the drug will be more targeted and the curative effect will be better.

9.2.2 External Treatment

9.2.2.1 External Application Method

According to the syndrome differentiation of anal fistula, select appropriate drugs and dosage forms and apply in the affected area to achieve the purpose of anti-inflammation and relieving pain, promoting local swelling and pain dissipation, or piercing drainage, removing pus, and generating muscles. The most commonly used methods are ointment, encirclement medicine, dusting power medicine, and so on.

Encirclement Medicine

This external treatment is when medicine powder is mixed with wine, tea, honey, egg white, and so on to make a paste. The medicine mixed with vinegar is to dissipate blood stasis and detoxify; with wine, is to enhance the drug; with egg white, is to ease irritation; with oil, is to moisturize the skin. With the gathering efficacy of encirclement medicine, the initial stage of sores can be dissipated; even if the poison has gathered, it can also promote the sore to shrink, limit its scale, and then break down the pus as early as possible. Even if the residual swelling does not disappear after the abscess has ruptured, the swelling can be eliminated by applying medicine, and the residual poison can be intercepted. Encirclement medicine is suitable for anal fistula patients with local redness, swelling, and heat pain. Commonly used prescriptions are Ruyi Jinhuang San, Yulu San, and so on. Jinhuang San and Yulu San are used for anal fistula with obvious redness, swelling, and heat pain; Huiyang Yulong San is used for Yin syndrome sores and ulcers; Chonghe San is used for semi-yin and semi-yang syndrome ulcers.

When applying, those with sores that are not ruptured should fill the entire red and swollen area; those with ulcers should apply around the affected area, but the ulcers should not be coated. When the hoop is dry after application, it is appropriate to wet with liquid from time to time so as to avoid local discomfort caused by drug spalling and dry hard plate.

Ointment

This is the medicine powder mixed evenly with Vaseline or something similar such as yellow wax, grease, and so on to make an ointment. This is then applied to the wound. It is suitable for patients with closed anal fistula or poor drainage and local redness, swelling, and heat pain. Commonly used drugs are Jinhuang ointment, Yulu ointment, red ointment, Shengji Yuhong ointment, and so on. Jinhuang ointment and Yulu ointment are suitable for those with red swelling and hot pain in the period of acute abscess of anal fistula, red ointment is used for all ulcers, and Shengji Yuhong ointment is used for all ulcers in which slough has not been removed, new muscles has not been developed, or when the wound cannot be closed for a long time. Shengji Baiyu ointment is used for ulcers in which slough has been cleaned and when sores have not converged.

When using ointment, we should apply a thick application when acute inflammation of anal fistula has not suppurated, and the range should be larger than the edge of the mass in order to reduce swelling. When there is a lot of purulent water, the ointment should be thin and frequently changed in order to avoid purulent water immersion in the skin and avoid converging sores. If patients are allergic to the drug, it should be changed to other medicine. When slough has been removed, new muscles grow, so the medicine should also be applied thinly. This is because too thick a coating can make granulation growth excessive and affect sore healing.

Dusting Power Medicine

Ancient Sanji, now simply known as powder, is the preparation of a variety of different drugs into a powder. According to the rule of preparation and drugs' different functions, a prescription of compatible powder is given. It is mixed with plaster or ointment, directly mixed with diseased tissue, or is inserted into the sores with a paper twist.

In the preparation of dusting power medicine, the drug should be ground to a fine powder, to the degree of silence. Among them, plant drugs should be ground and screened separately, and mineral drugs should be used for water flight. Musk, camphor, borneol, cinnabar, bezoar, and other spices and precious drugs should be ground separately, then mixed with other drugs evenly, and stored in porcelain bottles, with a plugged bottle cap, so as not to disperse the aroma.

Dusting power medicine can be divided into dispelling drugs, eliminating pus and necrotic drugs, corrosion drugs and flat pterygium drugs, regenerating and converging drugs, hemostatic drugs, and so on.

There are two kinds of drugs commonly used in anal fistula: (1) eliminating pus and necrotic drugs: suitable for when the abscess collapses, pus is not clean, slough is not removed, or fistula drainage is not smooth. Commonly used prescriptions include Jiuyidan, Baerdan, and Wuwudan. Most of these drugs are mercury-containing preparations, which are toxic drugs and should be used with caution; for those who have allergies to Shengdan, they should be banned; for large area wounds, eliminating pus and necrotic drugs should also be used cautiously to prevent mercury poisoning due to excessive absorption. (2) Regenerating and converging drugs: It's suitable for after operation. It can promote granulation and epithelial growth. The commonly used medicines are Shengji powder and Pinian powder.

When using dusting power medicine, we should pay attention to (1) wrapping the drug with cotton paper or mulberry paper to keep it wet so as to ensure full efficacy and also prevent it from falling out; (2) if the patient has itching, redness, rash, and blistering after medication, it is likely that the skin is allergic to the drug, so medication should be stopped immediately and cleaned. Other drugs or treatments should be employed instead. If necessary, local or systemic medication should be taken for allergies at the same time.

9.2.2.2 Drainage Method

This is a treatment that inserts the medicated thread into the fistula to make pus flow smoothly, decay and freshness, prevent the spread of poison, and relieve the disease. Medicated thread, commonly known as paper twist or medicine twist, mostly uses mulberry paper or silk cotton paper according to the needs of use. Directions are to cut the paper into a moderate width and length and rub it into different sizes. At present, twisted medicine thread is used after high-pressure steam disinfection to make it aseptic and more perfect. The use of medicated thread drainage and exploration has the advantages of convenience and less pain. Patients can change by themselves, and the depth of fistula can be detected by using it.

There are two types of medicated threads: external adhesive drugs and inner-wrapped drugs. At present, both of them are used in clinical practice. External adhesive drugs, mostly containing Shengdan or Heihudan, etc., have the effect of eliminating pus and necrosis. Inner-wrapped drugs mostly use Baijiangdan, withered hemorrhoids powder, etc. and have the effect of corroding tubes.

When inserting medicated threads into the fistula, a small part should be left outside, and the end of the thread should be folded to the side or below the fistula and then fixed with a plaster or ointment. When the pus has been exhausted, yellowish viscous liquid will flow out; even if the abscess cavity is still deep, there is no need to insert a medicated thread.

9.2.2.3 Fumigation and Washing Treatment

These are used before and after anal fistula operation. According to different conditions of the disease, drugs with the effects of heat-clearing and detoxifying, promoting flow of Qi and blood circulation, promoting dampness and insecticidal, softening hard lumps and dispelling nodes, reducing swelling and relieving pain, regenerating and converging, and dispelling wind and relieving itching can be selected. The drugs can be boiled to fumigate and wash the anus in order to play a corresponding effect. You can also use 1–5000 potassium permanganate sitting bath to clean the anus or surgical wounds.

Fumigation and washing treatment is generally carried out after defecation or before a dressing change. When using a sitting bath, adjust the temperature to about 50 °C with about 1000 mL of warm water and fumigation solution, place it in the bath basin, fumigate first by heat, and soak the buttocks in the basin for about 15–20 min after the temperature is suitable.

Prescription: Kushen decoction, Wubeizi decoction, Xiaofan lotion, and so on.

Commonly used drugs: Huangbai, Yinhua, Yejuhua, Yuxingcao, Lizhicao, Huzhang, Cangzhu, Kushen, Shechuangzi, Difuzi, Baixianpi, Shichangpu, Honghua, Wubeizi, Mingfan, Mangxiao, Qiancao, Bingpian, etc.

9.2.2.4 Flushing and Washing Treatment

The purpose of washing is to clean the pus or foreign body out of the wound or fistula. Commonly used washing drugs are hydrogen peroxide, normal saline, traditional Chinese medicine liquid, and so on. After washing, antibiotics, Shutaishu, and other drugs can be injected into the wound or fistula, which can inhibit bacteria and reduce inflammation, promote granulation growth, and close the lumen. It is suitable for local swelling, pain, and multiple external secretions of anal fistulas or after an operation on anal fistulas.

Fistula Flushing and Washing Method

Patients should be in a lateral position or lithotomy position, put the liquid into a 20-ml syringe, and connect with the ball infusion needle or fine plastic needle. Insert from the external orifice and extend into the fistula to flush. If the drug needs to be infused, the needle should be inserted into the fistula close to the inner orifice, the liquid should be slowly injected into the outer orifice, and the gauze should be covered with adhesive tape to fix it. Flushing may be carried out daily or every other day as appropriate. The infusion of drugs should be every 3–4 days.

Wound Cavity Flushing Method

Patients should be in a lateral position, then connect the syringe to a fine catheter, insert the front part of the catheter into the wound cavity for washing, and place a curved plate under the hip for the flushing fluid. The wound cavity should be washed and filled with a drainage strip each time.

9.2.2.5 Cotton Pad Drainage Treatment

Cotton or gauze is used to cover the fistula or wound from outside so that the pus in the fistula or wound can be removed after the thread is removed or dragged by pressure force. The skin and new muscles can be conglutinated to achieve the purpose of healing. Cotton pad drainage method is widely used in the anorectal department, and it is mostly used in anal fistula drainage or thread dragging operation.

When using the cotton pad drainage method, the cotton or gauze should be folded into pieces to be lined with the fistula or the wound after removing the thread or hanging the thread and fixed with rubber tape under pressure. The cotton pad bandaging of the skin bridge can promote the adhesion with the subcutaneous tissue so as to accelerate the tissue growth and shorten the wound healing time.

Due to the removal of residual fistula tissue after operation, traditional Chinese medicine is used to remove pus and generate muscles after an operation, and the cotton pad drainage method cannot be used until the wound is clean. It is reported in the literature that the cotton pad method should be used in about 10–14 days after operation. "Wai Ke Zheng Zong Yong Ju Nei Rou Bu He Fa" said that internal and external carrion of carbuncle, counterpart and big sore were exhausted, the inner muscles can not adhered to each other with scab pus. We can put on seven or eight layers of soft cottony which tie tightly with silk, and sleep on the affected area several times. The muscles inside and outside naturally adhere to each other, like new growth muscles.

This proves that the key time for the cotton pad drainage method is after "the carrion has run out" and when the new muscle is growing. Because the newborn wound contains a large amount of granulation tissue and is rich in blood supply, pressing the skin bridge and the wound at this time can make the skin adhere to the subcutaneous granulation tissue, promote the proliferation of fibrous tissue, and then the skin and subcutaneous tissue can grow into one. This is to achieve the purpose of speeding up healing.

Zhang Shaojun and Yang Wei found that if the fistula tissue was completely stripped off, the cotton pad drainage method could be used in advance so as to achieve better clinical results. Their study showed that early use of the cotton pad drainage method could shorten the adhesion time between skin bridge and subcutaneous tissue to about 7 days, which is significantly shorter than that of the usual 10–14 days, and there was no wound infection or recurrence after operation.

Attention should be paid to the following problems in the clinical application of the early cotton pad drainage method: (1) the fistula should be removed completely during the operation: after the fistula tissue is completely removed during the operation and the fresh granulation tissue is already under the skin bridge. Therefore, this fully meets the requirements of "carrion has been done" in the cotton pad drainage method. In this way, the cotton cushion can be pressed directly at the end of the operation, which avoids the trouble of removing the residual fistule through red oil ointment and other traditional Chinese medicine. (2) Selection of cases of anal fistula: the cases with obvious conduit and strip shape are generally selected. Through preoperative and intraoperative examination, we can obviously distinguish the fistule from the surrounding tissue, which is beneficial to the complete exfoliation of the fistula. If the anal fistula is in the stage of acute inflammation, this method is forbidden. (3) Notes for wound dressing change: when changing dressing, gently wipe the edge of the wound under the skin bridge, wipe all the secretions, but do not have to probe into the skin bridge; otherwise, it is easy to re-separate some of the tissues that have been adhered to. If the anal fistula cavity is small and there is not a lot of resected tissue, then the tension in the skin bridge is low; gentle pressure can be combined with the subcutaneous tissue. Early postoperative cotton cushion can make the skin bridge and subcutaneous tissue adhesion as quickly as possible; if the cavity is large and the wound is deep and large, then the skin bridge is more difficult to adhere to the subcutaneous tissue, and it is necessary to wait for the granulation hyperplasia of the wound to grow, so the wound can be gradually narrowed before it can be adhered to and healed. (4) The treatment of internal orifice and the selection of fistula incision are also important aspects in preventing recurrence and shortening the course of treatment.

Dressing change: the purpose of dressing change is to observe the condition of the sore, ensure smooth drainage, remove pus and necrotic tissue, prune abnormal granulation tissue, and promote the normal growth of granulation tissue in order to accelerate the healing of the sore. The method in changing the dressing is very important for the wound. In the case of proper operation, whether the anal fistula can be cured or not has a close relationship with whether the dressing change is appropriate or not. After the operation, if there is not a change in dressing or the change of dressing is not appropriate, the wound will be very difficult to heal and can even lead to the recurrence of anal fistula.

Common instruments for dressing change: two sets of tweezers, one close to the sore, the other sterile, clamping dressings and cotton balls, two bends or dressing bowls, one for sterile dressings, and the other for contaminated dressings. According to the condition of the sore, equipped with surgical scissors, curette, the surgeon should cut off the necrotic tissue and pterygium; in addition, deep sores or the formation of sinus should be equipped with probes and so on.

Commonly used dressings: disinfected dry cotton balls and iodine, alcohol, saline cotton balls to disinfect and clean sores; gauze, such as Vaseline, rhubarb gauze, to protect the sore surface, drainage, and hemostasis; gauze block or gauze cotton pad, adhesive tape or bandage to cover the sore and fix the bandage.

9.2.2.6 Dressing Change Method

The change of dressing is generally carried out after defecation and after the fumigation and sitting bath for the anus. According to the location of the sore, guide the patient to take an appropriate position in order to facilitate the operation. The left or right lying position is often used when changing dressing. First, disinfect the skin around the sore with iodophor cotton ball, then gently moisten the sore with iodophor cotton ball, remove the pus and secretion in the sore, and rinse the wound or fistula with normal saline or metronidazole if necessary. Do not scrub too hard or this will damage new tissue. After cleaning the sore, fill in the wound cavity or cover the wound with ointment gauze, cover the gauze and fix it with adhesive tape. When there is more early postoperative secretion, gauze cotton pads can be added, and finally, the dressings can be fixed with adhesive tape or bandaged with bandages. In the early stage after operation, because of the secretion from the wound, the dressing can easily become wet, so the dressing should be changed frequently; the interval between dressing change can be reduced in the middle and later stages of operation, and a cotton cushion can be used if necessary.

When changing the dressing, if the wound has pterygium higher than the skin or puffy granulation tissue, it can be cut off by operation, and if the necrotic tissue is not easy to fall off from the wound, a small amount of Jiuyi Dan, Baerdan, and other adulterants can be used and sprinkled on the sore surface. If the purulent water in the wound has been purified and the granulation tissue grows slowly, the wound can be covered with Shengji powder on the drainage strip to promote wound healing.

If the secretion increases when the wound is extruded in the middle and later stages after operation, the possibility of false healing should be considered and the false healing cavity should then be opened. In order to prevent the occurrence of false healing and cavity formation, when changing the dressing, the drainage strip should be placed at the base of the wound and attached to the granulation.

Sometimes the wound epithelium crawls slowly and the wound healing is poor. There are many reasons for this occurrence; anemia and malnutrition, diabetes, leukemia, Crohn's disease, ulcerative colitis, tuberculous anal fistula will all affect wound healing. It is therefore necessary to treat the cause in order to help wound growth return to normal.

The sores infected by tetanus, rotten furuncle, epidemic furuncle, and *Pseudomonas aeruginosa* or instruments used by patients with hepatitis or tuberculosis should be strictly disinfected, and the contaminated dressings must be burned so as not to cause cross-infection.

Suggested Reading

1. Gu Guoming, Zhang Yi. Examples of application of hoop medicine [J]. Journal of traditional Chinese Medicine, 2005, 23 (11): 2033–2034.
2. Tian Li, an Chao. Study on diagnosis and treatment of anal Fistula [J]. Journal of traditional Chinese Medicine, 2016, 31 (6): 795–798.
3. Mu Zhiyi, Xiao Huirong, Xie Changying, etc. Effect of anal lotion sitting bath and Shengji Yuhong ointment on wound healing after operation of tuberculous anal fistula. Bed study [J]. Clinical Application of Integrated traditional Chinese and Western Medicine, 2013, 13 (4): 34–36.
4. Song Minglin, Jia Guirong. 2000 cases of postoperative anorectal diseases were treated with Dangbai Shengji ointment [J]. Shaanxi traditional Chinese Medicine, 2008, 29 (5): 544.
5. Liu Shuxian. 5 cases of infantile anal fistula were treated with external treatment of traditional Chinese medicine [J]. Journal of external treatment of traditional Chinese Medicine, 2007, 16 (5): 40–40.
6. Tian Ying. Fumigation and washing prescription promoted wound healing after anal fistula operation in 80 cases [J]. Shaanxi traditional Chinese Medicine, 2009, 30 (9): 1157–1158.
7. Ai Meng, Qin Liguo. 37 cases of complex anal fistula were treated with different surgical methods combined with traditional Chinese medicine [J]. Modern distance Education of traditional Chinese Medicine, 2016, 14 (8): 89–90.
8. Zhang Shaojun, Yang Wei. Application of early cotton pad in postoperative drainage of anal fistula [J]. Hebei traditional Chinese Medicine, 2012, 34 (11): 1627–1628.
9. Zhen Jinxia, Cao Yongqing. Experience of dressing change after anorectal surgery [J]. Journal of practical traditional Chinese Medicine, 2008, 24 (3): 182–183.

Diagnosis and Treatment of Special Anal Fistula

Renjie Shi and Fang Liu

Abstract

The occurrence and development of anal fistula in Crohn's disease (CD) are different from those of common anal fistula, and CD anal fistula has its own special features in terms of diagnosis and treatment. For CD anal fistula, the most commonly used local examination methods are digital rectal examination and exploration under anesthesia (EUA), anorectal ultrasound (AUS), and magnetic resonance imaging (MRI). The treatment of Crohn's disease fistulas (CD fistulas) must be assessed using a combination of the commonly used standard Crohn's Disease Activity Index and the Perianal Crohn's Disease Activity Index. The purpose of CD anal fistula treatment is to cure anal fistula or reduce local symptoms on the basis of protecting anal function. Surgical treatment of Crohn's disease anal fistula must follow the principle of individualization, make judgment according to the severity of the disease and symptoms, and choose the appropriate surgical treatment plan. The purpose of treatment is to cure anal fistula or reduce local symptoms without affecting the anal control function. Asymptomatic Crohn's disease anal fistula could be not treated. Active intestinal inflammation should be treated systemically, combined with temporary or long-term drainage. Fistulotomy can be used for low intersphincteric fistula or trans sphincter fistula. High trans sphincter anal fistula, extra sphincter anal fistula, or suprasphincter anal fistula should be treated with seton therapy, skin flap pushing technique, or anal fistula plug.

Anal fistulas in infants and young children tend to develop within 1 year after birth and are definitely more common in boys than girls. Meanwhile, the anal fistulas mostly occur in the both sides of the anus, and they are relatively shallow and tend to heal spontaneously. The main etiological theories of infantile fistulas are immune insufficiency theory, sex hormone theory, anal crypt infection theory, diaper dermatitis theory, residual epithelium theory, and fecal compression theory. The treatment of infantile anal fistulas has been controversial, with differing views on whether to chooose conservative or surgical treatment, and the proper time of surgery. It is necessary to cut and discharge pus in time in the acute abscess stage. In China, the common surgical methods for the treatment of infant anal fistula include fistulotomy, fistulotomy and seton therapy, and thread-dragging therapy.

R. Shi (✉)
Department of Anorectal Surgery, Affiliated Hospital of Nanjing University of Traditional Chinese Medicine, Nanjing, Jiangsu, China

F. Liu
Sixth Affiliated Hospital, Sun Yat-sen University, Guangzhou, Guangdong, China
e-mail: liuf259@mail.sysu.edu.cn

Rectovaginal fistulas have a complex etiology and are very rare congenitally, often associated with malformations such as anus, urethra, or bladder. Most of the cases are posterity. The most common causes are birth injury or improper lateral incision, pelvic and pelvic surgery, rectal, perineal, vaginal, and cervical cancer and radiation injury, inflammatory bowel disease, and trauma. Rectovaginal fistula is generally divided into high and low, simple and complex types. Most of the rectovaginal fistulas need surgical treatment. In principle, rectovaginal fistula caused by fresh surgical trauma or trauma should be repaired immediately. Those with infection or chronic fistula should be repaired after tissue edema, and inflammatory reaction around the fistula subsided. The physical examination and auxiliary examination should be improved, and the perfection of rectal and perineal MRI, CT, ultrasound, colonoscopy, and enema contrast examination, etc. should be finished if possible. On the basis of the comprehensive assessment of the disease's condition, a relatively reasonable treatment plan should be carefully formulated. The common surgical methods include simple resection and suture repair, rectal mucosal flap covering repair, autologous tissue flap transfer and packing repair, transvaginal repair, transabdominal repair, and so on.

Tuberculous anal fistula is a specific infection caused by *Mycobacterium tuberculosis* in the perianal tissues and is relatively rare in clinical practice. In a typical tuberculous anal fistula, the redness and swelling are not obvious in the attack period, the local pain is not severe, and it takes a long time to break down. Purulent is the main symptom, with thin and clear pus, fistula not closing for a long time, persistent low fever, night sweats, and other symptoms. At present, atypical tuberculous anal fistula is more common, which is not characterized by obvious symptoms and can easily be missed or misdiagnosed. The diagnosis of tuberculous anal fistula depends on biopsy and mycobacterium culture. T-SPOT test has high sensitivity, specificity, and detection rate. In the case of tuberculous anal fistula, regular anti-tuberculosis treatment should be given promptly, followed by surgery if necessary, in the same way as for common anal fistulas. For the tuberculous anal fistula diagnosed after the surgery, rifampicin gauze and other topical medicine with anti-tuberculosis effect can be used in conjunction with systemic anti-tuberculosis treatment.

There is an increasing trend in the number of patients with AIDS and anorectal diseases. Regular screening for anorectal disease in patients with AIDS is essential for early detection, diagnosis, intervention, and treatment of anal fistulas and other anorectal diseases. The anal fistula associated with AIDS is not the absolute contraindication of surgery, and comprehensive assessment and communication are necessary before surgery. The main indicator for assessing the preoperative status of patients with HIV/AIDS is the blood CD4 lymphocyte count. For patients with a CD4+T lymphocyte count less than 200/μl, conservative treatment is recommended. For patients who are pre-surgical, preoperative antiviral medication routine and monitoring of HIV RNA quantification are recommended, and surgery should be performed after the viral load is below the lower limit of detection, if possible. The incidence of postoperative complications in AIDS patients is relatively higher, which needs to be taken into consideration. The medical staff should strictly protect themselves and strictly follow the operation rules during the contact process.

Keywords

Anal fistula · Crohn's disease anal fistula Treatment · Transrectal ultrasonography MRI examination · Perianal Crohn's disease activity index · Anal fistulas in infants and young children · Etiology · Sex hormone Immunity · Diaper dermatitis · Treatment Rectovaginal fistula · Pathogeny · Iatrogenic injury · MRI · Ultrasonic examination Assessment · Operation · Mucosal flap advancement · Tuberculous anal fistula

Biopsy · *Mycobacterium tuberculosis* culture
T-SPOT test · Anti-tuberculosis treatment
AIDS · Infectious diseases · Screening
Intervention · CD4 · T lymphocyte count
Antiviral · Occupational protection

10.1 Crohn's Disease Anal Fistula

Anal fistula is the most common and most difficult perianal lesion in Crohn's disease, often presenting as high complex anal fistula with extensive inflammation and scarring. Since Bissell first reported small intestinal colitis with perianal granulomatous lesions in 1934, Crohn's disease (CD) perianal lesions have received increasing attention from clinicians. Due to the development and potential pathological changes of Crohn's disease, the occurrence and development of Crohn's disease anal fistula are different from common anal fistula. Its diagnosis and treatment have its particularities.

10.1.1 Incidence and Epidemiology of Crohn's Disease Anal Fistula

Abundant lymphatic tissue around the anus may explain the high incidence of CD in the anus. It is reported that the incidence of anal fistula in CD patients is 17–43%. Hellers et al. reported that the incidence of anal fistula in CD patients in Stockholm, Sweden, from 1955 to 1974 was 23%. Schwartz et al. reported that the incidence of anal fistula among CD patients in Minnesota hospitals from 1970 to 1993 was 38%. After the diagnosis of intestinal CD, the incidence of anal fistula in 1, 10, and 20 years was 12%, 21%, and 26%, respectively. The location of intestinal inflammation significantly affects the occurrence of anal fistula. The incidence of anal fistula in patients with active colon lesions is significantly increased. When the rectum is involved, the incidence of anal fistula is 92%. Only 5% of CD patients first presented with anal fistula lack intestinal inflammation alongside it.

However, the exact etiology of CD anal fistula is not clear. Armuzzi et al. believe that chromosome 5 defects have a significant genetic predisposition to perianal lesions in CD patients. Low anal fistula in CD anal fistula can be regarded as glandular anal fistula. High complex anal fistulas with high internal orifices or complex fistulas are different from glandular anal fistulas in that they have complex interconnected canals. In Crohn's disease anal fistula, rectovaginal fistula is more common with an incidence of about 10%, and low fistula is also more common.

10.1.2 Diagnosis

10.1.2.1 Clinical Manifestations

The co-existence of multiple lesions is a typical feature of CD around the anus. CD anal fistula can be accompanied by perianal skin tags, anal fissure, anal incontinence, or anorectal stenosis, and local pain is mild or painless. Severe pain suggests an underlying infection and abscess formation.

Because CD is a chronic, inflammatory bowel disease and wall permeability disease, it can lead to internal and external sphincters and its progressive development of perineal body damage and rectal inflammation results in the decrease of rectal compliance. More severely, even moderate sphincter function can decline, and this may also be because of colon absorption moisture barrier, rectal volume, and the decline in compliance, which eventually results in anus incontinence. However, most anal incontinence is due to excessive surgical procedures.

10.1.2.2 Examination

At present, the most commonly used local examinations in the clinic include rectal touch, examination under anesthesia (EUA), anorectal ultrasound (AUS), and magnetic resonance imaging (MRI).

Digital rectal examination is simple and convenient. Whether an abscess has formed, the course of anal fistula and the location of the inner mouth can be determined by digital rectal examination. The characteristic changes of rectal mucosa thickening, anal and rectal strictures, and soft or thin fistula walls in Crohn's disease can be perceived by digital rectal examination. In addition, when abscess formation is suspected and MRI cannot be performed immediately, exploration under anesthesia (EUA) and abscess drainage are measures that can be taken and should not be delayed.

Ultrasound imaging of Crohn's fistula can distinguish Crohn's disease-related anal fistula from saphenous gland infected anal fistula. The positive predictive value and negative predictive value are 87% and 93%, respectively. As a complementary method, the accuracy of finding and classifying fistulas by transperineal ultrasound is comparable to that of intracavitary ultrasound. However, its diagnostic accuracy for deep abscess is low, but it may have certain advantages in the exploration of rectovaginal fistula (compared with MRI, 88.9% vs. 44.4%).

Magnetic resonance imaging can obtain ideal images from the sagittal plane, coronal plane, and cross section, fully showing the muscles around the anal canal and rectum, and accurate identification of fistula and scar with different imaging signals. This method has gradually become an important means of preoperative diagnosis of complex anal fistula. Pelvic MRI is a low invasive and high accuracy method in the diagnosis and classification of anal fistula in Crohn's disease.

The use of intracavity coils or body surface phased array coils helps to further improve the diagnostic accuracy. Intracavitary coils have advantages in distinguishing the position of the inner orifice; the accuracy of fistulas and abscesses is between 76 and 100%. However, it is thought that the coil in the rectum cavity is expensive and has similar disadvantages to ultrasonic probe, which is reported to be only 68% accurate. The application of body surface phasing front circle is simple, the patient has good tolerance, wide field of vision, and satisfactory image, and the lesions above the levator ani muscle can also be well displayed.

Much foreign literature reported that 1.0–1.5t MRI imager was used to evaluate anal fistula, and its accuracy was mostly within the range of 80–90%. Some scholars believe that the accuracy rate can reach 96%. In addition, it is believed that MRI can even show fistulas missed by surgical exploration. Some scholars have compared the accuracy of MRI and EUS in evaluating the anal fistula of the original CD, and the results between them are quite different. Reasons for this may be due to the different types of equipment used, patient selection criteria, and operator experience. Beckingham et al. believe that the sensitivity and specificity of dynamic enhanced MRI are better than AUS.

The scope and extent of intestinal inflammation affect the surgical management of CD anal fistula and the judgment of the prognosis of the disease. Therefore, patients should have regular fiber colonoscopy to evaluate the progress of intestinal inflammation. The whole digestive system contrast can be used to evaluate the degree of invasion of the small intestine.

10.1.2.3 Classification

As far as anal fistula is concerned, there is no universally accepted standard classification method. Park's classification is one of the most widely accepted clinical classification method, and this is also applicable to the classification of CD anal fistula.

10.1.2.4 Evaluation of CD Anal Fistula Activity

The correct evaluation of fistula activity is helpful for the clinical treatment of CD anal fistula. At present, there are several sets of classification criteria and scoring systems to quantitatively evaluate the extent and severity of anal fistula in Crohn's disease.

The anal fistula activity score of patients with Crohn's disease should reflect the severity of the disease and treatment effect to the clinician. The standard Crohn's disease activity index (CDAI) is useful for evaluating the degree of Crohn's disease activity, but not suitable for evaluating CD anal fistula. Perianal Crohn's disease activity index (PDAI) is commonly used to evaluate perianal activity. Standard Crohn's disease activity index and perianal Crohn's disease activity index are commonly used in clinical studies of anal fistula in Crohn's disease.

The perianal activity index (PDAI) is a Likert scale based on the quality of life assessment and the severity of perianal disease. The perianal lesions of CD patients were evaluated from five aspects: secretions, pain, difficulty in sexual activities, types of perianal lesions, and induration. PDAI scores greater than 4 were used as critical values for clinical evaluation (active fistula secretion and local inflammatory signs) with an accuracy rate of 87%. If fistulas are "closed," they are defined as having no exudate (even if pressed lightly with the fingers). Treatment response was defined as 50% or more reduction of fistula drainage after at least two consecutive follow-up visits. Fistula relief was defined as fistula without drainage after two consecutive follow-up visits. Although this clinical evaluation criterion has been applied in long-term randomized controlled trials, it has some disadvantages. "Finger pressure" is largely dependent on the observer, and this method has not been formally verified. Fistulas with persistent and no liquid secretions were assessed as "relieving"; the appearance of the outer opening of the fistula was substituted for the whole fistula internal conditions.

MRI studies have shown that fistula internal healing is delayed by 12 months (median) compared with clinical remission. The position of the original or residual fistula becomes the channel of least resistance, forming new fistula or recurrent fistula. In order to combine the anatomical position of anal fistula with imaging findings reflecting inflammatory activity, Van Assche et al. designed an MRI-based scoring system. Anatomical factors included the number and trend of fistulas, and inflammatory activity was reflected by MRI T2-weighted phase, fistula hypersignal, abscess, and proctitis.

Although the above scores are verified by PDAI, their correlation degree is relatively low ($r = 0.371$, $P = 0.036$). The disappearance of images after enhanced MRI is the only feature related to clinical remission. More recent studies have found that this score is not sensitive to changes in fistula diameter during long-term follow-up. The length of fistulas assessed by MRI is considered to be a predictor of current patient response to treatment.

10.1.2.5 CD Anal Fistula Canceration

Whether CD is a risk factor for colorectal cancer is debatable. Kersting et al. reported that among the 330 patients with CD treated by surgery, 10 were diagnosed with colorectal cancer, 3 of which were related to anal fistula. Ky et al. followed up more than 1000 CD patients with perianal lesions for 14 years, and 7 patients developed anal or rectal malignant tumors. The author believed that the canceration was related to anal fistula, and the canceration rate of CD anal fistula was 0.7%. In the 14 cases of anal fistula canceration reported by Gaertne et al., 10 cases were CD patients.

CD anal fistula canceration has a poor prognosis and difficult diagnosis, so it is necessary to guard against local canceration for CD patients with long-term complicated anal fistula. Complicated perianal lesions that result in narrowing, ulceration, inflammation, etc. limit local examination. MRI can provide an accurate and effective imaging basis for patients with suspected CD canceration, and it is necessary to explore it under anesthesia and conduct biopsy pathological examination. The treatment of CD anal fistula canceration is consistent with conventional tumor treatment. Squamous cell carcinoma needs radiotherapy and chemotherapy, while adenocarcinoma needs to be combined with radiotherapy and chemotherapy on the basis of surgery.

10.1.3 Treatment

The treatment of CD anal fistula aims to cure anal fistula or reduce local symptoms on the basis of protecting anal function. In principle, asymptomatic CD anal fistula does not need surgical treatment. For symptomatic CD anal fistula, drug treatment is usually the first choice. When there is abscess, it is necessary to cut open and discharge pus. In most cases, surgery is not taken as the main treatment measure.

It should be pointed out that the present study proves that traditional drug therapy cannot change the natural course of CD, and about half of patients eventually undergo surgery 10 years after diagnosis due to complications or medical treatment failure. In recent years, the issue of mucosal healing has received great attention. Biological agents can quickly obtain a higher rate of intestinal mucosal healing. Studies have shown that the mucosal healing rate is correlated with the clinical recurrence rate and surgical rate of CD. So, should mucosal healing be the target of CD therapy and should active drug therapy (so-called "step-down therapy") be given before CD progresses to the stage of irreversible intestinal injury (such as stenosis or penetration)? Might these change the natural course of CD? Can a range of predictors of poor prognosis be identified for early active treatment? These are the current research hotspots. Previously there were no clear answers; however, now it is recognized that risk factors of poor prognosis (such as anal fistula, infection or hormone therapy, patients less than 40 years of age) are associated with early active treatment.

10.1.3.1 Drug Therapy

Drug treatment of Crohn's disease anal fistula is the first choice. Since intestinal inflammation affects the activity degree and cure rate of CD anal fistula, it is necessary to use drugs to treat intestinal inflammation. When intestinal inflammation is relatively static, it can provide favorable conditions for the treatment of perianal lesions.

Currently, commonly used clinical drugs include antibiotics, 5-aminosalicylic acid or its drug precursor (such as sulfasalazine, azosalicylic acid, etc.), immunosuppressants (6-mercaptopurine, methotrexate, cyclosporine), antitumor necrosis factor-αmAb (infliximab), etc. Corticosteroids are not recommended. Steroids have no definite therapeutic effect on CD anal fistula, and they will affect the healing of anal fistula and lead to the formation of abscess.

Antibiotics

Metronidazole and ciprofloxacin are first-line drugs for CD around the anus. Metronidazole and ciprofloxacin should be used promptly when CD is accompanied by fistula or suppurative complications.

Although no RCT test has proved that metronidazole is effective in treating CD anal fistula, several nonrandomized clinical trials have proved that metronidazole is effective in treating CD anal fistula. The clinical application dose is usually 750–1000 mg/day, which takes effect 6–8 weeks later. Bernstein et al. reported 21 consecutive patients receiving 20 mg/kg metronidazole every day, and 83% of them had anal fistula closure. Reducing or stopping metronidazole can lead to activity, and one study showed that 78% of patients relapsed 4 months after stopping metronidazole, but the disease was quickly controlled when the dose was resumed. Adverse reactions associated with long-term use of metronidazole are usually oral metal taste, glossitis, nausea, and peripheral nerve inflammation.

Studies have shown that ciprofloxacin is effective in treating perianal CD by inhibiting the synthesis of bacterial DNA cyclocyclase. Through a double-blind placebo-controlled trial, West et al. confirmed that ciprofloxacin combined with infliximab was significantly better than infliximab alone in the treatment of CD anal fistula. As with metronidazole, randomized controlled clinical trials are lacking, and anal fistula may recur after withdrawal.

5-Aminosalicylic Acid and Its Drug Precursor

At present, 5-aminosalicylic acid and its drug precursor are widely used in the treatment of ulcerative colitis and intestinal CD, and 5-aminosalicylic acid local enema or suppository can significantly improve perianal CD. However, there are few reports on the exact efficacy of CD anal fistula.

Immunosuppressants

6-Mercaptopurine (6-MP) or its drug precursor azathioprine combined with metronidazole is the first-line drug for treating CD anal fistula. A meta-analysis of five randomized controlled clinical trials showed that fistula closure occurred in 22 (54%) of 44 patients with CD anal fistula treated with 6-mp or azathioprine, compared with

21% (6/29) of placebo patients. The American College of Gastroenterology recommends 6-mp 1.0–1.5 mg/(kg day) or azathioprine 2.0–3.0 mg/(kg day) for the treatment of CD anal fistula. Adverse reactions were reported in around 9–15% of patients and included mainly leukopenia, anaphylaxis, infection, pancreatitis, and drug-induced hepatitis.

Clinical trials have demonstrated that intravenous administration of cyclosporine in large doses is effective in the treatment of CD anal fistula. However, adverse reactions limit their clinical application, and symptoms often recur with oral maintenance doses. Present et al. reported that intravenous infusion of 4 mg/kg had an average onset time of 7.4 days, and followed by oral maintenance of 6–8 mg/kg had a clinical effective rate of 90%, and some patients relapsed at maintenance dose.

Tacrolimus is a powerful new immunosuppressant, which mainly inhibits the release of interleukin-2 (IL-2) and comprehensively inhibits the action of T lymphocytes, 100 times stronger than cyclosporine (CsA). In recent years, as a first-line drug for liver and kidney transplantation, it has been listed in 14 countries, including Japan and the United States. Tacrolimus is effective in the treatment of active anal fistula, and oral tacrolimus can avoid surgical ostomy in refractory patients. Because of its high renal toxicity, tacrolimus needs to be tested for its drug concentration at the time of application, and the dose should be reduced if necessary to minimize its toxic side effects. But there was no significant benefit compared with the topical use of tacrolimus.

Antitumor Necrosis Factor

Infliximab

Infliximab is a human and mouse chimerism monoclonal antibody that specifically blocks tumor necrosis factor-alpha (TNF-α). It is the first drug confirmed by RCT clinical trial to promote the closure of CD anal fistula and maintain symptoms for up to 1 year.

Its efficacy is to block TNF-α in the body of patients, reduce the inflammatory reaction caused by TNF-α value, and relieve the symptoms of the disease. It is mainly used in clinical practice for adult patients with moderately to severely active CD anal fistula so as to reduce the number of anal and rectovaginal fistulas and keep fistulas closed. Infliximab can reduce signs and symptoms, induce and maintain clinical response, and eliminate corticosteroid use in adult and child patients who do not respond to conventional treatment. However, it is not recommended for patients with Crohn's disease with tuberculosis, lymphoma, congestive heart failure, or gram allergy or other serious infections.

In an RCT trial at 12 centers in the United States and Europe, 94 patients with CD anal fistula received intravenous infliximab at 5 or 10 mg/kg at 0, 2, and 6 weeks. Fistula drainage was not required in 62% of patients (26% in the placebo group). Anal fistula symptoms disappeared completely in 55% of patients (placebo group, 13%). The mean onset time was 14 days, and 5 mg/kg was the optimal treatment dose. The ACCENT test confirmed these results and conducted long-term maintenance studies. In 306 patients with CD anal fistula, intravenous infusion of 5 mg/kg infliximab at 0, 2, and 6 weeks was effective for 69% (195 cases) at 14 weeks. Patients were randomized to receive 5 mg/kg infliximab maintenance therapy every 8 weeks, and 36% of patients had complete closure of fistulas at 54 weeks (placebo group, 19%). Infliximab maintenance treatment reduces the number of operations and length of hospital stay. Meanwhile, an RCT test confirmed that the efficacy of infliximab combined with ciprofloxacin in the treatment of CD anal fistula was significantly better than that of infliximab alone.

Application of infliximab saw 20–30% of patients having a transfusion reaction, mostly low thermal capabilities, flush on the face, and increased heart rate. These are examples of mild reactions, but about 2% of patients will witness a severe allergic reaction, difficulty in breathing, blood pressure drop, and rare lupus sample reaction. Recurrence of latent tuberculosis occurs in 10–35% of patients because the anal fistula mouth is closed and secondary crissum abscess can often be controlled through hanging line drainage. New or recurrent malignancies have been reported in patients using this drug in clinical trials. The incidence of lymphoma was higher than expected in the normal population. In an exploratory clinical trial that included moderate to severe chronic obstructive pulmonary disease (COPD) patients who smoked or had quit, more cases of malignancy were reported in the trial group than in the control group. The potential role of TNF inhibitors in malignant tumorigenesis is unknown.

Adalimumab
Adalimumab, a humanized monoclonal antibody against human tumor necrosis factor (TNF), is a dimer of human monoclonal D2E7 heavy and light chains bound by disulfide bonds. In the CLASSIC-1 and GAIN studies of adalimumab in the treatment of fistula Crohn's disease, there was no significant difference in the improvement and remission of fistula after 4 weeks of adalimumab treatment compared with the placebo group. The Phase III trial of CHARM was conducted to evaluate the results of adalimumab maintenance therapy that had responded to induction therapy after 56 weeks, and 33% of patients achieved complete healing of fistulas, compared with 13% in the placebo group ($P < 0.05$). The results of the open extension study of the trial showed that fistula healing remained in 90% of the patients during a 2-year follow-up. Long-term open studies have shown that adalimumab is effective in 23–29% of patients who lose response to infliximab or become resistant to it.

Cetuzumab
Cetuzumab is also a tumor necrosis factor inhibitor. A subgroup analysis of two large studies, PRECISE1 and PRECISE2, that assessed the response of cetuzumab to the treatment of moderate to severe Crohn's disease with fistulas showed that 36% of anal fistulas were completely closed at 26 weeks of cetuzumab treatment, compared with 17% in the placebo group ($P = 0.038$). However, there was no statistically significant difference between the two groups when fistula closure was more than 50% in two consecutive follow-up visits.

Anti-adhesion Molecule Antibody
Vedolizumab is an integrin receptor antagonist, which mainly inhibits the effect of adhesion molecules on the surface of immune cells, and is not appropriate to conventional treatment or response to TNF-α antagonist or is resistant to adult CD and CD anal fistula patients. It blocks the transport of lymphocytes involved in the immune response of cells in the digestive tract. It is suitable for patients who do not respond to glucocorticoids, immunomodulators, and tumor necrosis factor inhibitors. Originally, anti-adhesion molecule antibody preparation for bead sheet resistance (natalizumab) was used in the treatment of CD. However, due to the fact that some patients may have an increased risk of brain infection after using progressive multifocal leukoencephalopathy, vedolizumab has become an alternative therapy for natalizumab. This therefore plays an important role in curbing CD anal fistula patients with chronic inflammation.

Anti-inflammatory Cytokine Antibody
Ustekinumab (trade name: Stelara) is an anti-inflammatory cytokine preparation, which is a humanized monoclonal antibody against IL-12/23p40 subunit. It is an IL-12/23 antagonist. IL-12/23 is involved in inflammation and immune responses, while in vitro, ustekinumab disrupts IL-12/23-mediated signaling by disrupting cytokines that interact with shared cell surface receptors. Ustekinumab has therapeutic effect on CD and CD anal fistula patients who are not well treated by tumor necrosis factor inhibitors and can reduce the destructive effects of CD such as intestinal obstruction, abscess, fistula formation, bleeding, and intestinal perforation. There are also anti-inflammatory cytokines preparation of fontolizumab, tocilizumab, and other preparations.

10.1.3.2 Surgical Treatment
Surgical treatment of Crohn's disease anal fistula must follow the principle of individualization, making judgment according to the degree of disease and severity of symptoms, and selecting the appropriate surgical treatment plan. The aim of treatment is to cure anal fistula or reduce local

symptoms without affecting anal control function. Before surgery, the severity of perianal lesions, anal sphincter function, bowel control, concomitant rectal inflammation, number and complexity of fistulas, and nutritional status and symptoms of the patients should be comprehensively evaluated as part of the quality of life of the patients.

The principles of Crohn's disease anal fistula surgery are as follows: (1) no treatment for asymptomatic Crohn's disease anal fistula; (2) systemic treatment, combined with temporary drainage or long-term drainage, should be used for active intestinal inflammation; (3) fistulectomy can be used for low intersphincter fistula or transsphincter fistula; (4) high sphincter anal fistula, external sphincter anal fistula, or upper sphincter fistula should be treated by thread hanging technique, flaps of the upper sphincter flap technique, or anal fistula plug.

Incision and Drainage in Abscess Stage
Simple incision and drainage should be used for the first perianal abscesses in patients with Crohn's disease. Sphincter injury should be avoided as far as possible, and drainage should be adequate and unobstructed. If the abscess cavity is large and far from the anus, the mushroom head catheter can be placed into the abscess cavity through a small incision for continuous drainage, or the rubber band can be used for long-term drainage; the catheter can be placed for several weeks or months, until the formation of an anal fistula.

It has been reported that in seven patients who underwent perianal abscess incision and drainage, the rate of fistula healing was low, and four patients had postoperative recurrence. This suggests that simple incision and drainage of perianal abscess is difficult to play a full role in drainage; although the external fistula is healing, perianal tissue infection still exists.

Partial internal sphincterotomy can be used for recurrent abscesses to remove the infected anal epithelium, open the gap between sphincter muscles, and remove part of the internal sphincter muscle to fully drain the abscess cavity. Pritchardet et al. retrospectively studied the perirectal abscesses, 30 low abscesses, and 8 deep abscesses of 38 CD patients who received surgical treatment, and 53% (20/38) received simple incision drainage, 26% (10/38) received loose catheter drainage, and 21% (8/38) received mushroom head catheter drainage. The recurrence rates of the three groups were 42%, 46%, and 45%, respectively.

Fistulotomy
Because subcutaneous anal fistula, low sphincter interanal fistula, and low transsphincter anal fistula do not involve the muscles that are very important for anal parenthesis function, fistulotomy can be used, and the surgical safety is relatively high. Given the chronic course of the disease and its high recurrence rate, sphincter function should be preserved as much as possible. All risk factors, especially the severity of anorectal disease, sphincter function, rectal compliance, presence of active proctitis, history of anorectal surgery, and bowel coordination, should be considered before surgery.

Due to the particularity of this disease, the healing time of fistulotomy can be as long as 3–6 months or even longer, and this requires explanation and communication with patients. It has been reported that the cure rate of fistulotomy for Crohn's disease anal fistula patients with appropriate indications is 56–100%, and the rate of mild anal incontinence is 6–12%, suggesting that anal incontinence may be related to previous anal fistula operations.

Thread-Hanging Therapy for Anal Fistula
Complicated CD anal fistula should be treated with long-term (usually more than 6 weeks) string drainage. The purpose of long-term thread drainage is to continue the drainage and prevent the closure of the external orifice of anal fistula, in order to achieve the purpose of successful drainage and control of inflammation. Even so, repeated infection rates ranged from 20 to 40%, and 8 to 13% in patients who had varying degrees of fecal leakage. In addition to fistulotomy for low anal fistula, other CD anal fistulas should be treated with drainage and thread-hanging combined with drugs. Recent data have shown a heal-

ing rate of 24–78% after induction therapy with wire drainage combined with infliximab, with 25–100% of patients responding effectively to infliximab maintenance therapy.

Reconstructive Mucosal Flap/Flap Repair

If the rectal mucosa is generally normal, high rectal fistula without active proctitis or complicated Crohn's disease can be covered by mucous membrane flap metastasis. The key to successful surgery includes that the mucosal flap should include the mucosa, submucosa, and part of the internal sphincter and should be at least 1/4 of the total width of the rectum to ensure adequate blood supply. The length of the free flap should be longer than that of the anal fistula so as to ensure the tension-free suture after the internal mouth resection and debridement. Hemostasis must be carefully stopped during the operation. In complete fistula debridement or resection, adequate drainage should be maintained by proper expansion of the external orifice. The short-term cure rate is 64–75%. The short-term cure rate of Crohn's disease complicated by rectovaginal fistula is 40–50%. The recurrence rate was positively correlated with follow-up time. Patients who fail surgical treatment can be reoperated on. The success rate of prolapse mucous flap/flap repair in the treatment of CD anal fistula is closely related to intestinal inflammation, and the prognosis is poor when there is active rectal inflammation. The presence of rectal inflammation is a major factor in the failure of the operation. When there is rectal inflammation, suture drainage should be used, and the operation can only be accepted after the inflammation is controlled.

Whether it is necessary to perform enterostomy fecal diversion surgery in the treatment of complex anal fistula by patenting with elated mucous flap/flap is still controversial.

Treatment of Anal Fistula Suppository

Connor et al. applied an anal plug to treat CD anal fistula. Among the 20 patients, 16 cases healed (80%, follow-up time was 3–24 months, with an average of 10 months). However, Ky et al. treated 45 patients (20 of whom with complicated anal fistula) with this method, and the success rate was 84% at the follow-up of 8 weeks. However, the success rate decreased with the passage of time, and the success rate decreased to 54.6% at the mean follow-up of 6.5 months. The simple anal fistula was more effectively cured than complex anal fistula (70.8% vs. 35%), and the curative effect of non-CD anal fistula is better than CD anal fistula (66.7% vs. 26.6%). Christoforidis et al. compared the results of long-term follow-up of elapse flap and AFP in the treatment of complex anal fistula, the success rate of elapse flap was 63% (average follow-up of 56 months), and that of AFP was 56% (average follow-up of 14 months).

Rectal Resection and Permanent Ostomy Bypass

It is reported that 62–86% of CD anal fistulas are cured by effective surgery and drug therapy, and normal anal control function is maintained. However, in 31–49% of cases of extensively advanced complicated Crohn's disease, anal fistulas may require enterostomy or rectal resection in order to control perianal infection in cases where medication and thread drainage are not effective. The operation should be performed in an intersphincter approach to remove the rectal mucosa, submucosa, and internal sphincter and to preserve the external sphincter, and the branch tube should be incised, scraped, or drained through debridement.

Risk factors for permanent ostomy and rectal resection include colonic disease, persistent perianal infection, prior temporary ostomy, fecal incontinence, and anal stenosis.

Other Treatments

Ligation of Intersphincter Fistula (LIFT)
LIFT surgery can be performed when the fistula of the sphincter anal fistula has formed a fibrotic tube that can be ligated and transected. The surgery closes the internal opening and removes a partial fistula through the intersphincter plane. In a single-center small sample (40 cases), the reported success rate was 94%. Recent studies suggest that the efficacy is moderate (56% cure

rate after 1 year) and that all relapses occur within 2 months of surgery. Results of prospective large sample treatment for Crohn's disease have not been published.

Stem Cell Therapy

Mesenchymal stem cells have high plasticity and ability to regulate immune cells, so it is safe and feasible to inject autologous adipose stem cells or bone marrow stem cells into the fistula or around the fistula. Initial studies have shown that stem cells combined with fibrin glue can close fistulas in 56–82% of patients, with sustained relief rates of 53 and 30% at 1 and 3 years, respectively. Stem cell therapy seems promising, but it still needs randomized, placebo-controlled clinical trials of anal fistulas to treat Crohn's disease in the long term.

Gracilis Muscle Transplantation

In the case of gracilis muscle transplantation, a single-center retrospective study of 18 patients with Crohn's disease showed that gracilis muscle transplantation had a 64% success rate in treating complex anal fistulas and was effective in 50% of persistently unhealed sinus tracts.

10.2 Infant Anal Fistula

Infants and young children with anal fistula often have them on both sides of the anus, are shallower, and have a tendency of self-healing. Their occurrence, development, clinical manifestations, and treatment are significantly different with adult anal fistula.

10.2.1 Characteristics of Infantile Anal Fistula

10.2.1.1 Anatomical Features of the Anus of Infants and Young Children

Fujihara Akira et al. performed morphological studies on anal genital fossa, anal gland duct, anal gland, internal and external sphincter, and combined longitudinal muscle 7-month fetus to the anal specimens of all other ages. After aspect observation, infants and adults were compared and found to be significantly different.

Anal Crypt

Children's crypts and anal columns are more obvious than adults, and the anal crypts are well formed. As the age increases, both tend to flatten and become difficult to distinguish. The number of anal crypts is 6–11, with an average of eight, and there tends to be more in infants and young children. The measurement of the depth of the anal crypt is easily affected by deformation such as postmortem corpse treatment. The depth of the anal crypt is 0.1–1.5 mm, with an average of 0.65 mm. The average depth below 1 year of age is 0.62 mm, which is not significantly different from that of adults. In the position difference, the average of the posterior median is 1.0 mm, and the average in the anterior median is 0.7 mm. The difference between the left and the right sides is 0.4 mm. The adult cases and infant cases are deeper in the front and rear, two times that of other parts. The covered epithelium is mostly stratified columnar epithelium in neonates and gradually changes to stratified squamous epithelium as the age increases.

Cell Infiltration Centered on Anal Crypt

A total of 47.7% of patients have moderate or greater cell infiltration, including cells with infiltration only around the anal crypt, especially after 50 years of age. However, in the fetus, mild inflammatory cell infiltration can also be seen in neonates, but most of them are lymphocytic infiltration, and no clear signs of anal sinusitis can be seen.

Anal Glandular Duct and Anal Gland

When observing the opening of the anal crypt, the anal gland of the infant is thicker and more linear than in the adult. The length of the anus is long before and after the gland, and there is no big difference between the left and right. Most of the anal glands (67.6%) reached the submucosal layer and 21.6% reached the anal sphincter, but there was no age or part difference. Compared with adults, the covering epithelium of the anal glandular duct is mostly stratified columnar epithelium, and the gland is more tubular. However, the fetus, newborn, and pediatric duct tend to be simple, and the depth is not shallow compared with adults. There is no gender difference in morphology between the anal crypt and the anal gland, anal gland, and tissue surrounding the anus.

Anal Internal and External Sphincter

The external anal sphincter develops earlier than the internal anal sphincter and tends to shrink in the early stage. The external anal sphincter usually develops quite well from the early stages of infancy. In contrast, the gap between the muscle bundles of the anal sphincter can be seen. The boundary between the muscles of the anal sphincter can be seen about 9 months after birth when the muscle bundle is enlarged. It has a narrow loofah shape. The external anal sphincter is basically fully formed after 15 years of age. The thickest part of the width was observed to be approximately 30 mm wide after 25 years of age, and it is approximately 1/5 of that at 9 months after birth.

Combined Longitudinal Muscle and Subepithelial Muscle Fiber Group

The combined longitudinal muscle has a portion that is attached to the skin around the anus by the lower end of the internal and external sphincter and a portion that is meshed with each other through the anal and external sphincter muscle bundles and adheres to the skin around the anus. Both of these parts become elastic fibers in the vicinity of the attachment portion. The main body of the combined longitudinal muscle is the latter. There is almost no site difference in different age groups. The subepithelial muscle fiber group is a muscle fiber produced from the inner side of the upper part of the anal internal sphincter. In addition, there are muscle fibers from the rectal mucosal muscle layer and fibers penetrating the upper muscle bundle of the internal sphincter. The mucosal myocardium disappears near the tooth line, and the terminal part is mesh-like attached to the skin around the anus. There is no location differences for different age groups.

Perioral Space Around the Anus

About 9 months after the birth of a newborn, a rough interstitial space begins to appear around the internal and external anal sphincters and becomes more evident with age. However, the cord-like structure of the subcutaneous tissue is also thicker and stronger.

Distance from the Anal Margin to the Tooth Line

Compared with an average of 10.0 mm for adults, the average distance before 9 months after birth is 4.0 mm, which is 2/5 of that of adults. This becomes stable after 20 years of age.

Sun Lin and Wang Yanxia from China performed anal canal local dissection on 32 corpses of children from 1 day to 4 years old (male:female = 18:14). The cause of death of all corpses was nonanal rectal disease. The study identified (1) the form of the anal crypt: the storage of yellow-white mucus in the anus crypt of children, especially in newborns. The appearance of this is funnel-shaped, the mouth faces the inner upper part of the intestinal cavity, and the bottom of the socket extends outward and downward. (2) Distribution and number of anal crypts: the crypts are unevenly distributed, some are locally concentrated, and the distribution is irregular. The number of crypts ranged between 7 and 15, with a mode of 9–11. (3) The distance from the neonatal dentate line to the perianal skin edge is about 1 cm. (4) Correlation analysis is performed between the occurrence of anal fistula in male infants and the distribution of anal crypts in male infants (SPEARMAN method and KENDALL method), where the P value is greater than 0.05; therefore, there is no significant correlation between the location of anal fistula and the distribution of anal crypts.

10.2.1.2 The Clinical Characteristics of Infantile Anal Fistula

Incidence Rate

Sasaki et al. reported that infants and young children with anal fistula accounted for more than 10% of all children with anorectal diseases, second only to the incidence of anal fissure.

General Characteristics

The incidence of anal fistula in infants and young children occurs more than 1 year after birth, falls definitely more male infants than female infants. At the same time, anal fistulas are mostly located on both sides, most of which are not complicated (Fig. 10.1).

According to Arakawa's statistical analysis of 414 infants with anal fistula diagnosed over 23 years, infantile anal fistula has the following characteristics: (1) 38% of children develop it within 1 month after birth, and the earliest on the third day after birth. There were 13 cases of morbidity within 1 week, 49.8% (206/414) of cases were within 1 year of age, 12.6% (52/414) of cases from 1 to 5 years, and 7.7% (32/414) of cases from 5 to 10 years old. (2) Males account for an absolute majority (51:1). There was only one baby girl in the 414 cases. (3) It is prevalent on both sides. Among 414 cases of 590 fistulas, 296 occurred on the left side, 232 on the right side, 29 cases occurred on the anterior side, and 33 cases occurred on the posterior side. Those that occurred on both sides accounted for 528, 89%. (4) They mostly have fewer than two fistulas: 38.6% (160/414) had only one fistula, 32.1% (133/414) had two fistulas, 4.8% (20/414) had three fistulas, and 0.2% had four fistulas. (5) There are similar tendencies in the same family. There were nine groups of brothers with infantile anal fistula, two groups of fathers and sons, and the onset period is about the same age. In addition, the father or mother of 35 of the children had a history of surgery for adult anal fistula. Among them, 30 were fathers and 5 were mothers. (6) The fistula was simple, shallow, and opened in the anal crypt. (7) In the anal fistula resection specimens of adolescent recurrence cases, anal glandular tissue with inflammatory cell infiltration can be found. (8) A cure can be obtained by cutting the fistula or by removing the tube wall with a chloral emulsion. (9) Infants with anal fistula can be relieved for a long time until the onset of puberty.

According to Fujiwara's report, he treated 39 infantile anal fistulas in 9 years and 3 months, all of which were male infants, accounting for 9.2% of all anal fistula cases. In the case of 1-year-olds, 92% (36/29), 80% (31/39) had only one fistula, and the remaining 20% had two fistulas. The occurrence site was more on both sides: 39 cases had 48 fistulas and 73 (35/48) on both sides. The results support Arakawa's report.

Among the 64 cases reported by Tang Hanjun in China, there were 60 male infants and 4 female infants. There were 36 cases (56.25%) within 1 month after birth, and 58 cases (90.62%) occurred within 1 year. There were 44 cases (68.75%) with single anal fistula, including 22 cases in the low and high positions. There were 18 cases of multiple anal fistulas, including 9 cases with two fistulas, 7 with three fistulas, 1 with five fistulas, and 1 with six fistulas. A total of 64 children were diagnosed with an anal fistula.

He Yong and Han Yinghe reported that 41 cases of anal fistula in patients under 2 years old were treated in 10 years, all were male, with a median age of 9.5 months, and 75% (31 cases) were in those less than 1 year old. Eight cases suffered from gastrointestinal dysfunction due to improper feeding and irregular diet, and diarrhea occurred. In three cases, the diaper was rough and rubbed, and the infected skin around the anus caused an abscess to form. Symptoms in most of the children were accompanied by crying and fever. The examination showed local redness and swelling of the perianal area. Among them, 36 patients had initial symptoms of perianal abscess and five patients had anal fistula. The perianal abscess and anal fistula origin were carefully examined during operation, and 35 cases (85.4%)

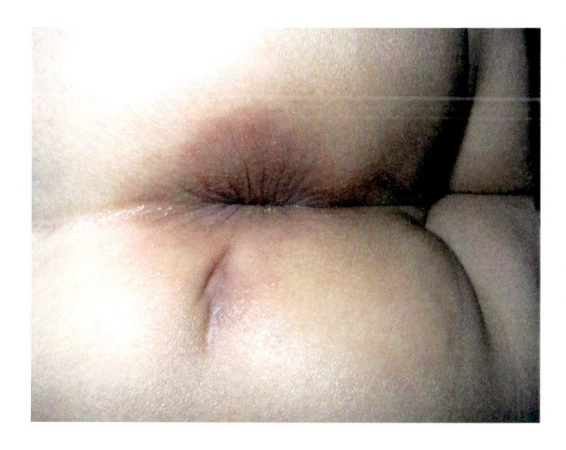

Fig. 10.1 Infant anal fistula

were identified as corresponding anal crypts. In addition, 19 cases (46.4%) found an abnormal development of the anal crypt (including anal crypts too deep, wall thickness, fusion, etc.). All the children had simple fistulas, and the sites were all behind the anus, including 22 cases on the left side and 19 cases on the right side. At the same time, it was pointed out that the source of perianal abscess and anal fistula could be accurately identified during surgery, and this is only 34.17% in adults but 85.14% in children.

Sun Lin and Wang Yanxia summarized 55 cases of male infantile anal fistula treated in Beijing Children's Hospital for 12 years. Of the 114 fistula cases, 79 (69.30%) were located at three o'clock and nine o'clock before the lithotomy. There were 34 cases (61.8%) with a single linear fistula. Whether it is simple or complicated, there is only one internal opening, and most of them are located in the anal crypt on the dentate line.

Zhang Sifen et al. treated 31 infants with anal fistula including 28 males and 3 females. The age of onset was 18 days to 11.5 months, including 21 cases within 3 months of birth, 6 cases from 4 to 6 months, and 4 cases from 6 months. The doctoral age ranged from 24 days to 2 and a half years, with an average of 1.1 years. Anal fistula classification (diagnostic criteria according to the 1975 National Surgical Conference unified standard classification method): 22 cases of low simple type, 6 cases of low complex, 1 case of high complex, and 2 cases of anal fistula. The position of the fistula is the most visible at the three, nine o'clock position, followed by the two, five, and seven points. Other locations are rare.

Have a Higher Self-Healing Tendency
Huang Naijian and others found that infantile anal fistula has self-healing cases. Screening Chinese medicine with the role of phlegm and blood stasis and promoting blood circulation, according to the requirements of processing ointment (referred to as anal fistula cream), this cream is injected into the anal canal of children. Under the action of drugs, the inner mouth closes by itself so as to cure the low anal fistula of the child. Through 62 clinical observations over 3 years, 60 cases were cured, and the cure rate was 96.8%. The results showed that this anal fistula cream is an ideal drug for nonsurgical treatment of low anal fistula in children. It has made breakthroughs in the study of drug application for treatment of anal fistula in children.

Huang Xiaoshan and other reports used the "immortal live drink" plus or minus (pangolin 4 g, Tianhua powder, honeysuckle each 9 g, licorice 6 g, frankincense, myrrh, tangerine peel 9 g, white peony, red peony, angelica, saponin each 6 g, Windproof, Fritillaria each 6 g), decoction concentrated to 100 ml, fumigation for 15 min, in the treatment of 25 children with perianal abscess. A total of 23 cases of anal fistula were treated using the local juice fumigation, sitting bath, and external application with Erhuang detoxification ointment to reduce swelling and detoxification, promote blood circulation, and remove muscles. Of the 44 patients who were followed up, 21 were cured, 11 still had pus, 2 had improved, 10 found it ineffective, and none had recurrent anal fistula. This proved that conservative treatment was effective. Moreover, some foreign scholars believe that the therapeutic treatment of anal fistula in infants and young children is better than surgery, and the recurrence rate is low.

10.2.2 Etiology of Infantile Anal Fistula

10.2.2.1 Immune Dysfunction Theory
The immunological doctrine of infantile anal fistula was first proposed by Yano. Yano believes that the local immunity of the intestine is mainly caused by IgA. The newborn does not have this IgA within 2 weeks of birth, and so it is in a state without IgA. IgA is gradually produced 3–4 weeks after birth and reaches a normal state in about 1 year. This change is more pronounced in the lower digestive tract than in the upper digestive tract. On the other hand, IgG from the mother is drastically reduced after birth, and the IgG produced by the newborn himself or herself begins to appear 1 month after birth and is insufficient from the beginning of birth to several months old. Yano believes that according to the above under-

standing of immunology, it can be explained that infantile anal fistula occurs during the period of immune dysfunction 1–2 months after birth, and the disease is reduced or naturally relieved after 1 year of age when the immune defense mechanism has stabilized.

A prospective study of 324 infants with anal fistula by Sasaki Chihiro found that the age of onset of infantile anal fistula is related to immune development and that more than 3 months after birth is just a weak period in immune function. A total of 27 patients in this group were fed with milk, and whether it is related to its secondary immune deficiency remains to be further studied.

Domestic doctor Tang Hanzhen proposed that the incidence of anal fistula in infants and young children is low, and infants' bodies are weak in the defense against infection and are also relatively weak in resistance to *E. coli*. Immunological studies have found that humoral immune IgM can control infection by Gram-negative bacilli such as *E. coli*. While the humoral immune IgM cannot be transmitted from the placenta from the mother, the neonatal IgM content is very low. The serum IgM levels in children of different ages in China were as follows: neonatal, 12 mg%;4 months, 57 mg%; 1 year old, 86 mg%; 3 years old, 80 mg%; 7 years old, 87 mg%; 12 years old, 72 mg%; and 18 years old, 85 mg%. Neonatal IgM is only 1/7 of that of adults. It can be seen that neonates are particularly vulnerable to Gram-negative bacilli, and they are easily infected by *E. coli*. In addition, due to some deficiencies in the neonatal complement system, the chemotactic response is weak, and neutrophils cannot fully exert phagocytosis, resulting in a situation where inflammation cannot be localized. According to this, it can be known that infants and young children have an infection in the perianal area. If this is not treated in time, it is easy for the inflammation to spread and form multiple anal fistula or complex anal fistula. Observations by Zheng Jinjuan and others found that IgG in the cord blood was close to the adult level, but the other values were extremely low. After birth, it increases with age. After birth, the IgG from the mother is rapidly destroyed, and the neonatal self-synthesis ability is poor, so it is reduced to the lowest level at around 6 months, and physiological temporary hypogammaglobulinemia occurs.

However, there are still many unclear explanations for infantile anal fistula with immunological insufficiency. For example, Arakawa believes that although the use of immune dysfunction can explain the characteristics of the onset of the disease, but if IgA is the main force of local intestinal immunity because breast milk contains more IgA, then infants not fed on breast milk should have a higher incidence of anal fistula, but this has not been found. In addition, this theory alone cannot explain why the infection of anal fistula in infants and young children develops around the anal crypt-anal gland. It also does not explain the phenomenon of infantile anal fistula occurring on both sides.

10.2.2.2 Sex Hormone Theory

Gao Yueshi believes that in infants and young children, especially male infants and young children, due to the action of androgens from the mother and the testis, the function of the anal sebaceous glands is hyperactive, and the secretion is extremely strong, which may lead to bacterial infection and anal fistula. Anal fistula in infants can be understood as a unique neonatal acne that occurs around the anus. However, it has been pointed out that the infection of the perianal sebaceous gland should be adenitis, and it cannot be regarded as an infection of the anal gland.

Arakawa also believes that it is true that infants and young children with anal fistula can be explained by anal sebaceous gland inflammation caused by sexual hormone imbalance. However, the abscess caused by inflammation of the skin appendage is different from the anal fistula caused by inflammation of the anal gland. The former can be cured with antibiotics or incision, and the latter often forms an anal fistula. The inner mouth is located in the anal crypt, which conforms to the theory of crypt infection. The clinical fact is that infantile anal fistula is the same as adult anal fistula. It is necessary to cut or remove the fistula including anal crypt to cure. Therefore, there is a difference between this understanding and clinical facts.

It is worth pointing out that some scholars in China have affirmed speculative aspects when citing foreign literature reports. As a result, the domestic anorectal community generally believes that infantile anal fistula is related to male hormones and is related to male hormones stimulating anal gland secretion. Studies have shown that (1) whether it is a baby boy or a baby girl, the level of sex hormones increases within 1 year after birth. In neonates, within 1 year of age, especially in newborns to 3 months, the negative feedback inhibition caused by the high concentration of sex hormones from the mother is no longer present, so the baby's own sex hormone secretion suddenly increases, reaching or even surpassing normal adult levels. These hormones include estradiol, progesterone, pituitary prolactin, etc. Some infants may even display galactorrhea, and there are significant differences compared with other age groups. After this, due to the gradual enhancement of the central nervous system's control ability, the hypothalamic–pituitary–gonadal axis is controlled by the negative feedback of sex hormones, so the level of sex hormones in the body rapidly decreases, in addition to PRL by the age of 1–3 years old. At the lowest level, the effect of this negative feedback can continue until puberty. (2) The male hormone content in male infants after birth to 3 years old is significantly lower than that of males aged 9–15 years, the former being 0.27 ± 0.31 and the latter being 0.38 ± 0.55. However, 9–15 years old is obviously not the peak incidence of anal fistula in infants and young children. (3) The multiple hormone levels of male infants (not just androgen, but also female hormones) are higher than those of female infants. Progesterone (P), testosterone (T), and pituitary prolactin (PRL) values were significantly different from those of females ($P < 0.05$). In the later growth and development process, the gender difference is more and more obvious. After entering puberty, the estrogens such as E2, P, and PRL in male children are decreasing year by year, and androgens and gonadotropins such as T, FSH, and LH are rising year by year, especially with T rising most significantly. At the age of 1 and 3 years of age, females are less affected by maternal sex hormones than men, and their changes in sex hormone levels are gradually distinguished from males of the same age in later growth and development. The greater the age, the greater the difference. After falling to the lowest level, female hormones such as E2, P, PRL, and gonadotropins such as FSH and LH in female children gradually increase. E2, P, and PRL in the 9–15 years old group were significantly different from those in the previous age group. There are also significant differences compared with males of the same age; male hormones in females also increase with age, but the extent is much lower than that of men of the same age, and there are significant differences. Therefore, it is suggested that the gender difference in infant and young children anal fistula is mainly due to the recognition of male hormones, but it seems that there is no theoretical or factual basis.

At the same time, the understanding of sex hormones leading to gender differences in anal fistula also lacks clinical support. For example, Chang Yilan and another 20 patients with adult perianal abscess were tested for serum testosterone and compared with normal controls. The results showed that the testosterone content in the serum of the observation group was not significantly higher than that of the normal control group ($P > 0.05$), and both were within the normal range. The fact that male hormones were not much higher should mean that there is no gender difference in anal fistula. However, in recent years, there have been two master's theses and one journal article related to the master's theses on this topic. The male hormone level in infants with anal fistula is significantly higher than that in normal children. In 2009, Liu Dewu found that testosterone levels in patients with anal fistula were higher than those in nonanal fistula and normal reference values. In 2013, Liang Wei et al. reported that serum testosterone levels and serum androstenedione levels in male patients with perianal abscess were significantly higher than those in the control group, and the difference was statistically significant. Serum dehydroepiandrosterone level was not significantly higher than that in the control group. However, there were only 11 cases in the control group used in the study, and they were not normal and were all children with inguinal hernia (no incarcerated history).

10.2.2.3 The Anal Crypt Is Easy to Infect

Some people think that the anus crypt in children has a funnel shape, which makes it easy to store dung. When diarrhea occurs, the mucus stored in the crypt is washed away. The lubrication of the mucus and the protection it offers against foreign body invasion also disappear, local immunity is therefore reduced, and it is easy to form cryptitis after bacterial invasion. In addition, the distance between the anus dentate line and the anal margin of the newborn is very short, and the anal sphincter of the child is relatively slack. When urine is soaked for a long time and the stool is smeared, the crypt is valgus damaged, and the crypt can easily become inflamed. The baby's external mouth is the skin, and this is temporarily closed after the formation of granulation. The internal mouth continues to be invaded by bacteria and fecal debris. After a period of time, due to poor drainage, a local abscess is formed. After ulceration and decompression, it heals again, but infectious granules can recur.

He Yong and Han Yinghe pointed out that the source of infection of perianal abscess and anal fistula can be accurately detected during surgery, and this is the case for 34.17% of adult cases and 85.14% of child cases. It is worth noting that there is usually a fusion crypt in the mouth or elsewhere in the child. There is no recurrence of anal fistula or abscess in the fusion crypt without other factors, suggesting that fusion of the crypt does not mean anal fistula and perianal but that abscesses must occur.

10.2.2.4 Diaper Dermatitis Pathology

Zhang Jinzhe believes that the neonatal anal sphincter is looser, and the anal mucosa can be turned out when rubbing the stool with a diaper. Especially when diarrhea is severe, anal skin eczema (diaper rash) is more prominent, and the anal mucosa can also be pulled out by itself. Because the anal mucosa often comes out, the diaper near the anal sinus can cause infection and form an anal abscess.

Tang Hanzhen believes that infantile anal fistula occurs on both sides of the anus. It may be easy to eversion with the mucosa on both sides of the anus. It is easily diaper-scratched and easily infected. The median mucosa on each side of the anus is relatively easy to be everted and not easily scratched by diapers. Infection can therefore easily occur.

According to Fuji's examination of diaper dermatitis on both sides of the anus, bacteriological examination was performed on the anus of the newborn, and the gender differences between males and females were studied, and significant differences were found. Quetta also reported that diaper dermatitis has a tendency to spread to both sides in both males and females, but for males, it covered with scrotum in the perianal area, so the degree of inflammation is more serious than that of baby girls. In addition, 3 months after birth, anal dermatitis is the most contaminated by feces and urine, which is consistent with the fact that there are more patients with anal fistula in infants within 3 months of age. Therefore, it is considered that from this point, the cause of the disease is appropriate. According to Gu Tian, a subcutaneous abscess is caused by an infection of the anus skin, an infection of the skin appendage, and damages to the skin of the anus and the like, and the abscess is sometimes connected to the anal crypt. Yi Zhaozhao believes that although this type of "diaper dermatitis" develops an abscess that will be encountered in daily life, such abscesses are completely different from abscesses caused by anal gland infection.

10.2.2.5 Residual Epithelium

In 1988, Shafik pointed out in his series of anorectal anatomy studies that the embryonic rectal neck mucosa extends downward, and the anus is inserted into the posterior intestine to form an anal sinus, covering the epithelial cells. Under normal circumstances, the anal sinus disappears after birth, but it can also persist under the mucous membrane, becoming an anal band, or there is epithelial cell debris, and it can form a tubular structure and become an anal muscle gland. In his 60 adult anal fistulas, 54 patients found epithelial cells in the vicinity of the fistula and between the muscles. It is believed that the presence of epithelial cells is an antigenic response to the perianal infection and causes the infection to become a recurrent chronic inflammatory process. In 1991, Klosterhalfen et al. performed immunohistochemical examination on 62 cadaveric specimens and found that 90% of the anal sinus were present. More than half of the fetuses, newborns, and children had anal intermuscular glands. In adults, this was rare. Epithelial cells were found in all three cases of anal fistula, indicating that there appears to be some anatomical association between the anal muscle glands and anal fistula.

Wang Jun et al. serially sliced the anal canal from nine cases of neonates and infants and three cases of fetal corpses (both nonperianal infections) from the sagittal, coronal, and horizontal planes and routinely stained for histology. It was found that 10 cases showed anal sinus, and three cases showed epithelial cells under the mucosa near the dentate line. The columnar epithelial cells existed in the form of acinus or debris. Pathological examination of anal fistula resection specimens in infants and young children revealed that among the 27 children who developed symptoms within 3 months after birth, 22 (81.48%) found epithelial cells in the vicinity of the fistula and between the muscle tissues, and 5 cases did not. Epithelial cells were observed in six pathological sections from 6 to 11.5 year olds. These epithelial cells are cubic epithelial cells, columnar epithelial cells, or stratified squamous epithelial cells. They exist in the form of acincin-like structures or fragments with inflammatory cells accumulating around them. According to this, they believe that the anal sinus has a self-improving process during the development from the fetal period to the postnatal period. In this process, a small number of children have embryonic residues, that is, epithelial cells or epithelial cell debris with acinar-like structures. Because the rectal longitudinal muscles form multiple interstitial spaces during the extension of the perianal skin, the epithelial cell debris is interspersed. Once diarrhea, eczema, anal fissure, and other predisposing factors are present, abscess formation occurs. The presence of rectal submucosal and intermuscular epithelial cells near the dentate line is the root cause of recurrent episodes of perianal infection and prolonged unhealing and is the main pathological basis for anal fistula formation. As for the pathological section, the five cases where epithelial cells were not found may be related to the formation of abscess after infection. The range of the abscess is large, the circulation is smooth, and the epithelial cells are destroyed and excreted. According to the operation, the fistula is thicker and the central part has a spherical cavity.

Zhong Shiqing et al. found an anal sinus in 58 children during operation. Among them, 50 cases of anal fistula are located in the anal sinus, indicating that the anal sinus is a susceptible site. When diarrhea occurs, red buttocks and anal fissures are infected, it becomes easy to form an anal infection. Among the 45 children who developed symptoms within 3 months after birth, 36 found epithelial cells in the vicinity of the fistula and between the muscle tissues. In the children who developed the disease after 1 year of age, the presence of epithelial cells was found in the pathological sections. According to this, the presence of perianal epithelial cells may be the pathological basis for repeated episodes of infection and prolonged unhealing.

10.2.2.6 Fecal Compression

This theory has long been proposed by the Ikeuti and the Sakane. It is believed that the formation of the humerus in infants and young children is insufficient, from the rectum to the anal canal is nearly linear, and because the anal sphincter does not have enough tension, the feces directly compress the mucosa, especially that the mucosa of the rectal nodules on both sides is more strongly compressed, further contributes to the invasion of bacteria due to abrasions and inflammation, and finally leads to anal fistula. In addition, the reason why infants and young children have less anal fistula is that the uterus of female infants is in a state of dorsiflexion. This kind of compression forms a shape similar to that of a rectum in adults. Because the direction of fecal compression is changed, anal fistula is difficult to occur.

This kind of theory explains why the characteristics of infants and young children make them more prone to anal fistula than women and also more prone to getting them on both sides. However, if it is only because of such physical reasons, as mentioned above, infantile anal fistula should be a disease with a high incidence. It is also important to know when the humeral curvature is formed and whether the age of onset of infantile anal fistula is synchronized.

Regarding the reasons why they occur on both sides, some people think that it is because the anus is perpendicular to the rectum of infants and young children, and both sides are easy to be compressed, and the anal crypts on both sides are well developed. However, Fujihara's report that the anal crypts in the anterior and posterior parts are two times deeper than in other parts, which is contrary to the fact that Ventero said that the anal crypts on both sides develop better. It is believed that the cause of anal fistula in infants and young children should be related to the depth of the anal crypt and the sex of the child.

10.2.3 Treatment of Infantile Anal Fistula

10.2.3.1 Principles of Treatment

The treatment of anal fistula in infants and young children has been controversial, and there are different opinions on whether to choose conservative treatment or surgical treatment and when to perform surgery.

Yi Yanshi advocated conservative treatment for infantile anal fistula within 1 year of age and then switch to surgery if there is no nonsurgical cure. Because of the various theories of the onset of anal fistula, it is possible to see the complete formation of the tibia curvature at around 1 year of age, and the production of IgA in the blood is close to that of adults. Yi Xiaoshi believes that the anal fistula of infants and young children is different from adult anal fistula in terms of their location and gender differences, and most of the anal fistula of infants and young children are subcutaneous fistulas and have a tendency to heal naturally. They can rely on simple fistula incision to cure. Most of the pathogens are *Escherichia coli* and *Streptococcus faecalis*. In the early stage of abscess formation, the antibiotic effect is not obvious. It is necessary to cut the abscess for adequate drainage during the formation of abscess. Sometimes the pus can be gently wiped when changing the diaper. Although there are many kinds of disinfectants for cleaning, sometimes there are concerns about causing drug dermatitis, so it is thought that it can be achieved by simply washing with warm water. Surgical treatment should be performed for those who are considered to be incapable of achieving healing after the above treatment. In addition, another reason for the conservative treatment is that infants and young children have poor compatibility and that diarrhea tends to increase after surgery.

Arakawa believes that longer-term conservative treatment of infantile anal fistula will bring obstacles to the well-being of the child and may increase the risk of mental health caused by emotional disorders. In addition, mothers usually strongly urge surgery over longer-term conservative therapy. It also has a certain adverse effect on the doctor's reputation, so conservative treatment should only last for about 8 months, and it should later be treated with fistula incision.

Regarding the operation period of infantile anal fistula, many advocate for early active surgery. Ming Haishi believes that there is no reason for conservative treatment and advocates early active surgical treatment. Sanchi believes that although there are benefits to nonsurgical methods, if conservative treatment is used in all cases, the timing of surgery for some patients will be delayed. Therefore, in order not to delay the optimal operation period, it is better to choose surgery early on.

10.2.3.2 Surgical Methods

Anal Fistula Incision

Yi Zhao believes that it is not necessary to remove the fistula in the same way as an adult anal fistula. It is only necessary to cut the fistula including the anal crypt. The specific method is to probe it from the outer mouth, puncture it from the inner mouth, and then cut it along the probe. After the bowel movement, wipe the wound clean and put on the sterile gauze.

Tang believes that the anal fistula should be thoroughly treated in infants and young children, and second-stage surgery is recommended. Seven to 10 days after the anal abscess is cut, when the redness is basically subsided, the anal fistula can be cut or sutured. It is not advisable to perform a one-time radical surgery during incision and drainage of the perianal abscess because it is easy to damage excessive inflammatory cellular loose tissue, making the scar tissue too large after surgery, and may continue to spread the inflammation that has not yet been fully controlled.

He Yong et al. advocated an open radical cure for infantile anal fistula. They believe that infantile perianal abscess and anal fistula are usually simple and that the origin is mostly the corresponding anal crypt. They recommend performing an operation to cut the abscess and carefully search for the source of infection. If the source of infection can be determined, it should be removed together. If the source of infection cannot be determined, the anal crypt with the same part of the abscess should be removed. Such an operation can cure the anal fistula, shorten the course of treatment, and alleviate the pain of the child. Infants with low anal fistula can be cut in local anesthesia while the sphincter tissue hanged with rubber bands in high anal fistula. This is the same as the treatment principles for adult anal fistula. However, the baby's muscles are delicate and the hanging line should be looser. Even so, the time for the rubber band to fall off is shorter than that of the adult. According to their observation, there were 34 cases that were (89.47%) off-line in 3–5 days.

Zhang Sifen and others believe that although some infants have an tendency to heal themselves after clinical treatment, due to improper care and other reasons, the condition may be repeated or aggravated in others, and most of the infantile anal fistula is low anal fistula, and the surgical treatment is relatively simple. The effect is exact, and the complications are few, so the author believes that surgery should be appropriate. The surgical approach is based on direct incision. Because the growth and development of children are rapid, not too much tissue should be removed, and generally it is not needed to remove the fistula so as not to prolong the healing time and damage the anal sphincter function. For a few patients with a higher position of the fistula, the thread can be treated, but the muscles of the child are young, and the hanging line should not be pulled too tightly so as not to break the muscles too early, and the function of protecting the anal sphincter cannot be achieved.

Cut the Hanging Line

He Ping believes that the development of anal sphincter in children is imperfect. The anal straight ring is narrower and thinner than in the adult, and the anal canal is short. Therefore, in infants, doctors should avoid cutting the fistula directly. If one accidentally cut off too much anal sphincter, it will lead to anal incontinence and deformity. After the sequelae, if multiple fistulas are cut open, it will affect the normal bowel reflex of the anus. The use of hanging thread has the following advantages: (1) during the process of gradual incision, the basal wound is gradually healed, and the sphincter is cut off, but the broken end has been fixed by the tissue so that the separation is not too large. After healing, the scar is small and will not cause anal deformation and incontinence. (2) Less bleeding due to surgical injury. (3) When the rubber band is not falling off, the wound generally does not undergo bridge healing. (4) Convenient dressing change. (5) The rubber band continues to drain, reducing the number of dressing changes and reducing postoperative care.

Pang Wenbin and others advocated for the use of the incision and hanging line method to treat children with anal fistula. They believe that "anal fistula incision" is not suitable for children with anal fistula. Although there is no anal incontinence after the low anal fistula is cut, the sick child is not well matched, and it is not easy to change the medicine. Sometimes the wound is forced to take off the drainage strip, and it will not be able to get rid of the drainage. If the drainage strip is not placed, the simple bridge-shaped adhesion forms a false healing, so it is better to cut and tie the hanging line.

Therefore, it is advocated that for children with anal fistula, whether it is low or high, it is better to cut the hanging line. It is believed that the use of hanging wire therapy has the following advantages: (1) smooth drainage can prevent wound infection and adhesion. The rubber band used for hanging the thread not only can cut the fistula chronically but also has a good drainage effect. Although the wound is often contaminated by feces, it does not cause infection. The incision of the hanging line forms an ulcer wound, which is not easy to adhere, and after the rubber band is detached, the gauze may not be drained. (2) The pain is mild, and the sick child can bear it. The sensory nerve receptors of the anus are mainly distributed in the skin layer, and the pain perception of the subcutaneous tissue and the muscular layer is less sensitive. When the thread is hung, the skin of the anal canal has been incision-cut, and the thread is hung on the incision to avoid the pain-sensitive skin, so the pain is mild and there is no need to use analgesics. (3) Wound care is simple. Because the drainage is smooth, the wound is not easily infected and adhered. After each stool, the anus can be washed with potassium permanganate solution. Except for a few older children, most of the children with postoperative dressing are treated by parents and all are cured. (4) The wound of the hanging thread is narrower and smaller, and the scar is small after healing, and anal deformation does not occur. It is worth noting that the pediatric tissue is soft, the sphincter bundle is small, the fistula is easy to cut, and the off-line period is shorter than that of the adult. Therefore, for children with high anal fistula, the principle of the second-stage incision should be followed when hanging the thread so that the off-line should not be too fast so as to avoid anal incontinence.

The surgical point of the incision hanging line method is that the soft round tip probe is gently passed through the fistula from the outer mouth of the anal fistula into the inner mouth. If the inner mouth is not found, it is pierced from the thinnest part of the anal mucosa. The needle cuts the skin and subcutaneous tissue between the inner and outer mouths, and draws the 7th silk thread and the rubber band (single strand) with the probe, tightens the rubber band, closes the skin around the anus, clamps it with a hemostat, and uses it under the hemostatic forceps. The No. 7 silk thread was double-ligated, embedded in the skin incision, the hemostatic forceps removed, and the excess rubber band cut, and the end was kept 1–2 cm to prevent slipping.

He Ping used the incision and hanging line method to treat 30 infants with anal fistula and all recovered. Postoperative anal defecation function was normal. There was no anal deformation, stenosis, and incontinence. No recurrence occurred within 3 years.

Dragline Therapy

Wang Minghua and others advocated the use of the tow line method to treat anal fistula in infants and young children. The basic method is to use three to four strands of No. 10 silk thread to hang between the inner and outer mouths. After the dressing change, apply the traditional Chinese medicine "Jiuyi Dan" on the silk thread and drag it into the anus. When the pus is reduced for about 4–6 days, the thread is gradually removed, one per day, and the cotton filling method is used for 3–4 days. It is believed that the internal anal fistula of infants and young children is mostly low-grade simple anal fistula. The degree of fibrosis of the fistula wall is not high, and it is easy to stagnate and de-pipe and this provides favorable conditions for the implementation of the towline method. Compared with the traditional incision and expansion, the tow therapy has the advantages of simple operation, less damage to the tissue, effective protection of the anal function, less postoperative pain, short course of disease, and long exposure time of the drug after dressing change.

10.2.3.3 Nursing and Dressing Points

It is generally believed that infant wounds have a strong ability to heal and heal and usually heal within 2 weeks of surgery. However, according to Down's report, only 36 cases (56.25%) of the 64 cases healed in 12–16 days, and most wound healing was delayed. The reasons may be as follows: (1) too much friction to the wound. Due to postoperative diarrhea, it is necessary to wipe the wound after each stool and increase the number of dressing changes, and this affects the growth of wound epithelium and delays wound healing. (2) Too much pressure used during wound dressing change. Parents worry about the wounds being not clean enough and often scrub too heavily. The baby's skin is delicate; rubbing too heavily affects healing. (3) Infants are young, and parents fail to master the main points of dressing change, resulting in poor drainage of the wound, excessive growth of granulation, or improper use of cotton, thus affecting wound healing. (4) Infant eczema, perianal allergic dermatitis, etc. will also affect wound healing time. It is considered that the nursing and dressing change after anal fistula in infants and young children is extremely important.

Infants with anal fistula are prone to diarrhea or increased stools. For this, 9–15 g/day of yam can be used, boiled into a paste to feed, or Chinese herbal medicine fried Atractylodes, medlar, fried six koji, and fried malt each 9 g. The decoction can also be applied to the abdomen at the same time.

10.3 Rectal Vaginal Fistula

The rectal vaginal fistula refers to the pathological pathway formed between the anterior wall mucosa of the rectum and the posterior epithelium of the vagina. It is manifested as gas, pus, or feces in the vagina, long-term repeated intravaginal infection, accompanied by itching and pain in the perineum, often causing sexual life disorders and causing a heavy psychological burden on patients. The disease requires surgery, but the recurrence rate is high, which seriously affects the quality of life of patients. The disease is often described as "the most depressing, embarrassing, and most discouraging thing a woman has ever experienced."

10.3.1 Cause

The causes of rectal vaginal fistula are complicated and divided into congenital and acquired. Congenital is very rare, and often complicated by anal, urethra, or bladder deformities, so treatment is more difficult. Acquired is divided into iatrogenic and noniatrogenic. The iatrogenic causes of rectal vaginal fistula include the following:

1. Injury or improper side-cutting during childbirth is the most common cause of rectal vaginal fistula. A 1994 study in Germany suggested that this condition accounted for 88% of total causes, accounting for 0.1% of all vaginal delivery. At present, in areas with underdeveloped medical conditions, such as developing countries, childbirth injury is still the most significant cause of rectal vaginal fistula.

2. Intrapelvic uterine attachment tumor resection, intraoperative injury of the rectum or reproductive septum, especially in the lower rectum, or reproductive compartment endometriosis resection is likely to cause rectal vaginal fistula.

3. Surgical pelvic floor surgery, such as retroperitoneal tumor resection and low rectal tumor resection: injury to the posterior wall of the vagina when the tumor is removed, or when the rectum is closed with the stapler, the posterior wall of the vagina is not completely pushed open and the posterior wall of the vagina is mistakenly cut. Especially when using double staplers, it is more likely to appear. In recent years, the wide application of the double stapler has led to an increase in rectal vaginal fistula. According to the literature, the proportion of rectal vaginal fistula in low rectal cancer surgery is as high as 10%. Local anal canal or low rectal mass resection and more than three degrees of internal hemorrhoids sacral circumcision can also cause rectal vaginal fistula. In addition, perianal abscess incision, improper drainage, or anal sphincter repair may also be complicated by rectal vaginal fistula.

4. Malignant tumors of the rectum, perineum, vagina, and cervix: local high-dose radiotherapy can directly damage the rectal reproductive septum, causing chronic necrosis, perforation, and formation of rectal vaginal fistula. Studies have suggested that radiation

injury is a risk factor for the failure of rectal vaginal fistula treatment.

Lin Guole et al. retrospectively analyzed the clinical data of 52 cases of iatrogenic rectal vaginal fistula. Results: occurred in 22 cases (42.3%) after gynecological surgery, 14 cases (26.9%) after birth injury (impaired delivery). 13 patients (25.0%) after rectal surgery and 3 patients (5.8%) due to other causes.

Noniatrogenic causes of rectal vaginal fistula include the following:

1. Inflammatory bowel disease, accounting for 0.2–2.1% of cases, such as crypt disease and Crohn's disease, is also a high risk factor for failure of rectal vaginal fistula repair.
2. Rectal vaginal tumor directly infiltrating the reproductive septum, necrosis caused by rectal vaginal fistula, although rare, but the treatment is tricky.
3. Abscesses in the perianal and perineal areas, such as the perianal abscess not cut in time, or the spread of the abscess of the papillary gland, invading the deep fascia.
4. Mechanical external force directly crossing the area causing injury.

10.3.2 Categories

Rectal vaginal fistula is generally divided into two types: high and low. The lower rectal vaginal fistula is located in the lower third of the rectum and halfway below the vagina. The high rectal vaginal fistula is located in the rectum in the upper one-third part of the vagina. According to the diameter of the mouth, it is divided into three types, of which less than 0.5 cm is called small sputum; 0.5–2.5 cm is called scorpion; and more than 2.5 cm is called big sputum.

According to the degree of difficulty in treatment, it can be divided into two types: simple and complex: middle and low position, diameter less than 2.5 cm and previous history without surgery are generally considered as simple sputum; relatively high position, diameter greater than 2.5 cm, presence of two or more fistulas, and previous history of repair surgery or local radiotherapy, and those caused by crypt gland disease, Crohn's disease, or tumor invasion are considered complex sputum.

10.3.3 Diagnosis

The patient's clinical symptoms, including gas, feces, pus, etc., are all present in the vagina, together with local itching, tingling, and other manifestations. The low rectal vaginal fistula is examined under direct vision of a proctoscope, colposcope, or vaginal speculum. It can be seen that the rectum and the vagina are separated by a fistula, and the size, height, and even biopsy pathology can be determined. Methylene blue can also be infused through the rectum, and the gauze dressing preset in the vagina can be verified. It is important to collect the history of patients with complicated recto-vaginal fistula, including the cause of the disease, the details of previous treatment, the surgical procedure, the time interval, and performance before and after each onset. Auxiliary examinations include pelvic MRI and CT, transrectal or intravaginal ultrasound and colorectaloscopy (Fig. 10.2), cystoscopy, and laparoscopy. Simple low rectal vaginal fistula diagnosis is easy; for complex high rectal vaginal fistula, especially inflamma-

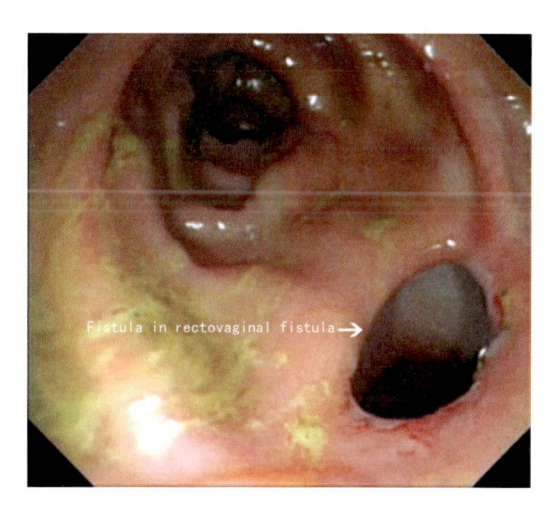

Fig. 10.2 The fistula of the rectovaginal fistula seen under the colonoscope

tory bowel disease, endometriosis, pelvic floor rectal vaginal surgery, direct tumor invasion or high polysinus, and more recurrent rectal vaginal fistula after subsurgical treatment, a careful and comprehensive evaluation of systemic and local conditions is required before surgery to help develop a surgical plan.

10.3.4 Treatment

Rectal vaginal fistula is rarely self-healing, conservative treatment is also difficult to achieve, and most require surgery.

Rectal vaginal fistula caused by fresh surgical trauma or trauma should in principle be repaired immediately. Rectal vaginal fistula caused by perianal infection or inflammatory disease, due to congestion and edema of surrounding tissues, is difficult to find the correct level between the rectum and vagina and is not suitable for immediate surgical repair. The intestinal function of the patient should be improved while strengthening the anti-infective bathing and nursing to actively control the inflammatory response. From the clinical practice point of view, for patients with rectal vaginal fistula and rectal vaginal abscess, drainage can be used to fully drain the abscess in the deep gap, creating conditions for the final radical surgery. Generally, after 3–6 months of conservative treatment, the tissue edema around the fistula and the inflammatory reaction should have subsided and then repaired.

The patient's medical history should be comprehensively and accurately understood before surgery. Whether there are possible risk factors such as Crohn's disease, local radiotherapy, diabetes and taking immunosuppressive agents, course of disease, treatment, and whether there are other basic diseases should all be taken into account. For the surgical treatment of rectal vaginal fistula, it is necessary to know in detail the previous surgical methods and analyze the possible causes of failure. Doctors should improve physical examination and auxiliary examination, as far as possible to improve the rectal perineal MRI, CT, ultrasound, and colorectal and enema angiography, to determine the level of sputum, size, local inflammatory edema control, whether or not there is anal sphincter dysfunction and sexual dysfunction, and a psychological assessment if necessary. On the basis of a comprehensive understanding of the disease, and through a multidisciplinary discussion, doctors should prudently formulate a relatively reasonable treatment plan.

10.3.4.1 Commonly Used Surgery

Simple Resection and Suture Repair

Simple and low rectal vaginal fistula can be repaired by hand suture. The main point of surgery is to fully expose the surgical field through the vaginal speculum or rectal hook, through the rectal side or the vaginal side, or bilaterally combined with direct vision to remove the scar tissue around the fistula, and then use layered suture to close the fistula (Fig. 10.3). Absorbable sutures are preferred for suturing to reduce localized foreign body reactions and inflammatory responses. Anal sphincter reconstruction should be performed at the same time as an anal dysfunction or when there is a large diameter of 2.5 cm or more in order to prevent postoperative loss of control or incontinence.

Before the operation of this surgery, adequate preoperative preparation should be done. Preoperative control of diabetes and autoimmune diseases should be taken out so that the nutritional status of the system is relatively good.

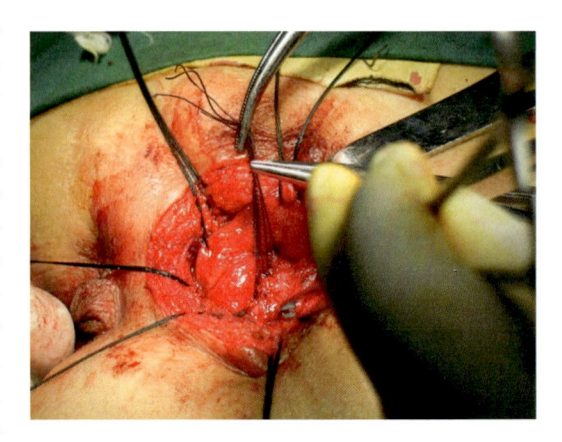

Fig. 10.3 Transrectal repair of rectovaginal fistula

For a large diameter, high position, recurrence, and inflammatory bowel disease caused by sputum, direct suture repair is not recommended; in this case, the failure rate of rectal vaginal hernia repair is very high. If surgery is rushed, once failed, it will be extremely difficult to treat again.

In 2012, Ommer et al. conducted a meta-analysis of 39 studies of rectal repair of primary rectal vaginal fistula between 1978 and 2011. The results showed that the success rate of surgery was low, about 50–70%. There was a large difference in the success rate of surgery. The success rate of repair in young women was higher than that in the elderly or those post-radiotherapy. There was no significant difference in the success rate between the transrectal and the transperineal approach. At the same time, anal sphincter reconstruction can greatly reduce postoperative re-operation and the incidence of anal sphincter dysfunction. However, this meta-analysis did not include studies of recurrent rectal vaginal fistula. Lowry et al. reported a single-center experience with a success rate of 88%, and the success rate of recurrent rectal vaginal fistula was reduced to 55%. Tsang et al. reported the same situation, with a success rate reduced from 45 to 25%.

Rectal Mucosal Flap Replacement Repair

At present, for the middle and lower rectal vaginal fistula, most surgeons tend to use the valvular valve repair method. This procedure is mainly to use a healthy epithelial tissue to cover one end of the ankle to eliminate rectal vaginal fistula, including transanal or vaginal valvular valve repair. Most surgeons choose transanal valvular valve repair because of the high-pressure area of the rectum. If the opening of the rectum is repaired satisfactorily, it can prevent bacterial contamination in the high-pressure area.

The operation procedure of the valvular valve repair is as follows: 20 ml of adrenaline sodium chloride solution is infiltrated around the mouth and the rectal mucosa to reduce bleeding, and a narrow and wide rectal mucosa muscle is made from the distal end of the fistula to the proximal end. The flap (bottom width is two times the width of the top), about 4.0 cm long, includes mucosa, submucosa, and part of the ring muscle layer to ensure blood supply and suture without tension; remove the part of the rectal flap containing the fistula, first with 2-0 so that it can absorb the suture to suture the defect of the sacral muscle layer, then pull the rectal flap downward to cover the fistula, and suture the top and both sides of the rectal flap with 3-0 absorbable suture.

Rectal push valve repair or anal push flap repair for simple rectal vaginal fistula has the following advantages: (1) no need to cut the vaginal body, less pain, and quick healing; (2) no need to cut the sphincter, will not cause anal incontinence; (3) avoids keyhole deformity; (4) no need for protective stoma.

Looking back at the relevant literature for nearly 30 years, the success rate of valvuloplasty for rectal vaginal fistula varies widely, ranging from 43 to 100%. In 1998, Tsang et al. retrospectively analyzed the rectal valvuloplasty for the treatment of 52 cases of mid-low rectal vaginal fistula caused by birth injury. The study found that patients with anal sphincter injury before surgery were treated with simple rectal valvuloplasty. The success rate was only 33%, and the success rate of combined sphincter angioplasty was 88%. In addition, for simple rectal valvuloplasty, patients with a history of preoperative repair had a surgical success rate of only 25%. Therefore, the middle and low rectal vaginal fistula combined with sphincter injury and surgical repair history is an important factor affecting the success of the surgery. The key to the success of the operation is good blood supply to the valvular flap and the in-situ suture covering the fistula without tension after sufficient dissociation. The injury of the external anal sphincter causes the support of a good blood supply to be lost between the rectum and the vagina, and the preoperative repair history leads to the formation of scar tissue around the fistula, which affects the compliance of the rectal wall.

However, the success rate reported in recent years has not improved significantly, especially for recurrent rectal vaginal fistula, and the recurrence rate is still high. Studies have reported recurrent rectal vaginal fistula with rectal mucosal flap replacement repair for 21 patients and the recurrence rate of up to 56.8%. Therefore, some scholars do not agree with this method as the preferred method for the treatment of recurrent rectal vaginal fistula.

Autologous Tissue Flap Transfer Tamponade Repair

In the early 1990s, the use of autologous tissue with vascular pedicles including flaps, myocutaneous flaps, fat flaps, bulbar muscle fat pads, gracilis muscles, gluteus maximus, tibia rectus, omentum or small intestine flaps, etc. began to be used in filling and repairing the rectal vaginal fistula. The most common of these is the labia fat pad (also known as the Martius flap, which is the labia majora fat pad tissue flap), which was first reported by Martius in 1928.

The principle of surgery is the following: (1) increase the thickness of the rectal vagina (urethra) interval and play a role of isolation; (2) isolated tissue has a healthy blood supply; its anti-infective ability is only two layers weaker than the original. This tissue is much stronger, and it is not easy to cause infection. (3) The presence of the isolated healthy tissue increases the ability of local healing and makes it not easy to relapse. The advantages of using autologous blood for tissue isolation: (1) to ensure the success of surgery without improving the prophylactic stoma and to improve the quality of life of patients; (2) not limited by the timing of surgery for traditional surgery. Traditional surgery generally advocates that patients who do not recover after conservative treatment should consider surgery only 6 months after the onset of sputum. (3) Generally, it is not necessary to consider the size of the fistula and the inflammatory scar around the fistula.

The procedure of Martius operation is as follows: an arc-shaped incision is made in the perineal vaginal opening, the rectal vaginal septum is separated from the genital side to the upper 2 cm of the fistula, the rectal side is sutured, the vaginal side is removed, and a vertical incision is made in the labia majora. Free up the labia fat pad and bulb sponge muscle, and protect the blood supply under the lower part, implant the rectal vaginal septum through the subcutaneous tunnel, and suture the vaginal side (Fig. 10.4). The literature reports that the success rate of surgery is 60–94%.

There are also reports of treatment of rectal vaginal fistula and rectal urethral fistula with femoral muscle transfer. Large chunks of thin muscle transfer can increase the thickness of the rectal vaginal septum so that the rectum and vagina are completely separated, but the complications are relatively high due to the large separation and metastasis of the femoral muscle. The surgical procedure for the transfer of the gracilis muscle is as follows: first the perineal incision is made, the rectal vaginal septum is separated to the 2 cm healthy tissue above the fistula, the rectal side and the vaginal side are respectively repaired, and the free gracilis muscle (Fig. 10.5) is passed through the subcutaneous tunnel. Rotate into the rectal vaginal septum, be careful not to twist, suture fixed at the top of the rectal vaginal septum, and then suture the perineal incision. The literature reported a success rate of 53–92%. Retrospective large-scale clinical data from Pinto et al. showed that the success rate of massive gracilis transfer in the treatment of rectal vaginal fistula was 79%.

Cui Long et al. summarized the experience of autologous blood supply for metastasis and tamponade repair of rectal vaginal fistula: (1) selection of incision length: generally 3–5 cm. (2) Special attention should be paid to the separation of the rectal vaginal septum. First, the upper edge of the sphincter should be separated from the

Fig. 10.4 Transvaginal repair of rectovaginal fistula. (**a**) Make an arc-shaped incision near the vagina. (**b**) Separate the rectovaginal septum upward to 2 cm above the fistula. (**c**) Suture to repair the rectum side, and remove the fistula on the vaginal side. (**d**) Make a vertical incision in the labia majora to free the labia majora fat pad and bulboma. (**e**) The already made labia majora flap with vascular tissue. (**f**) Insert the labia majora tissue flap into the rectovaginal septum through a subcutaneous tunnel and suture and fix it. (**g**) The labia majora tissue flap is packed behind the rectovaginal septum and has been sutured and fixed. (**h**) After the labia majora tissue flap is packed to repair the rectovaginal septum, before the incision is not sutured. (**i**) Suture the labia majora incision and the incision near the vagina

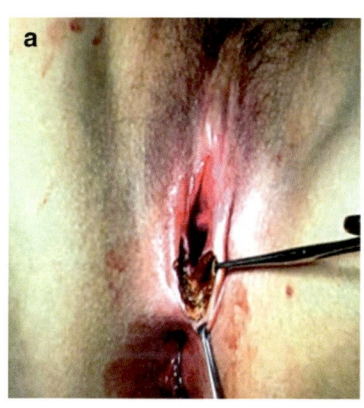

10 Diagnosis and Treatment of Special Anal Fistula

a Make an arc–shaped incision near the vaginal

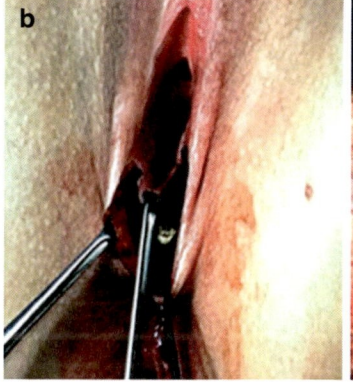

b Separate the rectovaginal septum upward to 2cm above the fistula

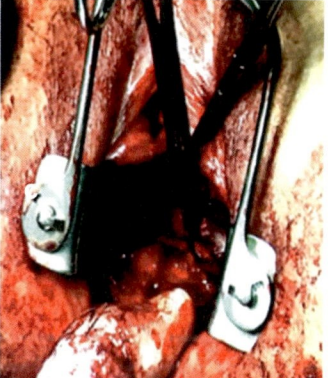

c Suture to repair the rectum side, and remove the fistula on the vaginal side

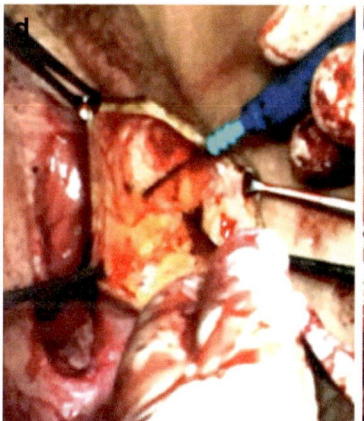

d Make a vertical incision in the labia majora to free the labia majora fat pad and bulboma

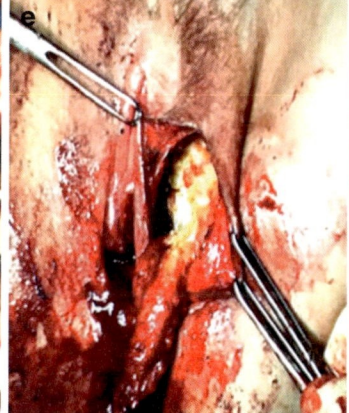

e The already made labia majora flap with vascular tissue

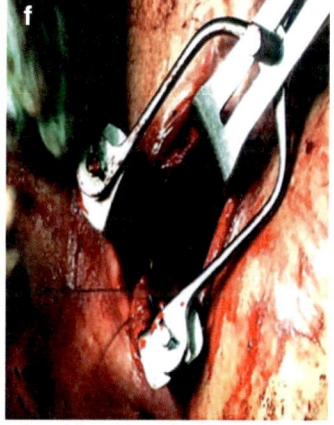

f Insert the labia majora tissue flap into the rectovaginal septum through a subcutaneous tunnel and suture and fix it

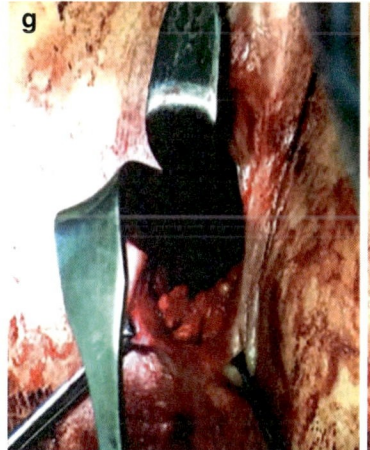

g The labia majora tissue flap is picked behind the rectovaginal septum and has been sutured and fixed

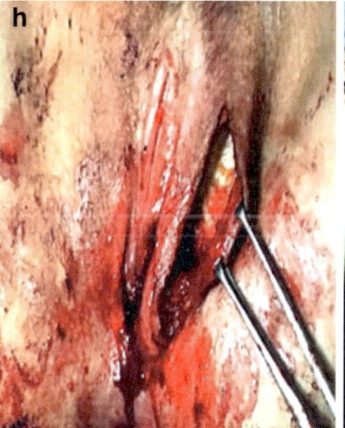

h After the labia majora tissue flap is packed to repair the rectovaginal septum, before the incision is not sutured

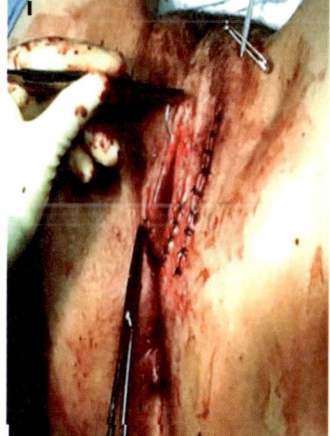

i Suture the labia majora incision and the incision near the vaginal

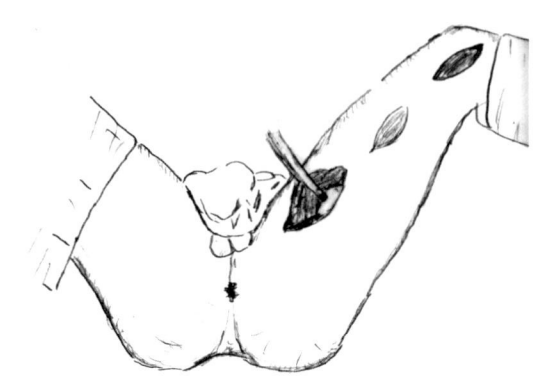

Fig. 10.5 Free indication of gracilis

sphincter; the second is to find the boundary of the interval. Generally, there will be no bleeding. (3) The free tissue flap should be paid attention to so as to protect the blood supply of the tissue, generally starting from the top in the separation process, carefully identifying the tissue supply blood vessels to protect. Freely isolate the tissue before repairing the fistula, thus ensuring that there is a certain period of time to observe the blood supply of the tissue, and at the same time ensure that the free tissue has sufficient length, and the method of measuring the length by pulling and separating the tissue can be adopted. It is also necessary to ensure that the tissue has sufficient thickness so that the blood supply can be effectively ensured and that the thickness of the interval can be made standard. (4) When the same tissue is isolated, care should be taken not to leave dead space; during the suturing process, the blood supply to the original end of the tissue cannot be blocked to avoid tissue necrosis. (5) When closing the perineal body, pay attention to the drainage. You can use a rubber piece to pull out from the incision. Generally, the drainage piece can be removed after 48 h. (6) After the operation, enteral nutrition is generally used to control defecation for 1 week, so it is completely unnecessary to make a preventive stoma.

Transvaginal Repair

Transvaginal surgery is used by most gynecologists and has certain advantages in some special cases. For patients who have failed multiple rectal valvuloplasty or patients with unhealthy rectal mucosa (Crohn's disease with proctitis), the injection of sclerosing agent will cause the rectal mucosa to be hardened. Transvaginal valvular valve repair or fistula resection combined with stratified suture can also achieve good results.

Surgical methods: (1) good exposure of the posterior wall of the vagina, the surgeon should stick a finger into the anus to jack up the mouth. Dilute adrenaline fluid is injected under the vaginal mucosa around the fistula. A circular incision should be made 0.5 cm from the edge of the fistula with a curved scalpel blade, deep to the vaginal fascia. (2) The vaginal margin of the incision is to be pulled with a tissue forceps, and the vaginal mucosa and the rectal wall are to be centrifuged about 2 cm around the mouth with a curved blade. The vaginal mucosa of the mouth should be slightly separated from the center by about 2 mm, and the scar of the mouth should not be removed. (3) The suture is to be sutured along the edge of the mouth with a No. 1 silk thread, and the suture should not pass through the rectal mucosa. The larger mouth (>2 cm) will be interrupted by suture. (4) The vaginal submucosal connective tissue should be sutured with a No. 1 silk thread to reinforce the front of the fistula. (5) The vaginal mucosa should be sutured intermittently with a 3-0 absorbable line. The vagina is to be filled with an iodov gauze roll.

Tang Jie et al. used this procedure to treat 13 patients with rectal vaginal fistula. The postoperative vaginal defecation symptoms disappeared, and patients were discharged. The hospital stay was 11–16 days, with a median of 12 days. All patients were followed up for 0.5–7 years, with an average of 2.5 years. All 13 patients were able to defecate normally. There was no venting and defecation in the vagina. The rectal examination and vaginal speculum were well examined. The rectal vaginal fistula healed well. There was no recurrence of rectal vaginal fistula. No symptoms such as vaginal stricture occurred.

Transperitoneal Repair

Transabdominal repair is often used for vaginal bladder fistula or vaginal colon hernia repair and rectal vaginal fistula after rectal cancer surgery. Laparoscopic surgery is sometimes used, and laparoscopic direct vision helps to identify the structure and facilitate separation.

Wang Gangcheng et al. reported the method of colonic transanal extraction combined with pedicled omental packing. The specific methods are as follows: (1) the patient takes the lithotomy position. After the anesthesia is successful, the perineal group of surgeons expand the anus, revealing the flushing rectal anastomosis, vaginal and rectal vaginal fistula. Then, they should disinfect and remove the ulcerated tissue around the vaginal fistula. (2) Open the abdominal cavity along the original incision and extend the incision upward to expose the greater omentum, transverse colon, and left colon. Free the descending colonic peritoneum, spleen colon ligament, gastric colon ligament, broken submucosal vein, and descending colonic first-class ovoid arch traffic branch, so that the left colon is completely free from the middle of the transverse colon, and pay attention to protect the arteries and veins in the colon. (3) Separate the pelvic adhesions and free the colon above the anastomosis. Care should be taken to protect the bilateral ureters and mesenteric vessels and completely detach the pelvic intestines. (4) The intestinal clamp should block the proximal intestinal tube, prevent the intestinal contents from being contaminated and contaminate the abdominal pelvic cavity, and the intestinal tube is freed from the anastomosis to the lower rectum. The anastomosis is 3.0 cm below the rectum, and the stump stops bleeding. (5) Again, the rectal stump, vaginal and rectal vaginal fistula should be rinsed and disinfected. (6) The left colon is to be pulled out of the body through the rectal stump and the anus and is fixed to the skin. When fixing the intestine, avoid suturing the mesenteric vessels and preventing intestinal necrosis. (7) Free the omentum. The large omentum with the right aortic vein of the gastric retina is completely freed from the left aortic vein of the gastric retina to the root from the abdomen and avascular zone of the stomach. (8) Isolation and repair. The pedicled omentum is passed through the transverse colon and the small mesenteric avascular zone (vertical distance) to the pelvic floor, and the omentum is placed under the vaginal opening. The perineal group should use the absorbable line to suture the vaginal fistula together with the underlying omentum while avoiding the omental inclusions in the vaginal incision so as not to affect the healing of the fistula. (9) After 3–4 weeks, after the adhesion between the colon and the anus is firm, remove the extraintestinal tube outside the anus.

Wang Gangcheng and others treated 12 patients with this method. The operation was successful, and the median operation time was 95 min. The median amount of bleeding was 250 ml. Eight patients recovered well after operation, and the anus was drained from 5 to 8 days. Among the other four patients, two had pulmonary infection and two had incisional fat liquefaction. Eight to 12 days after surgery, the anus was drained. Nine of the 12 patients underwent vaginal examination at 3 weeks post-surgery. The posterior vaginal wall was dense, with no emptiness, and a pelvic CT examination was carried out. There was no fluid in the vaginal rectal space, and the intestine was removed. In the other three cases, vaginal examination was performed 3 weeks after operation. The posterior vaginal wall was loose and emptied. The posterior wall of the vagina and the omentum were not adhered tightly. After 6 weeks under a pelvic CT examination, there was no effusion in the vaginal rectal space. The limp was removed from the intestine. All 12 patients were followed up for 3 months. Among them, five patients developed anal stenosis 1 month after operation and were cured by intermittent anal sphincter. There was no intestinal retraction and vaginal discharge of intestinal contents or venting, which were all successfully repaired. Barium enema indicates that the rectal vaginal fistula disappears.

Some literature reports the use of sleeve segmental resection of the rectal intestine and suture of the fistula, the proximal intestine, and anal dentate line anastomosis for the treatment of rectal vaginal fistula. However, this method is complicated to operate and may affect the function of the anal sphincter, so it has few clinical applications.

Kraske Posterior Approach

In 2009, Schouten et al. reported the use of the Kraske posterior approach in the treatment of eight patients with recurrent low-grade rectal vaginal fistula, through the sleeve resection of the rectum, proximal rectum, and dentate line direct anastomosis, and achieved a better effect. The patient takes the folding position, corresponding to the left end of the tailbone area from the junction of the appendix to the anal external sphincter for longitudinal incision, the distal end of the tailbone is removed, the pelvic floor is exposed, and the lower part of the posterior wall of the rectum is cut longitudinally to expose the anterior wall of the rectum. The truncated section of the rectum is cut to ensure a sufficient range of resection. Identify the enlarged fistula, remove the scar tissue, layer the suture of the vaginal and rectal muscle layer, open the drainage of the vaginal mucosa, pull the proximal rectum and the dentate line to manually suture the anastomosis, close the pelvic floor peritoneum, drain the wound, and close the layer incision.

The method reported by Qiu Huizhong is that the patient takes the prone position, the hips are raised as much as possible, and the sides of the buttocks are stretched to the sides with a wide tape to expose the perineum as much as possible. From the appendix joint, make a midline incision to the anal margin, about 12 cm long, and cut the skin and subcutaneous layer. Determining whether to remove the tailbone should be done according to the distance from the anal margin of the mouth. If the distance from the anal margin is greater than 6 cm, the tailbone should be removed; otherwise, it may not be removed. The anal external sphincter and the puborectalis muscle were cut off in groups, and the posterior wall of the rectum should be cut upward from the anal margin until the fistula of the anterior wall of the rectum is revealed. After revealing the fistula, first remove the scar around the fistula, then lift the rectal wall at the edge of the fistula to carefully dissect the inflammatory adhesion between the rectum and the vaginal wall. After separation, the rectal wall and the vaginal wall are free. The edge is preferably greater than 2–3 cm to minimize the tension during stitching. Then, the vaginal wall and the rectal wall of the fistula should be sutured intermittently. Finally, the incision on the posterior wall of the rectum is to be sutured, and the anal external sphincters should be cut to repair the suture. If the tailbone is removed during the operation, a drainage is placed in the coccyx at the end of the operation. Qiu used this method to treat 23 cases of rectal vaginal fistula, and 3 cases of wound infection occurred after operation. The wounds healed after a dressing change. The 23 patients were all hospitalized 8.0 ± 1.0 days. After being followed up for more than 3 months, some were admitted to the hospital again. After examination, 19 cases (82.6%) healed, and 4 cases (17.4%, including one case of loss of follow-up) were not healed. All patients were followed up for 3 months to 7 years with an average of 20.8 months. The 23 patients had no postoperative anal dysfunction except for possibly one who did not follow up. Nineteen patients who were successfully repaired had no recurrence of rectal vaginal fistula after colostomy.

The author believes that this method is slightly complicated, traumatic, technically demanding, easy to infect, and needs a high level of attention.

By Perineal Incisional Repair (Musset)

Perineal rectal incision through the perineal approach has a unique advantage in the treatment of middle and lower rectal vaginal fistula with anal sphincter injury. The main point of the perineal rectal fistula is to convert the recto-vaginal fistula into a grade IV perineal laceration and then suture the laceration layer by layer. The biggest advantage of this procedure is that the surgical field is wide, the surgical path is shallow and straight, and it can fully enter the fistula and sphincter defects so as to carry out adequate sphincter folding and perineal reconstruction. However, incision of the anal sphincter has the risk of postoperative anal incontinence.

Musset uses a surgical method that directly cuts the perineal body from the rectum and the vagina to the rectal vaginal fistula, sutures the rectal wall, the levator ani muscle and the external sphincter, and finally sutures the vaginal wall. The main points of the procedure are as follows:

fully revealing the fistula, the morphological changes are made to the full layer of the vaginal body, and the skin, the subcutaneous, the lower sphincter of the fistula, and the fistula are directly connected (Fig. 10.6). After the infection and necrotic tissue are removed, the vagina is separated sharply. The interstitial tissue between the posterior wall and the anterior wall of the rectum is freely distributed upward to the proximal side of the fistula by 2–3 cm and is released to the lower edge of the external sphincter and levator ani muscle. After complete hemostasis, the upper layer of the rectal wall is to be first sutured with the strong absorption of Weishengwei 4.0, and then the levator ani muscles and the external sphincter muscles are to be sutured with absorbable lines. The suture of the muscles is not suitable for knotting. Finally, the vaginal full layer and perineal incision are sutured (Fig. 10.7). Antibiotics should be used for 5 days to prevent infection. After fasting for 3 days, patients were fed on the fourth day, and solid food was taken after 1 week. After the anal canal was placed for 3 days, the catheter was kept for 1 week. Avoid premature defecation, and take a bath with 1:5000 potassium permanganate solution after defecation.

According to foreign reports, the success rate of Musset in the treatment of rectal vaginal fistula is 87–100%. Shen Zhen et al. used this method to treat 20 cases of rectal vaginal fistula. All patients underwent surgery successfully. The operation time of the whole group was 30–50 min. Six patients had perineal incision redness and purulent exudation. Healing and physiotherapy healed well; hospitalization time was 10–15 (average 12.1) days. All patients were followed up for outpatient and telephone follow-up, with an average follow-up of 7.0 ± 2.6 months; no recurrence occurred.

In 2011, Hull et al. retrospectively analyzed 87 patients with rectal vaginal fistula and found that the success rate of perineal rectal incision and rectal valvuloplasty was similar, but postoperative sexual function and control in patients with perineal rectal incision was significantly improved.

Transanal Endoscopic Minimally Invasive (TEM) Surgery

Transanal endoscopic minimally invasive (TEM) surgery is a new method for repairing rectal vaginal fistula. It has the advantages of being minimally invasive, having clear visual field and accurate mouth recognition. The disadvantage is that it is difficult to conduct the operation and its application range is limited. It is limited to the rectal mucosal flap. Covering the endoscopic operation of the repair, some of this still needs to be done manually.

Synthetic Materials Repair Spells

Since 2004, more and more research groups have reported the use of biological patches in recto-

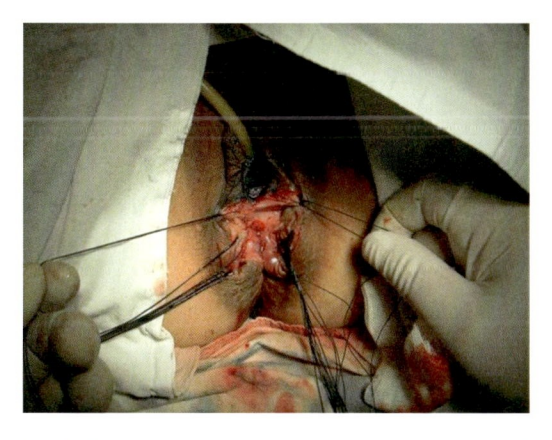

Fig. 10.6 Transperineal repair of congenital rectovaginal fistula

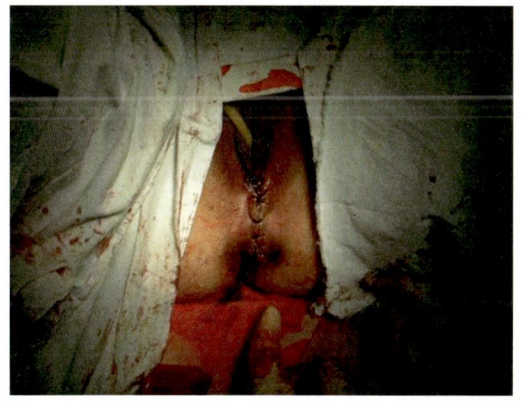

Fig. 10.7 After transperineal repair of congenital rectovaginal fistula

vaginal fistulas. The decellularized dermal graft patch retains the biological scaffold mainly composed of collagen and extracellular matrix by removing the antigen component. After being implanted into the body, due to the reticular framework structure, the host cells can be induced and promoted to grow on the scaffold, and the degradation products of the host are absorbed by the normal tissues, thereby completing the regenerative reconstruction of the defect tissue. In 2006, Shelton and Welton reported that the use of acellular dermal patch for reoperation of two patients with recurrent rectal vaginal fistula was successful. Other repair methods, such as fibrin glue closure and Surgisis Biodsign fistula, have been gradually applied to the treatment of rectal vaginal fistula since the 1990s, but due to the limited number of studies, the failure rate is high, and currently, it is almost not used as the first line of treatment for rectovaginal fistula.

10.3.4.2 Preoperative Management

Preoperative bowel preparation: 3 days before surgery, patients should halt the intake of food, oral laxatives, and no slag diet 1 day before surgery. Oral parenteral antibiotics should be taken to keep the intestinal tract relatively clean after surgery, delaying postoperative formation of feces, and ensuring there is no high pressure and high tension in the early rectal area.

Postoperative management: patients should stay in bed after surgery, indwelling catheterization, and maintaining a slag-free diet for about 1 week to avoid increasing the traction in the operating area. It is recommended to inject intravenous metronidazole and cephalosporin antibiotics on the first day before surgery and change oral antibiotics or antibiotics after surgery. Avoid constipation and sexual life within 3 months after surgery.

10.3.4.3 Others

There has been a great deal of controversy about the role of proximal colostomy in the repair of rectal vaginal fistula. In 2016, Lambertz et al. found through retrospective studies that proximal colostomy did not help to improve the recurrence rate after rectal vaginal hernia repair, which coincided with the views of Jones et al. However, Corte et al. performed a total of 286 surgical procedures on 79 patients with rectal vaginal fistula and found that temporary fecal diversion surgery significantly improved the success rate of repair.

Peng Hui and others believe that for the lower rectal vaginal fistula with good general condition and small wound inflammatory reaction, the fecal diversion ostomy should not be routinely performed. However, if the diameter of the fistula is larger and the position is higher, multiple repair failures have occurred, and for rectal vaginal fistulas with difficult to control inflammatory responses, or those with poor general tumors, radiotherapy, and Crohn's disease rectal vaginal fistula, the suggestion is a proximal colostomy to control infection. Definitive repair surgery is performed on the basis of nutritional support.

The stoma is usually performed after clearing when the rectal vaginal fistula has healed for 3 months. There are also studies that do not make a stoma by extending the fasting time, total parenteral nutrition support, etc.

10.4 Tuberculous Anal Fistula

The rectal anus is prone to getting fistulas. Before the discovery of modern anti-tuberculosis drugs, most anal fistulas were caused by tuberculous. Since the widespread use of anti-tuberculosis drugs in recent times, tuberculous fistulas have been greatly reduced. At present, tuberculous anal fistula accounts for 3–4% of extrapulmonary tuberculosis, which is the sixth most common infection point of extrapulmonary tuberculosis. The disease is more common in men and is often associated with tuberculosis. At present, it is relatively rare in clinical practice, and there are many atypical cases that are easy to misdiagnose and mistreat.

10.4.1 Cause

Tuberculous anal fistula is a specific infection formed by *Mycobacterium tuberculosis* around the anus. The traditional classification of tuberculosis is a type of skin cavity. It is thought to be a tuberculosis lesion inside the body or tissue, or ingested with bacteria or sputum, so that *Mycobacterium tuberculosis* is brought to the skin near the cavity through the natural cavity to form an infection. *Mycobacterium tuberculosis* can also enter the bloodstream and reach the anus through blood circulation, causing tuberculosis. Skin and mucosal trauma can also be followed by primary inoculation of mycobacteria.

Chinese medicine believes that the occurrence of tuberculous anal fistula forms mostly due to patients' diet, heat and heat endogenous, damage to the lung and spleen, blockage of the large intestine or anus, or due to anal damage, meridian obstruction, or blood stasis. The syndrome type is mostly yin deficiency internal heat, or both humid and hot blockage and lack of blood flowing smoothly.

10.4.2 Clinical Manifestations

The typical local manifestations of tuberculous anal fistula are special. Redness and swelling in the attack period are not obvious, local pain is not severe, and ulceration is long-term. Pus is the main symptom, it is more dilute, and the mouth is not closed for a long time. Skin lesions begin with brown-red papules, which can then develop ulcerative plaques called tuberculous sputum. There are many external mouths, irregular, with large openings, fusiform shape, often curled at the edges or subcutaneously, and the surrounding skin is dark. The granulation tissue is pale and swollen and slightly flooded. There are many branches of the fistula, pus is thin, the color is yellowish, or there are rice water and cheese-like secretions. The wall of the tube is soft, the lumen is large, and the inner port is larger than the common fistula. Most tuberculous anal fistulas do not follow Goodsall's laws. Local lymph nodes often have swelling. If it is not diagnosed as tuberculous anal fistula before surgery, the wound will not heal for a long time after surgery.

Typical tuberculous anal fistula patients often have more or less systemic manifestations of *Mycobacterium tuberculosis* infection, such as long-term persistent low fever, sometimes even high fever, night sweats, cough, hemoptysis, chest pain, fatigue, irritability, anorexia, etc.

At present, atypical tuberculous anal fistula is more common, and its symptoms are similar to those of nontuberculous abscess or anal fistula. Douglas's research shows that most patients with tuberculous anal fistula do not have convincing symptoms of systemic tuberculosis. Because there is no systemic tuberculosis, missed diagnosis and misdiagnosis are likely to occur.

According to Wang Zhigang and Lu Weijian, the current clinical features of tuberculous anal fistula are the following: (1) patients are more likely to be young and middle-aged men, and they occur more often because of perianal abscess, pain, or stool with blood. (2) The symptoms of the respiratory system and tuberculosis poisoning are often not obvious. Patients can often find tuberculosis after a chest X-ray examination. (3) Laboratory examination: the positive rate of acid-fast staining of sputum and purulent secretions is higher. (4) There is a long history of misdiagnosis. Because the anal fistula does not heal, tuberculosis is usually found only after repeated diagnosis. (5) Compared with the clinical symptoms of other nonspecific infectious anal fistulas, tuberculous perianal abscess is softer in texture, but the tenderness is not obvious, and there is a sense of fluctuation. After the formation of anal fistula, there is often a depression in the outer mouth, which is a cylinder mouth, no induration, irregular, not fresh, easy to bleed, and at the same time, the surrounding skin is often dark purple, granulation tissue is grayish-white, and it can be seen as cheese-like necrosis. The pus is usually thin, is pale yellow in color, and quite like the water after washing rice.

10.4.3 Inspection and Diagnosis

The early diagnosis and correct treatment of tuberculous anal fistula are difficult, and doctors need a certain level of experience and high vigilance against this disease. When the anal fistula is not healed for a long time, a biopsy should be performed and pathological examination and bacterial culture should be performed to exclude tuberculosis infection.

Tuberculous anal fistula needs to rely on biopsy and tuberculosis culture to diagnose. Biopsy tissue acid-fast staining (Ziehl–Nielsen staining) found that mycobacteria, or positive guinea pig vaccination, or skin-like pathologically visible caseous necrotic granuloma, all contribute to the diagnosis of tuberculosis. Since the culture takes 4 weeks, some new methods are more useful such as PCR amplification to detect bacterial DNA, which takes only 48 h.

However, many times, sputum secretions were taken for acid-fast staining, and no mycobacteria were found. The chest X-ray, PPD test, and erythrocyte sedimentation test were also found to be normal. When this happens, the fistula tissue is used for disease detection, and Xerox staining to find acid-fast bacilli is an effective diagnostic method. Pathological examination can confirm the diagnosis. However, it is not easy to obtain tuberculosis lesions in fibrosis, and small lesions of varying depths and typical tuberculosis lesions can only be found in local lymph nodes.

Colonoscopy does not help the diagnosis of tuberculosis because the morphology of the mucosa and mucosal biopsy lack specific performance, making it difficult to rule out other lesions. However, if the biopsy pathology has tuberculosis, it can be diagnosed.

Patients with tuberculous anal fistula must be diagnosed with or without tuberculosis. The methods for diagnosing tuberculosis include the following: (1) sputum smear for tuberculosis: it is simple, fast, and inexpensive, and the results are available on the same day, but the type of bacteria cannot be distinguished; the sensitivity is low, usually 5000–10,000 and the bacteria/ml can obtain positive results; the specificity is poor, and various acid-fast bacilli can be colored, and further tests are needed to determine whether it is tuberculosis. (2) Tuberculosis culture of sputum is a reliable method for identifying live bacteria and is known as the "gold standard." The shortcoming is that it takes a long time, it takes several days to 2 weeks to report results, and the sensitivity is low. Only about 80% of the smear-positive specimens are culture-positive; the specificity is poor, and various mycobacteria can grow, and a drug sensitivity test needs to be combined. Identification of mycobacterial species can determine whether it is tuberculosis. (3) Mycobacterium species identification: based on the physicochemical properties of different mycobacteria, mainly biochemical methods. Different strains of mycobacteria can be accurately identified, but the operation is complicated, and the drugs used in individual tests have certain risks. (4) Chest X-ray or video and CT examination. Tuberculosis of the lungs can often be found. (5) Tuberculin skin test positive is more common, has a certain reference significance, but there are also false-positive or false-negative cases. (6) T-SPOT test: there are specific effector T lymphocytes in the infected patients, and the effector T lymphocytes secrete various cytokines (IFN-γ) when stimulated by the antigen again. Therefore, examination of effector T lymphocytes can be used for the diagnosis of tuberculosis or potentially infected persons with tuberculosis. That is to say, the cytokine secreted by the cells in the culture is captured by the antibody and expressed by enzyme-linked spot color development. The T-SPOT assay is a C-interferon release assay that uses TLR to detect T cells that respond to 6 kD early secreted target antigens and 10 kD cultured filter protein–peptide pools to diagnose tuberculosis infection. It has high sensitivity and specificity and is not affected by the immunity of the body and BCG vaccination. According to US FDA data, its sensitivity is 95.6%, and the sensitivity of domestic clinical data report is 95.3%. There is a high rate of detection in patients with extrapulmonary tuberculosis. A negative result suggests that there are no effector T cells specific for *Mycobacterium tuberculosis* in the patient. Negative results may be related to different stages of infection, a small number of patients with immune system dysfunction or disease, and abnormal operation of the experiment. Negative results suggest that there are effector T cells specific to *Mycobacterium tuberculosis* in the patient, and the patient has tuberculosis infection. However, whether it is active tuberculosis, it is necessary to combine clinical symptoms and other examinations and examination indicators to comprehensively judge the situation. When *M. kansasli*, *M. szulgai*, *M. marinum* (sea), and *M. gordonae* (Gordon) are infected with four environmental mycobacteria, the T-SPOT test also has certain false positives. This test method is used by more and more researchers to identify active tuberculosis and latent tuberculosis infections and to predict the risk of tuberculosis.

Tuberculous anal fistula needs to be differentiated from Crohn's disease, actinomycosis, anal fistula, gelatinous carcinoma, sarcoidosis, and other skin diseases. It should be noted that tuberculosis is rarely considered in the differential diagnosis of perianal ulcers. Some tuberculous anal fistulas were initially diagnosed as Crohn's disease, so attention should paid to the medical history and to whether the patients have had contact history such as epidemic areas. In the absence of evidence of tuberculosis, at least for Crohn's disease, the fistula should not be easily diagnosed and treated, but a tuberculin test and long-lasting ulcer tissue should be first cultured.

10.4.4 Treatment

Once tuberculous anal fistula is diagnosed, regular anti-tuberculosis treatment should be done promptly. After anti-tuberculosis treatment for a period of time, if necessary, surgery should be performed. Surgical treatment should be performed after the local and systemic symptoms have subsided, and the symptoms will continue to alleviate for several months. If the incision does not heal for a long time after surgery, the tuberculous anal fistula should be diagnosed after an examination, and anti-tuberculosis drugs should be treated as soon as possible. Local anti-tuberculosis drugs can be used to help the sore surface healing.

10.4.4.1 Anti-tuberculosis Treatment

The Principle of Treatment
The key to anti-tuberculosis treatment is to control systemic and local tubercle bacilli infection. A reasonable and regular chemotherapy regimen must have two or more bactericidal drugs, a reasonable dose, a scientific method of use, a sufficient course of treatment, and a standard and early medication to cure tuberculosis. In order to thoroughly treat tuberculosis, we must follow the above five principles: early, joint, appropriate, standardized, and full-course. We must ensure that the rule must be ruled out, and the rule must be thorough. The lack of any of the above components can lead to treatment failure.

1. Early
   Early treatment can help the lesions absorb and dissipate without leaving traces.
2. Combination
   Patients with initial treatment or re-treatment should be combined with drugs, and the cause of clinical failure is often refractory to single medication. Combination therapy must be combined with two or more drugs to prevent or delay the development of drug resistance and can improve the sterilization effect. There are both intracellular bactericidal drugs and extracellular bactericidal drugs, as well as bactericidal drugs suitable for acidic environments so that the chemotherapy regimen achieves the best effect. This can also shorten the course of treatment and reduce unnecessary waste of resources.
3. Moderate
   Be sure to use appropriate doses under the guidance of a specialist. If the dose is too large, the blood drug concentration is too high, and it may cause a large toxic side reaction in the digestive system, nervous system, or urinary system, especially to the liver and lung. When the dose is insufficient, the blood concentration is low, and the antibacterial effect is not achieved. Sterilization is therefore not achieved, and it is easy to develop drug resistance.
4. Specification
   Because tuberculosis is a stubborn bacteria with a long split cycle, slow growth, and reproduction, it is difficult to kill. In treatment, the medication must be standardized. If the medication is improper, symptom relief will not be achieved, which will inevitably

lead to the occurrence of drug resistance, resulting in treatment failure, and it will be more difficult to treat in the future. Therefore, medication must be strictly regulated.

5. Full course

One course of treatment is for 3 months. The full course of treatment is 1 year or 1 and a half years. Short-term treatment should not be less than 6 or 10 months.

It should be noted that the drug resistance of tuberculosis has increased year by year. The WHO 2008 report showed that the global tuberculosis total resistance rate was 20%, and the multidrug resistance rate was 5.3%. China is one of 27 countries with high MDR-TB and high-drug-resistant tuberculosis. The treatment of severe drug-resistant tuberculosis is more complicated. At present, in addition to standard treatment, chemotherapy, intervention, and immune treatment have been gradually adopted.

Traditional Chinese medicine plays an important role in the treatment of tuberculosis. Chinese medicine treatment of tuberculosis is mainly aimed at the body's own resistance, by strengthening the body's immune function and resistance, to achieve the role of inhibition of tuberculosis. At the same time, in the treatment of tuberculosis, traditional Chinese medicine can also inhibit and reduce the side effects of western medicine on the stomach, liver, and kidney.

Medication Plan

This is generally divided into the intensive treatment phase (intensive phase) and consolidation therapy phase (consolidation phase). Standard in the intensive chemotherapy regimen is four drugs in combination for 2 months, while that in the consolidation phase is two or three drugs in combination for 4 months.

1. Recommended treatment plan for initial treatment of dysentery and/or vaginal tuberculosis

    2HRZE/4HR (H: isoniazid, R: rifampicin, Z: pyrazinamide, E: ethambutol).

    The intensive phase should be treated with the HRZE regimen for 2 months and continued with the HR regimen for 4 months. The course of treatment is generally 6 months. For patients with severe disease or comorbidities that affect prognosis, the course of treatment may be extended appropriately.

2. Recommended treatment plan for retreatment of tuberculosis

    2SHRZE/6HRE or 3HRZE/6HRE (S: streptomycin, H: isoniazid, R: rifampicin, Z: pyrazinamide, E: ethambutol).

    The intensive phase should be treated with the SHRZE regimen for 2 months, and the duration of treatment with the HRE regimen for 6 months, or the intensive phase with the HRZE regimen for 3 months, and the extended phase with the HRE regimen for 6 months. After obtaining the results of the patient's anti-tuberculosis drug sensitivity test, a reasonable treatment plan should be selected according to the drug resistance spectrum and the history of previous treatment. The course of treatment is generally 8 months. For patients with severe disease or comorbidities that affect prognosis, the course of treatment may be extended appropriately.

3. Recommended treatment plan for multidrug-resistant tuberculosis

    6 Z Am(Km,Cm)Lfx(Mfx)Cs (PAS)Pto/18 Z Lfx(Mfx)Cs(PAS)Pto Scheme (Lfx: levofloxacin, Mfx: moxifloxacin, Am: amikacin, Km: kanamycin, Cm: capreomycin, Pto: prothionamide, PAS: p-aminosalicylic acid, Cs: cycloserine).

    The Z Am (Km, Cm) Lfx (Mfx) Cs (PAS) Pto regimen should be used for 6 months during the boost period and continued for 18 months using the Z Lfx (Mfx) Cs (PAS) Pto regimen (alternative medicines in brackets).

    The course of treatment is generally 24 months. For patients with severe disease or comorbidities that affect prognosis, the course of treatment may be extended appropriately. For special patients, such as children, the elderly, pregnant women, those on immunosuppression drugs, and those with adverse drug reactions, doctors can adjust the drug dose or drug based on the above program.

10.4.4.2 Surgical Therapy

After regular anti-tuberculosis treatment, after reviewing tuberculosis, the patient should then be treated with surgery. By this time, the surgical treatment is the same as that for common anal fistula.

10.4.4.3 Topical Treatment

For postoperative tuberculous anal fistula, rifampicin and some topical anti-tuberculosis drugs can be used at the same time as systemic anti-tuberculosis treatment.

10.5 AIDS Associated with Anal Fistula

Acquired immunodeficiency syndrome (AIDS) is a sexually transmitted disease (STD) caused by human immunodeficiency virus (HIV) infection and characterized by severe immunodeficiency. Patients often contract lymphadenopathy, anorexia, chronic diarrhea, weight loss, fever, fatigue, and other systemic symptoms, and opportunistic infections or secondary tumors can gradually develop and ultimately lead to death. In recent years, the number of patients with AIDS complicated with anorectal diseases has gradually increased. According to the survey, the incidence of anorectal diseases in AIDS patients is 92.7% (204/220), including 179 cases of acne (87.7%) and 15 cases of perianal eczema (7.4%)—18 cases of anal papilloma (accounting for 8.8%), 5 cases of anal condyloma acuminata (2.5%), 3 cases of perianal folliculitis (1.5%), 4 cases of anal fissure (2.0%), and 6 cases of anal fistula (2.9%). Some patients had two or more anorectal diseases. There was no significant correlation between the incidence of anorectal diseases in AIDS patients and gender, age, ethnicity, drug use, and CD4+ T cell count. It indicates that the incidence of anorectal diseases in AIDS patients is high and the diseases are diverse. Therefore, AIDS patients should pay attention to regular anorectal examinations for early diagnosis and treatment of anorectal diseases.

10.5.1 Diagnosis

Regular anorectal disease screening is important for AIDS patients, especially gay men. Moreover, the screening method for anorectal diseases is more convenient. More than 90% of anorectal diseases can be found through anal examination, anal finger examination, and anal microscopy. The method is simple, and the patient spends less, and it is easy to be clinically popularized. During the AIDS treatment, clinicians should strengthen the regular screening of patients with anorectal diseases, so that early anorectal diseases, early diagnosis, early intervention, and treatment can be found to improve the quality of life of patients.

Anorectal surgeons should consider the possibility of HIV infection for severe, long-term treatment, recurrent episodes of hemorrhoids, perianal eczema, anal condyloma acuminata, perianal folliculitis, anal fissure and anal fistula, or anorectal symptoms in high-risk groups. It is necessary to screen all patients with anal fistula for HIV before surgery. If HIV infection is suspected, a further examination should be carried out and reported to the local CDC.

10.5.2 Treatment

In the AIDS Prevention and Control Regulations, China stipulates that medical institutions may not refrain or refuse treatment of other diseases of AIDS patients. In recent years, the number of HIV/AIDS patients requiring surgery has increased, and hospitals have encountered such patients, but most hospital surgeons will shut out such patients or push them to the so-called "specialized hospitals," but some specialized hospitals do not have the conditions to carry out certain operations of this disease.

HIV/AIDS is not an absolute contraindication to surgery, and reasonable surgical treatment is the only effective way to save some HIV/AIDS patients. Medical staff should take a positive attitude toward the operation of HIV/AIDS patients and conduct a comprehensive assessment and communication. As long as strict occupational protection during surgery and strict adherence to operating procedures, medical staff can avoid iatrogenic infections. The primary measure of preoperative status assessment in HIV/AIDS patients is blood CD4 lymphocyte counts. Some scholars have reported that CD4 lymphocyte count as a direct method for measuring immune function is the most clear indicator of immune system damage in HIV-infected patients. Many domestic scholars believe that HIV/AIDS surgical indications are based on the number of CD4 lymphocytes. For people with HIV infection, if the CD4+ T lymphocyte count is normal, they can tolerate all kinds of major surgery.

For patients with CD4+ T lymphocyte counts below normal and >400/μl, if the nutritional status is good, they can tolerate various operations. For patients with CD4+ T lymphocyte counts between 200 and 400/μl, if the nutritional status is good, the patient can tolerate the trauma of moderate surgery, but active antibacterial and antiviral therapy should be performed after surgery. Before any major surgery, a comprehensive assessment should be taken out to determine if the patient is able to undergo such a procedure.

For patients with CD4+ T lymphocyte count <200/μl, conservative treatment is the main option, some scholars believe that the proportion of postoperative complications in such patients is significantly increased, hospitalization time is significantly extended, but there are also patients that successfully undergo major surgery. If CD4+ T lymphocyte count is <50/μl, it is considered a contraindication for surgery. However, for some critically ill patients, when surgery is the only way to save lives, you can take active surgery without considering the CD4 lymphocyte count.

For patients undergoing preoperative surgery, it is recommended to routinely take antiviral drugs, monitor HIV RNA quantification, and perform surgery as much as possible after the viral load is below the lower limit of detection. For patients who require limited surgery (such as patients with malignant tumors) or emergency surgery, it is difficult to require patients to achieve the above criteria for antiviral therapy. Such patients are potentially more contagious and pose a greater threat to the surgeon. Therefore, the surgical staff must attach great importance to staying safe during surgery and must do professional protection during the operation.

HIV/AIDS is not a contraindication to general surgery. When performing surgery on HIV/AIDS patients, as long as adequate preoperative preparation and preoperative evaluation are made, strict occupational protection is undertaken during surgery, and strict adherence to operating procedures if followed, it is possible to avoid iatrogenic infections. However, the incidence of postoperative complications in patients with AIDS is relatively high, as reported in the literature to be as high as 10.1%, and the postoperative complications will be higher for open surgery or emergency surgery.

10.5.3 Self-Protection in the Treatment of AIDS Patients

The vast majority of surgeons at home and abroad are still very concerned about such surgeries, and some even talk about "Ai" color change. The reasons may be complicated: (1) the surgeon fears he or she may become infected; foreign data reported that the infection rate of intraoperative needlestick injury is 0.3–0.6%, and the intraoperative glove rupture exposes the unbroken skin directly to the patient's blood. The possibility of infection is relatively small, but the infection rate of skin damage during surgery can reach 5–6%; (2) it is considered that the risk of surgery is large, and the expected benefit is low, especially given the patient's own poor condition and short life expectancy.

Surgery personnel must strictly abide by the below operating procedures in the operation of AIDS patients, which clearly requires the surgeon to (1) wear isolation suits, gloves, and rubber shoes with anti-penetration properties; (2) wear double-layer gloves, anti-penetration masks, and face shields; (3) surgical medical personnel should pay special attention to the correct use of syringes, needles, and sharp objects. Sharp instruments should be transmitted indirectly through the instrument tray. Face masks, gloves, and anti-seepage equipment should be worn during the cleaning and disinfection of contaminated products to ensure safety.

Bleeding, exudate, and pus in the field are sucked up with a suction device. Do not contaminate the eyes and skin of the surgeon. All disposable items should be wrapped and burned. The scalpel and the vascular clamp should be immersed in disinfectant for a long period of time and then sterilized at high temperature. After the operation room is disinfected, it should be closed and further operations should be suspended for at least 1 day. (4) Minimize the wound surface during surgery to avoid excessive wound size because this will be difficult to heal and bleeding must be stopped in time. (5) Do a good job in communication between doctors and patients, family signatures, case records, and patients' privacy protection should all be strictly followed. (6) Do a good job in protection work and avoid nosocomial infections, especially when there are suspected cases of infectious diseases that cannot be diagnosed.

In the treatment of some emergencies, such as major bleeding, the surgical staff must be calm and should not panic; otherwise, occupational exposure might occur and the consequences will be very serious. Once occupational exposure occurs, it should be treated according to standard. For those who have a needlestick injury or a knife scratch, the medical staff must remain calm and collected, immediately remove the gloves, sag the finger, and immediately squeeze the wound from the proximal end to the telecentric end so that the wound blood flows out of the body and rinse it with running water. Disinfect the puncture site with 0.5% iodophor or 75% alcohol. Do not squeeze locally on the wound. For those exposed to the ocular mucosa, rinse immediately with plenty of water or saline. For complete skin exposure, wash immediately with soap or hand soap. Immediately after the emergency treatment of the exposed area, the hospital's preventive health department should be reported, and the expert group should conduct an exposure level assessment to determine whether antiviral drugs are needed. If you need medication, try to take it within two hours of exposure. There are multiple HIV blocking regimens, and anti-HIV is detected at 0, 6, and 12 months after occupational exposure.

Suggested Reading

Crohn's Disease Anal Fistula

1. Yang Bo-lin, Zhu Ping, Sun Guidong, et al. Crohn's disease of the diagnosis and treatment of anal fistula [J]. *World Chinese Journal of Digestology*, 2009, (20):2058–2063.
2. Li Youran (translated), Gu Yunfei, Lian Lei (review), et al. Expert consensus on Crohn's disease anal fistula of the World Gastroenterology Organization [J]. *Chinese Journal of Gastrointestinal Surgery*, 2015, (7):726–729.
3. Li Wenru, Yuan Fen, Zhou Zhiyang, et al. Imaging diagnosis of anal fistula in Crohn's disease [J]. *Chinese Journal of Gastrointestinal Surgery*, 2014, 17(3):215–218.
4. Yang Bolin, Lin Qiu, Chen Hongjin et al. Clinical efficacy of infliximab combined with surgery in the treatment of Crohn's disease anal fistula [J]. *Chinese Journal of Gastrointestinal Surgery*, 2013, 16(4):323–327.
5. Hu Pinjin. Multidisciplinary combined treatment of Crohn's disease and anal fistula [J]. *Chinese Journal of Internal Medicine*, 2013, 52(5):359-361.
6. Huang Fuda, Li Tianzi. Monoclonal antibody targeting preparation and its new progress in treatment of Crohn's disease anal fistula [J]. *Youjiang Medical Journal*, 2015, 43(3):353–356.
7. Ren Donglin, Zhang Heng. Several key issues that need attention in the diagnosis and treatment of complex anal fistula [J]. *Chinese Journal of Gastrointestinal Surgery*, 2015, 18(12):1186–1192.
8. Hu Jiancong, He Xiaosheng, Zeng Yang et al. Comprehensive treatment of Crohn's disease with anal fistula [J]. *Chinese Journal of Digestive Surgery*, 2013, 12(7):516–519.
9. Zhou Acheng. Research progress in the diagnosis and treatment of Crohn's disease with anal fistula [J]. *Medical Recapitulate*, 2014, 20(1):97–99.
10. Hu Pinjin. Difficulties in diagnosis and treatment of Crohn's disease [J]. *Chinese Journal of Gastrointestinal Surgery*, 2013, 16(4):301–303.

Infant Anal Fistula

11. 富士原彰,宮崎治男,秦堅.形態学的にみた乳児痔ろうについて.大腸肛門誌, 1978, 31:432–437.
12. Sun Lin, Wang Yanxia. Discussion on the prevalence and etiology of anal fistula in children. *Journal of Clinical Surgery*, 1994, 2(6): 306–307.

13. 佐佐木一晃,中山豊,後藤幸夫,早坂滉,他.小児における肛門疾患の検討.大腸肛門誌, 1984, 37:741–744.
14. 荒川健二郎,荒川二郎.乳児痔ろう414例の検討.大腸肛門誌, 1978, 31:438–443.
15. Huang Naijian, Liang Xincheng, et al. Clinical study of anal fistula cream in the treatment of anal fistula in children. *Chinese Journal of Coloproctology* , 2002, 22(5): 8–9.
16. Tang Hanjun. Prevention and treatment of infant anal fistula (with a clinical analysis of 64 cases). *Shanghai Journal of Traditional Chinese Medicine*, 1985, (10): 17–19.
17. He Yong, Han Yinghe. Characteristics and surgical treatment of anal fistula and perianal abscess in male infants. *Journal of Chinese Physician*, 2002, 4(1): 27–29.
18. Zhang Sifen, Yuan Hanxiong, Luo Zhanbin, Ren Donglin. 31 Cases of Infant Anal Fistula Treated by Integrated Traditional Chinese and Western Medicine. *Chinese Journal of Surgery of Integrated Traditional and Western Medicine*, 1998, 4(1): 17–19
19. 矢野道博ほか.痔ろう.肛門周囲膿瘍, 特に発生病理と外科的療法について.小児外科, 1977, 9:26–272.
20. Zheng Jinjuan, Li Shennong, Chen Hong, Zhou Ning. Jiangsu Medicine, 1981, (10): 10–13.
21. 高月晋.痔ろうへの新しいアプノーチ.大腸肛門誌, 1985, 38(3):401–406.
22. Xu Jiachang, Jiang Xiaorong, Feng Li. Investigation of normal children's sex hormone levels in Jiangsu and Anhui. *Journal of Radioimmunology*, 1998, 11(4): 205–206.
23. Zhen Yilan, Qu Lixia, Niu Hong. Determination of serum testosterone in patients with perianal abscess. *Chinese Journal of Coloproctology* , 1995, 15(3): 13–14.
24. 佐佐木志朗.乳児痔ろうの成因に関する研究.日本小児外科学会雑誌, 1988, 24(8):1101.
25. Zhang Jinzhe. Treatment of anal fistula after perianal infection in children. *Chinese Journal of Surgery*, 1979, 17(3): 203–204.
26. 貴田誠,他.教室における乳幼児痔ろうの臨床的検討.大腸肛門誌, 1973, 26(1):76–77.
27. Shafik A. A new concept of the anatomy of the anal sphincter mechanism and the physiology of defecation. XXXI. "Strainodynia": an etiopatholoigc study [J]. *J Clin Gastroenterol*, 1988, 10(2):179–184.
28. Klosterhalfen B, Offner F. Vgel P, et al. Anatomic nature and surgical significance of anal sinus and anal intramuscular glands. *Dis Colon Rectum*. 1991, 34:156.
29. Wang Jun, Yu Shiyao, Shi Chengren, et al. The etiology of acquired perianal infection and anal thinness. *Chinese Journal of Pediatric Surgery*, 1996, 17(1): 28–3.
30. Zhong Shiqing, Li Shanbo. Clinical analysis of 58 cases of acquired anal fistula in children. *Hua-xia Medicine Journal*, 2004, 17(6): 942–943.
31. 衣笠昭.乳児痔ろうの治療方針について.大腸肛門誌, 1978, 31(5):429–431.
32. He Hongyan, He Ping, Li Zhipeng et al. Thread-drawing therapy for the treatment of infant anal fistula (a report of 30 cases) [J]. *Journal of Colorectal & Anal Surgery*, 2008, 14(2):95–96.
33. Li Ruiji. Experience in the treatment of anal fistula in children. *Chinese Journal of Coloproctology*, 1984, 4(4): 23.
34. Wang Minghua, Tang Yiduo, Guo Xiutian, Cao Yongqing. 21 cases of simple low-position anal fistula in infants treated with thread-drawing method. *Journal of Chinese Integrative Medicine*, 2005, 3(3): 231–232.
35. Wang Longfeng, Cao Yongqing. Study on the treatment of infant anal fistula [J]. *Jilin Journal of Traditional Chinese Medicine*, 2014, 34(3):246–248.

Rectal Vaginal Fistula

36. Zhe Zhanfei, Lv Yi. Clinical research progress of rectovaginal fistula [J]. *Chinese Journal of Gastrointestinal Surgery*, 2014, (12):1250–1254.
37. Lin Guole, Qiu Huizhong, Meng Jiaxing et al. Cause analysis and treatment of iatrogenic rectovaginal fistula [J]. *Chinese Journal of General Surgery*, 2006, 15(9):685–688.
38. Peng Hui, Ren Donglin. The status of diagnosis and treatment of rectal-vaginal fistula [J]. *Chinese Journal of Gastrointestinal Surgery*, 2016, 19(12):1324–1328.
39. Shao Wanjin. Diagnosis and surgical treatment of rectovaginal fistula [J]. *Chinese Journal of Gastrointestinal Surgery*, 2016, 19(12):1351–1354.
40. Tang Jie, Zhang Juanjuan, Du Min, et al. Discussion on transvaginal surgical treatment of rectal-vaginal fistula [J]. *Chinese Journal of Minimally Invasive Surgery*, 2014, (8):683–685, 691.
41. Cui Long, Liu Qi, Yu Zhige et al. The treatment of complicated rectovaginal (urethral) fistula with autologous tissue flap internal grafting [J]. Chinese Journal of Gastrointestinal Surgery, 2007, 10(6):589–590.
42. Qiu Fang, Wang Shaochen, Huang Danian et al. Analysis of 20 cases of congenital rectal-vaginal fistula treated by modified vaginal surgery [J]. *Journal of Colorectal & Anal Surgery*, 2009, 15(5):345.
43. Wang Gangcheng, Han Guangsen, Ren Yingkun, et al. The treatment of high rectal-vaginal fistula after anterior resection of rectal cancer with colon transanal dragging and pedicled omentum packing [J]. *Chinese Journal of Gastrointestinal Surgery*, 2012, 15(10): 1080-1081.
44. Qiu Huizhong, Lu Junyang, Zhou Jiaolin et al. Repair of rectovaginal fistula through anal sphincter approach [J]. *Chinese Journal of Gastrointestinal Surgery*, 2015, (4):358–360.
45. Shen Zhen, Zhang Haishan, Liu Tongjun et al. Clinical analysis of 20 cases of rectovaginal fistula treated by Musset operation [J]. *Chinese Journal of Gastrointestinal Surgery*, 2014, (12):1241–1242.

Tuberculous Anal Fistula

46. Colon and rectal surgery (5th edition). Beijing: People's Medical Publishing House, 2009, 577.
47. Cao Jixun. New edition of Chinese Hemorrhoids and Fistula. Chengdu: Sichuan Science and Technology Press, 2015, 217–218.
48. Zheng Zhitian. Gastroenterology (3rd edition). Beijing: People's Medical Publishing House, 2000, 582.
49. Lin Jie, Yao Zhicheng. The status quo of diagnosis and treatment of tuberculous anal fistula with Chinese and Western medicine [J]. *Chinese Journal of Misdiagnostics*, 2011, 11(13):3046–3047.
50. Wang Zhigang, Lu Weijian. Clinical analysis of 11 cases of pulmonary tuberculosis with tuberculous anal fistula [J]. *Chinese Journal of Antituberculosis*, 2014, 36(7):597–598.
51. Zhao Zenghu, Wang Liling, Ding Ruiliang et al. Treatment of 12 cases of atypical tuberculous anal fistula with integrated traditional Chinese and western medicine [J]. *Chinese Journal of Surgery of Integrated Traditional and Western Medicine*, 2002, 8(4):309.
52. Tian Jinfeng. Clinical analysis of operation plus anti-tuberculosis treatment of tuberculous anal fistula [J]. *Guide of China Medicine*, 2016, 14(17):17–17, 18.
53. Li Yufang. Experience in the treatment of 30 cases of pulmonary tuberculosis with tuberculous anal fistula [J]. *The Chinese and foreign health abstract*, 2012, 09(16):130–130.

AIDS Associated with Anal Fistula

54. Qing Yong, Zhang Yi, Su Chen et al. Screening and analysis of anorectal diseases in 220 patients with acquired immunodeficiency syndrome [J]. *Chinese Journal of Experimental and Clinical Infectious Diseases* (Electronic Edition), 2015, 9(6):18–20.
55. Zhao Dong, He Qing, Tao Hongguang et al. Analysis of clinical diagnosis and treatment of HIV/AIDS combined with general surgical diseases [J]. *Chinese Journal of Experimental and Clinical Infectious Diseases* (Electronic Edition), 2015, (3):355–358.
56. Li Zhigang. Experience in surgical treatment of 26 cases of high anal fistula complicated with HIV infection [J]. *Chinese Community Physician* (Medical Major), 2011, 13(36):133.
57. Xie Shouyong, Lin Mao, Lei Yan et al. Analysis of 68 cases of anorectal diseases with HIV/AIDS [J]. *Chinese Archives of General Surgery* (Electronic Edition), 2016, 10(6):452–453.
58. Hu Xianfang, He Xiangdong, Yuan Dan et al. A case of complex anal fistula complicated with AIDS [J]. *Heilongjiang Journal of Traditional Chinese Medicine*, 2011, 40(5):15–16.
59. Liu Xin, Liu Baochi. A case of surgical treatment of AIDS complicated with tuberculous anal fistula [J]. *Chinese Journal of Clinical Infectious Diseases*, 2015, (3):282–282.
60. Li Dongmei, Fu Yan, Gao Meixia, etc. Perioperative nursing care of HIV infection combined with anal fistula [J]. *Health Required* (Mid-term Journal), 2013, 12(8):455–455.

11. Controversial Problems in the Diagnosis and Treatment of Anal Fistula

Renjie Shi and Yu He

Abstract

There are still some different opinions in the diagnosis and treatment of anal fistula: the controversy over whether complex anal fistulas should be based on shape or difficulty of treatment; the controversy over whether it is better to perform the first-stage surgery for anal fistulas at the abscess stage or to perform the second-stage surgery after incision and drainage; the controversy over whether to conduct active anal fistula surgery or to allow patients to "live with fistulas" without surgery; the controversy over the origins of seton therapy in China; and the controversy over whether anal fistulas cause cancer or cancer causes anal fistulas. At present, the lack of uniform criteria for evaluating the efficacy of anal fistula surgery leads to different or even contradictory findings of the same method in the literature, which suggests that it is necessary to establish the worldwide uniform criteria for diagnosis and efficacy evaluation.

Keywords

Anal fistula · Complex anal fistula · Simple anal fistula · First-stage operation · Second-stage operation · Minimally invasive · Seton therapy · The evaluation criteria of efficacy

11.1 Definition of Complex Anal Fistula

Complex anal fistula often appears in both the clinic and literature, but its definition is still controversial.

At present, the guidelines for the diagnosis and treatment of anal fistula developed by the Society of Traditional Chinese Medicine in 2012 still follow the classification standards developed in 1975. They state that anal fistulas with two or more internal orifices, fistulas, or external orifices are referred to as complex anal fistulas. That is to say, the criterion for judging whether anal fistula is complex or not is whether there are more than two internal orifices, fistulas, or external orifices.

When Yu Dehong described the concept of complex anal fistula in Huang Jiazhong surgery, he pointed out that there are only one external orifice and one internal orifice in simple anal fistulas. If the external orifice is temporarily closed and pus is not flowing smoothly, it will gradually appear red and swollen, forming

R. Shi (✉)
Department of Anorectal Surgery, Affiliated Hospital of Nanjing University of Traditional Chinese Medicine, Nanjing, Jiangsu, China

Y. He
People's Hospital of Suzhow New District Hospital, Suzhou, Jiangsu, China

© Chemical Industry Press 2021
R. Shi, L. Zheng (eds.), *Diagnosis and Treatment of Anal Fistula*,
https://doi.org/10.1007/978-981-16-5804-4_11

an abscess again, and the closed external orifice can be broken again, or another external orifice can be formed elsewhere. After repeated attacks, the result is that the scope of the lesion expands, or the formation of multiple external orifices and internal orifices connects. This kind of anal fistula is then becomes complex anal fistula. The complexity Yu expounds contains three conditions: recurrence, more than one external orifice, and the expansion of the scope of the lesion.

Some people think that complex anal fistula should not be divided by the number of external orifices. Alternatively, they believe that complex anal fistula should be associated with refractory, postoperative incontinence, recurrence, and other factors. The main fistula also involves an anorectal ring. Although this kind of anal fistula has only one external or internal orifice, it is difficult to treat and should also be called a complex anal fistula. On the contrary, although some anal fistulas have more than two external orifices or more than two branches, their diagnosis and treatment are not particularly difficult, so these anal fistulas are not really complex anal fistulas.

The formulation of complex anal fistula is rare in foreign literature. High transphincter fistula, superior sphincter fistula, and partial intersphincter fistula are difficult to cure because they involve the deep part of external sphincter and levator anus. They are equivalent to the complex anal fistula in the clinic.

11.2 Basis for One-Stage and Two-Stage Operation of Anal Fistula in Abscess Period

Many scholars believe that acute inflammation of the perianal abscess is serious, and it is difficult to fully understand the expansion direction and scope of the abscess cavity. Because of this, the operation will cause great damage to normal surrounding tissues, and it is difficult to protect anal function well. Especially in this case, it is difficult to determine the location of the inner orifice and therefore it cannot be dealt it, so we advocate the second-stage operation. The Japanese scholar Ghost Bundy thinks that it is like clearing the silt of a pond. When the pond dries up, one can clearly see where the water source (inner orifice) lies and it becomes easier to deal with. Therefore, it is advocated to first perform incision and excretion of pus in the abscess period and then surgery after the formation of fistula so that the difficulty and scope of the operation become smaller, the injury smaller, and subsequently it will be easier to get a radical cure.

At present, there are relatively more scholars who advocate the second-stage operation, but there are still some scholars who advocate the first-stage radical operation in the stage of the abscess. It is believed that it can relieve patient's pain in one operation, avoid the ordeal of a second operation, shorten the course of treatment, and reduce the economic burden to patients.

Because operating at the abscess stage of phase I or phase II is controversial, there is no unified consensus at present. In the author's opinion, there are no absolute advantages and disadvantages between the first- and second-stage operations. The former operation does not necessarily reduce the pain; at best, it reduces the pain of the second operation. In these cases, the perianal abscess was treated by simple incision and drainage, and anal fistula was not observed afterward.

Accordingly, which operation to take should be based on the patient's specific illness. If the stage of abscess has a definite inner mouth or can be probed with a probe, it is better to do a one-stage operation. Because the tube wall is not formed, there is no need to remove the hardened tissue during the operation. No tube wall means that tissue blood supply is good and healing ability is also strong, so postoperative recovery will be faster. However, if the internal mouth is not clear, the scope of the abscess is large, the lumen wall is thick, or it is tuberculous venereal disease, Crohn's anal fistula, ulcerative colitis, severe diabetes, and other systemic complications, or the systemic condition is extremely poor, or the patient requires a second operation, then the second operation should be chosen. It is safer to cut and drain the pus first and then operate after the abscess cavity is reduced.

11.3 "Minimally Invasive" and "Invasive" Anal Fistula Surgery

With the progress of medical technology, the concept and techniques of minimally invasive surgery have been increasingly applied in anal fistula surgery. "Sphincter preserving surgery," endoanal advancement flap (ERAF), and ligation of intersphincteric fistula tract (LIFT) are often recommended as the main surgical methods for the treatment of anal fistula. Although "minimally invasive" and other technologies are the trend now in anal fistula treatment, it does not mean that "minimally invasive" or other technologies must become the only choice in future treatment strategies. Remember that minimally invasive treatment is not based solely on the size of the wound. The essence of the so-called "minimally invasive" surgery is to minimize damage to the patient's body and achieve a better curative effect. Therefore, the author believes that as far as anal fistula surgery is concerned, it can reduce the damage to the anal sphincter and reduce postoperative complications and sequelae. No matter how big the wound is, such a surgery can also be considered a "minimally invasive" surgery in essence.

For some of the most complex cases, such as primary fistula that has spread over a long distance to glutes maximus, subcutaneous space of buttock, urogenital organs, retroperitoneal space, space around the inguinal canal, groin and thigh subcutaneous space, and repeated reoccurrence after operation, the pelvis rectum gap remains scared, and with acute infectious abscess, in order to ensure good vision, entire debridement and adequate drainage, and appropriate incision wound, a wide range of double thread-drawing drainage is necessary. Sometimes even the abdominal and perineal approach combination surgery should be considered. This relatively "massively invasive" surgery is mainly aimed at the sphincter complex in vitro soft tissue and coccyx, etc., with large wound surface, which is necessary to create the conditions for curing anal fistula. Although the wound is large, the damage to the sphincter is not necessarily great.

Therefore, we should not confine ourselves to "minimally invasive" surgery, and only take the size of the incision as the starting point to make surgical plans and carry out surgery. According to this principle, under the premise of maximizing the protection of anal function, surgeons should choose the most suitable treatment to each particular case of anal fistula. If only for the purpose of being "minimally invasive" and emphasizing the protection of tissues, the thorough treatment and drainage of lesions will be affected, thus leading to anal fistula recurrence. In this case, even if the wound surface is minimal, the treatment itself is meaningless.

At present, the contradiction between minimally invasive and radical treatment rate of anal fistula has not been well resolved. It has been reported that although minimally invasive surgery has some advantages, it has certain costs in terms of cure rate compared with traditional fistulectomy or incision and hanging, endoanal advancement flap (ERAF), ligation of intersphincteric fistula tract (LIFT), and other surgical procedures have better protection of anal function. The cure rate is significantly lower than traditional surgery, and postoperative anal function is still damaged and decreased to some extent. Endoanal advancement flap (ERAF) is the oldest "sphincter retention" technique in clinical practice. According to relevant reports in different pieces of literature, the median cure rate of this operation method is about 70%. In the process of dissociating the rectal flap, the internal sphincter will be damaged and anal function will also be affected. Some literature reported that the rate of decline of anal function after operation can reach about 35%. At the same time, ERAF is also a skills-dependent surgery. Postoperative complications such as rectal valve hematoma and dehiscence or necrosis are often closely related to the operator's experience and surgical skills. Ligation of intersphincteric fistula tract (LIFT) is seen as the most promising of all sphincter sparing procedures for the treatment of transsphincteric anal fistula. In a meta-analysis of LIFT surgery, the median follow-up period was 10 months, with a cure rate of 76.5%, a decrease in anal function of 0, and a postoperative complication rate of 5.5%.

After stratified analysis, LIFT had a cure rate of only 50% for high-complexity transsphincter anal fistula and only 33% for recurrent fistula.

Although "minimally invasive" surgery and "sphincter preservation" methods are the trend in anal fistula surgery, it does not mean that "minimally invasive" surgery is the only choice in anal fistula treatment. The choice of surgery should depend on the patient's specific situation and the doctor's ideas and technical level.

11.4 The "Survival with Fistula" of Anal Fistula

Because anal fistula is a benign lesion, the primary purpose of treatment should be to relieve pain and improve the patient's quality of life. However, if the operation damage is too large, the anus cannot fully function or offer effective protection and postoperatively there will be anal leakage, leakage fluid, gas leakage and other discomfort, and bring new pain. This will in turn reduce the quality of life in patients and anal fistula may even still relapse.

Therefore, "survival with fistula" can be selected as a principle when there is insufficient confidence in the surgical cure and functional protection, or the expected success rate of treatment is very low, or if patients cannot tolerate surgery due to constitutional reasons. Anal fistula is a benign disease, and although there is certain pain, after all, it does not affect everyday life. If the operation will endanger one's life or cannot improve the quality of life, we should not blindly pursue radical surgery.

At present, Crohn's disease anal fistula and some incurable anal fistulas are often treated by draining and hanging threads. Among them, Crohn's anal fistula with long-term or even lifelong drainage hanging threads is the most common situation. For those "incurable" or extremely complex cases where the cost is too high, long-term drainage and hanging can prevent the expansion of the infection focus point, control the formation of acute stage abscess, and thus improve the quality of life in the patient.

"Stabilizing" fistulas are as important to these cases as healing them. Therefore, for the colon and anorectal surgeon, the "life with fistula" method in some cases is not a failure but a success in treatment. On the contrary, continuing multiple "radical" surgeries in the overzealous pursuit of a cure can have disastrous consequences for a patient. This should be of great concern to all colorectal and anal surgeons.

11.5 The Origin and Evaluation of Anal Fistula Hanging Therapy

The exact origin of surgical hanging is unclear. In 600 BC, Sushruta, an Indian surgeon, first applied hanging therapy by inserting it into a fistula. In 460–377 BC, Hippocrates advocated the cutting seton method. Albucasis underwent a fistulectomy after hanging in the eleventh century. In 1376, Arderne proposed a modified second-stage hanging procedure for the treatment of anal fistula. In 1873, Vietnamese Dittel first reported the advantages of Indian rubber ligation in treating anal fistula, and 18 months later, St. Mark Hospital's William Allingham was inspired by Dittel. The experience of elastic ligation in the treatment of 60 cases of anal fistula was officially published in the London Medical Association in 1875. Pennington was the first surgeon to reinstate the technique in the twentieth century (1908).

In the literature of traditional Chinese medicine (TCM), the earliest record of hanging therapy appeared in the Ming Dynasty's "Gu Jin Yi Tong Da Quan" (AD 1556), in which there were clear records on the production of medical line, the operation method, curative effect, mechanism, and so on. In China, hanging therapy has been promoted as a characteristic therapy of TCM. However, it is true that the earliest records of "hanging therapy" in China are many years later than those in India and the West, and there is a lack of clear records in Chinese medicine literature before "Yong Lei Qian Fang," so the origin of "hanging therapy" in China is still unclear.

11.6 Cancer of Anal Fistula

Anal fistula is a common and frequently occurring disease in the clinic. Occasionally, anal fistula is accompanied by canceration. However, one has to ask, is the cancer tumor evolved from the anal fistula, or is the anal fistula just a clinical manifestation of cancer? Or are they just incidental and not causally related? There are different views on these issues at present, and they are always controversial.

Currently, it is believed that the relationship between anal fistula and anal carcinoma is clinically manifested in four forms as follows. (1) Anal fistula and anal carcinoma exist simultaneously, but there is no causal relationship between them. (2) Anal carcinoma penetrates and ruptures, presenting the anal fistula; that is, anal fistula is a manifestation in the development process of anal carcinoma, which is the most common clinical situation. (3) Canceration occurs on the basis of long-term chronic anal fistula, and the existence of anal fistula is much earlier than the occurrence of cancer, which is relatively rare in clinical practice. Since Rosser first reported this in 1934, no more than six cases have been reported in the literature. (4) Perianal Crohn's disease is malignant, and much foreign literature has reported this kind of disease. It is believed that patients are often delayed in seeking treatment due to the coverage of Crohn's disease symptoms. Once diagnosed, most patients are in the advanced stage, with a worse prognosis than the primary tumor. As for the relationship between anal fistula and cancer, most scholars believe that anal fistula and its related perianal abscess can exist for many years, even decades, before the discovery of cancer, indicating that the long-term existence of fistula and chronic inflammation eventually leads to malignant transformation, excluding the possibility of anal fistula secondary to anal cancer. Getz et al. firmly believed that cancer came from the anal fistula itself, which may be caused by tissue canceration due to long-term stimulation. They suggest that chronic inflammation destroys lymphoid structures in areas long stimulated by chronic inflammation and reduces immune surveillance against intercellular and malignant changes, leading to cancer. Some scholars also believe that chronic anal fistula cancerosis is a manifestation of primary perianal mucinous adenocarcinoma (anal fistula type), and perianal mucinous adenocarcinoma grows slowly in the deep, with unclear boundary between the two, and no clear distinction has been reported at home or abroad. At the same time, there have been many reports of exfoliated colorectal cancer cells being transplanted into the anus, leading to mucosal damage. Exfoliated cancer cells do not grow on normal mucosa but can be grown in open or ulcerated areas. For implant metastasis, the proximal colon must also be cancerous, while the anal fistula cancer has no manifestations. Postoperative pathological types of metastatic tumor and primary tumor are the same. Immunohistochemistry was very helpful in distinguishing cancer generated on the basis of chronic fistula and implantation metastasis of colorectal cancer. CK20(+) and CK7(−) are typical manifestations of colorectal cancer, while the anal tumor is the opposite.

The exact pathophysiological process of anal fistula complicated with mucinous adenocarcinoma is unknown. It is often believed to be secondary to chronic inflammatory changes, similar to Marjolins ulcers secondary to chronic ulcers. Rudolf Virchow first established the correlation between inflammation and tumor in 1863, believing that chronic and invasive inflammatory pathological processes can induce malignant transformation and progression of cells. It has been found that the fistula at different anatomical sites can be cancerous, with their own histopathological characteristics. The normal cell components of the common affected areas in the tumor, adenocarcinoma, and squamous cell carcinoma can all be generated in the wall of the uncured fistula. The pathogenesis of anal cancer is controversial, and it is difficult to identify the exact origin of such tumors histologically. Because cancer is often found late, normal anatomical relationships have been severely disrupted already. Although the WHO recommends that extramucosal adenocarcinoma be divided into two groups according to whether the tumor originated from residual glands or fistulas, current laboratory methods cannot be used to make a definitive distinction.

Western scholars proposed three points as the diagnostic criteria for the carcinogenesis on the basis of chronic anal fistula: (1) the existence of anal fistula for several years (usually more than 10 years), excluding the occurrence of malignant tumor before anal fistula; (2) no simultaneous detection of colorectal cancer; and (3) no tumor cells were found in the anal fistula.

Japanese scholars have also proposed similar diagnostic criteria: (1) a history of anal fistula more than 10 years, (2) severe perianal pain with induration, (3) the fistula secretes mucus, (4) external oral hyperplasia and hypertrophy are found in the anal canal and anal fossae, and (5) no tumor is found in the anal fistula.

Cancers secondary to chronic anal fistula are different from general anal rectum cancer, usually without diarrhea or constipation in the early stage; complaints of the early rectal irritation and bloody situation are also relatively rare. There is also generally no damage or lump of rectal mucosa during the rectal examination. The early manifestations are often covered by perianal abscess or fistula symptoms, so its early diagnosis is difficult. Common characteristics are (1) worsening of fistula symptoms, increased local secretions, and no signs of temporary pseudo healing. (2) Local perianal pain is persistent and tends to be progressively aggravated, with abnormal hyperplasia of wounds and eczema-like changes in the surrounding skin. (3) The characteristics of the fluid excreted from the fistula change with jelly-like fluid and/or bloody fluid, sometimes mixed with coffee-colored necrotic tissue with a special foul odor. (4) The mass in the perianal fistula was progressively enlarged, but there was no obvious manifestation of acute inflammation such as red or heat. In the later stage, the mass could spontaneously burst, with mixed necrotic tissue flowing out, accompanied by fetid odor. (5) In the late stage, there was a progressive enlargement of lymph nodes in the inguinal region, which do not subside after anti-infection treatment, and the pain gradually worsens perianal mass, and the nature of fistula discharge also changes.

In such cases, digital rectal examination, colonoscopy, barium enema, and other examinations were all negative, and the diagnosis depended on multipoint and deep biopsies of fistula and perianal mass. Because of the superficial biopsy surface of external fistula, it is easy to be misdiagnosed, especially when scar formation or fibrosis occurs. Therefore, patients with long-term anal fistula should be regularly and closely followed up. If the fistula is prolonged and does not heal, doctors should be alert to the possibility of cancer. If malignancy is highly suspected, the fistula should be opened under anesthesia, and the fistula wall should be removed to obtain enough tissue samples for pathological examination. All excised tissues should be sent for pathological examination. A more prudent measure is to take secretions for the examination of cancer cell coating before surgery, and biopsy should be done at the induration, and as many and deeper locations as possible, so as to reduce the possibility of misdiagnosis. If a single biopsy does not yield a diagnosis of malignancy, biopsy and curettage cytology must be repeated, at least once every 4–6 months. Mucin corpuscles found in post-anal fistula specimens are often helpful for pathologists to make early diagnosis of mucinous adenocarcinoma.

There are few reported cases of mucinous adenocarcinoma of anal fistula diagnosed by MRI, but MRI can accurately display the perianal anatomical relationship and determine the preoperative anal fistula. This is considered the most accurate perianal imaging diagnostic technique.

Transrectal three-dimensional ultrasound (EAUS) can accurately diagnose perianal diseases and is a good auxiliary examination for recurrent anal fistula. At the same time, accurate biopsy samples can be obtained under ultrasound guidance. Intraoperative EAUS can be used to evaluate the depth of tumor invasion in order to determine the surgical method. EAUS can also be used as a long-term follow-up for patients after surgery.

The most common pathological type of chronic anal carcinoma was mucinous adenocarcinoma (44%), followed by squamous cell carcinoma (34%) and adenocarcinoma (22%). It has been suggested that the incidence of anal cancer is 0.1%. From 1995 to 2010, Beijing Erlong Road Hospital treated a total of around 50,000 patients with anal fistula. In 1995, 2008, 2009, and 2010, a total of four male patients with mucinous adenocarcinoma were found. Their ages ranged from 52 to 69, with an average age of 58.6. All of the four patients had chronic perianal fistula with repeated rupture and no recovery and with pus and blood and mucus-like substance spillage. The medical history was 7–15 years, with an average of 10.2 years. Two to six anal fistulas were performed before diagnosis. The common clinical features are long-term postoperative wound nonhealing, abnormal hyperplasia of granulation tissue, mucus-like secretion from the wound, and occasionally eczema-like changes in the skin around the wound. The final diagnosis was confirmed after 4–5 biopsies, the pathological interval of biopsy was 2–4 months, and the final pathological report was mucinous adenocarcinoma. All the four patients were excluded from intestinal and extra-intestinal tumors by colonoscopy, chest radiograph, and abdominal ultrasound before surgery. No tumor tissue was found in the anal fistula during operation, and the primary colorectal anal tumor could be excluded, meeting the diagnostic criteria for secondary cancerization of anal fistula.

For patients with anal fistula cancer, the preferred operation is combined abdominal and perineal resection, but this method is more invasive and postoperative quality of life will be reduced. Local resection is also an option, but no tumor cells should be left at the cutting edge. Postoperative radiotherapy and chemotherapy help control the local recurrence and metastasis.

The canceration of chronic anal fistula grows slowly, and metastasis occurs late. The tumor is usually carried out in the form of lymphatic metastasis, and the inguinal lymph node is the first place of metastasis of anal fistula cancer. However, inguinal lymph node dissection is performed only when the inguinal lymph nodes are invaded, and inguinal lymph node dissection is not a routine operation.

Mucinous adenocarcinoma produced on the basis of chronic anal fistula has a slower development, lower degree of malignancy, and better prognosis than primary rectoanal mucinous adenocarcinoma. It has been reported that the pathological type of chronic anal fistula canceration is mucinous adenocarcinoma, which progresses slowly and has a better prognosis than squamous cell carcinoma.

11.7 Evaluation of the Curative Effect of Anal Fistula Operation

More studies have also found that many trials are rarely comparable and repeatable. An important reason is that these studies lack the same criteria, whether in the grouping of anal fistula or in the judgment of postoperative healing, incontinence, and other indicators. Therefore, the establishment of unified diagnostic criteria and postoperative observation indicators should be the foundation of further research on the treatment of complex anal fistula.

On anal fistula incision and anal fistula resection: Belmonte et al. found that anal fistula resection was more likely to lead to internal and external sphincter defect than anal fistula incision in RCT through postoperative ultrasound examination. Kronborg also suggested that the healing time of patients undergoing anal fistula incision was significantly shorter (34 days vs. 41 days).

Anal fistula hanging: there are few randomized controlled articles that study the role of hanging in the treatment of anal fistula, especially the comparison between hanging and the gold standard therapy—anal fistula incision. A multicenter study in India found that the healing time of drug thread was longer than anal fistula resection, but the recurrence rate was lower (4% than 11%). Compared with anal fistula incision with the same drug thread, Ho et al. found that there was no difference in healing time and complications, but the postoperative pain was more obvious, especially in the first 2–4 days after the operation, and there was a significant difference on the 7th day after operation.

Bag suture of wound after resection of anal fistula: this refers to the curl suture of exposed or rough tissue into a bag after the incision of anal fistula, which can generally reduce postoperative bleeding and speed up wound healing. Ho et al. compared the incision of anal fistula with the suture of locking edge after incision and confirmed that the healing speed of locking suture was faster. After comparing 46 patients, Pescatori found that locking edge suture could reduce postoperative bleeding and accelerate the speed of wound reduction.

Suggested Reading

1. Ren Donglin, several questions about the treatment of high complex anal fistula Guangdong Medicine, 2001, 22 (12): 1093–1094.
2. Ren Donglin. Several valuable questions in the treatment of high complex anal fistula. Department of surgery of Colorectal anal Disease, 2002. 8 (3): 136–137.
3. Zhu Ping, Gu Yunfei, Yang Bolin, etc. Existing problems and countermeasures in surgical treatment of complex anal fistula [J]. Journal of Integrated traditional Chinese and Western Medicine, 2009 Journal 7 (12): 1101–1103.
4. Chen Chaowen. Treatment of complex anal fistula [J]. Chinese Journal of basic and Clinical General surgery, 2010 Journal of General surgery 17 (2): 119–121.
5. Li Ruiji. Experience in the treatment of anal fistula in children. Chinese Journal of anorectal Diseases. 1984 4 (4): 23.
6. Shi Renjie. The focus of thread-drawing therapy for anal fistula. Chinese Journal of Modern traditional Chinese Medicine. 2005 Journal 1 (2): 136–138.
7. Gu Yunfei, Shi Renjie. Modern clinical application of thread-hanging therapy. Chinese Journal of anorectal Diseases. 1996 16 (1).
8. Hu Bohu, Li Ninghan, editor. Chapter VII anorectal fistula. Practical hemorrhoids and fistulas. 1st edition, Beijing: science and Technology Literature Publishing House. 1988; 244–249.
9. Yu Baodian, Cao Lei, Yao Yujie, Liu Chen, Lin Hui. Simultaneous treatment of high complex anal fistula with multiple thread hanging: a clinical analysis of 19 cases. Chinese Journal of surgery of Integrated traditional Chinese and Western Medicine, 2001 focus 7 (6): 378–379.
10. Cao Lei, Yu Baodian. Clinical exploration of simultaneous multi-lateral thread-drawing operation for high complex anal fistula. Journal of external Therapy of traditional Chinese Medicine, 2001 Journal 10 (6): 18
11. Gu Yunfei, Shi Renjie. Professor Zhu Bingyi's experience in treating anal fistula. Journal of Nanjing University of traditional Chinese Medicine. 2000 and 16 (4): 240–241.
12. Xiong Lagen, Xiong Jinlan. Clinical analysis of incision and suture drainage in the treatment of complex anal fistula. Miscellaneous Chronicles of surgery for Colorectal and anal Diseases. 2002 minute 8 (3): 186–187.
13. Li Chunyu, Jiao Fang, Nie Min. 118 cases of high complex anal fistula were treated by incision and suture drainage. Surgical Chronicles of Colorectal and anal Diseases, 1999 5 (3): 32–34.
14. Li Jingxiang, Liu Xinbin. Observation on the efficacy of suture tightening in the treatment of 41 cases of high anal fistula. Shandong Medicine, 2003. 43 (12): 51–52.
15. Guo Yi, Li Yunxia, Chen Xia. Li Bainian's experience in the treatment of high anal fistula. Journal of practical traditional Chinese Medicine, 2004. 20 (7): 38–12.
16. Wang Jianxin, Lu Yanfeng, Ding Ke, etc. Canceration of chronic anal fistula: a case report and literature review [J]. Shandong Medicine, 2008. 48 (35): 84–85.
17. Du Jiming, Gong Aimin, Chen Xilei, etc. Analysis of 1 case of canceration of anal fistula [J]. Chinese Journal of misdiagnosis, 2008 8 (25): 6278.
18. Zhang Zhanjun. Diagnosis and treatment of canceration of chronic anal fistula [J]. World's latest Medical Information Abstracts (continuous Electronic Journal), 2014, (23): 87–87.
19. Wu Yao, Liu Liancheng, Chen Xilin, etc. Diagnosis and treatment of mucinous adenocarcinoma secondary to chronic anal fistula (report of 4 cases) [J]. Department of Colorectal and anal surgery, 2011 quot; 17 (2): 96–97.
20. Dou Hongman. Clinical and pathological analysis of perianal mucinous adenocarcinoma [J]. Chinese Journal of surgery of Integrated traditional Chinese and Western Medicine, 2011.
21. Chen Zhikang, Chen Zihua, Wu Shaobin. Canceration of chronic anal fistula: clinical analysis of 6 cases [J]. Chinese Journal of General surgery, 2012, 1015 669–771.

Printed by Books on Demand, Germany

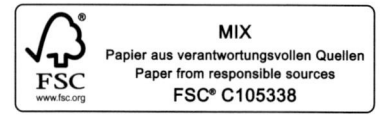

Diagnosis and Treatment of Anal Fistula